ATLAS OF
Endoscopic Sinus and Skull Base Surgery

ATLAS OF
Endoscopic
Sinus and
Skull Base Surgery

SECOND EDITION

Editors:

Alexander G. Chiu, MD
Russell E. Bridwell, MD Endowed Chairman and Professor
Department of Otolaryngology—Head and Neck Surgery
University of Kansas School of Medicine
Kansas City, Kansas

James N. Palmer, MD
Professor and Director, Division of Rhinology
Co-Director, Penn Center for Skull Base Surgery
Department of Otorhinolaryngology:HNS
Department of Neurosurgery
University of Pennsylvania
Philadelphia, Pennsylvania

Nithin D. Adappa, MD
Associate Professor
Division of Rhinology
Department of Otorhinolaryngology—Head and Neck Surgery
University of Pennsylvania
Philadelphia, Pennsylvania

ELSEVIER

ELSEVIER

1600 John F. Kennedy Blvd.
Ste 1800
Philadelphia, PA 19103-2899

ATLAS OF ENDOSCOPIC SINUS AND SKULL BASE
SURGERY, SECOND EDITION   ISBN: 978-0-323-47664-5

Previous edition copyrighted 2013.

Library of Congress Cataloging-in-Publication Data
Names: Chiu, Alexander G., editor. | Palmer, James N., 1967- editor. |
  Adappa, Nithin D., editor.
Title: Atlas of endoscopic sinus and skull base surgery / editors, Alexander
  G. Chiu, James N. Palmer, Nithin D. Adappa.
Description: Second edition. | Philadelphia, PA : Elsevier, [2019] | Includes
  bibliographical references and index.
Identifiers: LCCN 2018013446 | ISBN 9780323476645 (hardcover : alk. paper)
Subjects: | MESH: Paranasal Sinuses--surgery | Paranasal Sinuses--anatomy &
  histology | Skull Base--surgery | Skull Base--anatomy & histology |
  Endoscopy--methods | Otorhinolaryngologic Surgical Procedures | Atlases
Classification: LCC RF421 | NLM WV 17 | DDC 616.2/120597--dc23
LC record available at https://lccn.loc.gov/2018013446

Senior Content Strategist: Belinda Kuhn
Content Development Specialist: Angie Breckon
Publishing Services Manager: Catherine Jackson
Senior Project Manager: Daniel Fitzgerald
Designer: Bridget Hoette

Printed in China.

Last digit is the print number: 9 8 7 6 5 4 3 2 1

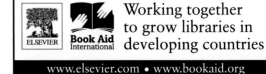

To my beautiful wife, Michelle, and my sweet, sweet boys, Nicolas and Aidan.

Alexander G. Chiu, MD

To my coauthors—Alex and Nithin—thank you so much for your friendship, guidance, and making this second edition comprise all the advancements we wanted to have in the first. To all the colleagues and trainees that make academic rhinology such an exciting, satisfying field—thank you for your interest and dedication. To my family—Amy, Sam, and Zoe—time with you is always better than time at work!

James N. Palmer, MD

This book is dedicated first and foremost to the three lovely ladies in my life: my daughters, Aryana and Maya, and my wonderful wife, Jyoti. Without their unconditional love and support, I would not have been able to spend the time needed for teaching the field I love day in and day out. I also want to dedicate this book to my amazing parents, Usha and Vijay, as they continue to cheer me on through my life endeavors both in and outside of work. Thank you all for helping me make this edition better than the first!

Nithin D. Adappa, MD

CONTRIBUTORS

Nithin D. Adappa, MD
Associate Professor
Division of Rhinology
Department of Otorhinolaryngology—Head and Neck
Surgery
University of Pennsylvania
Philadelphia, Pennsylvania, United States

Robert T. Adelson, MD
Albany ENT & Allergy Services
Albany, New York, United States

Marcelo Antunes, MD
The Piazza Center for Plastic Surgery
Austin, Texas, United States

Leonardo Balsalobre, MD
PhD Student
Department of Otolaryngology and Head Neck
Surgery
Federal University of Sao Paulo
ENT Center of Sao Paulo
Sao Paulo, Brazil

Henry P. Barham, MD
Sinus and Nasal Specialists of Louisiana
Baton Rouge, Louisiana, United States

Daniel G. Becker, MD, FACS
Clinical Professor
University of Pennsylvania
Sewell, New Jersey, United States

Samuel S. Becker, MD
Clinical Assistant Professor
University of Pennsylvania
Sewell, New Jersey, United States

Benjamin S. Bleier, MD
Associate Professor
Department of Otolaryngology
Massachusetts Eye and Ear Infirmary
Harvard Medical School
Boston, Massachusetts, United States

Rakesh Chandra, MD
Professor of Otolaryngology
Chief—Rhinology, Sinus & Skull Base Surgery
Vanderbilt University
Nashville, Tennessee, United States

Alexander G. Chiu, MD
Russell E. Bridwell, MD Endowed Chairman and
Professor
Department of Otolaryngology—Head and Neck
Surgery
University of Kansas School of Medicine
Kansas City, Kansas, United States

Garret Choby, MD
Division of Rhinology and Endoscopic Skull Base
Surgery
Department of Otolaryngology—Head and Neck
Surgery
Stanford University School of Medicine
Stanford, California, United States

Martin J. Citardi, MD, FACS
Professor and Chair
Department of Otorhinolaryngology—Head and Neck
Surgery
McGovern Medical School
University of Texas
Health Science Center at Houston
Houston, Texas, United States

Noam Cohen, MD, PhD
Associate Professor of Otorhinolaryngology—Head
and Neck Surgery
Veterans Administration Medical Center
Director
Rhinology Research
University of Pennsylvania
Philadelphia, Pennsylvania, United States

David B. Conley, MD
Associate Professor of Otolaryngology
Otolaryngology—Head and Neck Surgery
Northwestern University—Feinberg School of Medicine
Chicago, Illinois, United States

Samer Fakhri, MD, FACS, FRCS(C)
Professor and Chair
Department of Otolaryngology
Head and Neck Surgery
American University of Beirut Medical Center
Beirut, Lebanon

Elisabeth H. Ference, MD, MPH
Clinical Assistant Professor
Rick and Tina Caruso Department of Otolaryngology
Keck School of Medicine of the University of Southern California
Los Angeles, California, United States

Satish Govindaraj, MD, FACS
Associate Professor
Department of Otolaryngology—Head and Neck Surgery
Mount Sinai Medical Center
New York, New York, United States

Jessica Grayson, MD
Otolaryngology Head and Neck Surgery
University of Alabama Birmingham
Birmingham, Alabama, United States

Griffith R. Harsh, MD
Professor and Julian R. Youmans Chair
Department of Neurosurgery
University of California, Davis
Sacramento, California, United States

Richard J. Harvey, MD, PhD, FRACS
Professor
Division of Rhinology & Skull Base Surgery
Department of Otolaryngology
St. Vincent's Hospital
Sydney, Australia

Peter H. Hwang, MD
Professor and Chief
Division of Rhinology & Endoscopic Skull Base Surgery
Department of Otolaryngology—Head and Neck Surgery
Stanford University School of Medicine
Stanford, California, United States

Alfred Marc C. Iloreta, MD
Assistant Professor
Department of Otolaryngology—Head and Neck Surgery
Mount Sinai Medical Center
New York, New York, United States

Stephanie A. Joe, MD, FACS
Professor
Rhinology, Sinus & Skull Base Surgery
Department of Otolaryngology—Head and Neck Surgery
University of Illinois at Chicago
Chicago, Illinois, United States

Todd T. Kingdom, MD
Department of Otolaryngology
Department of Ophthalmology
University of Colorado, Denver School of Medicine
Aurora, Colorado, United States

Edward C. Kuan, MD, MBA
Fellow
Rhinology and Skull Base Surgery
Division of Rhinology
Department of Otorhinolaryngology—Head and Neck Surgery
University of Pennsylvania
Philadelphia, Pennsylvania, United States

Jivianne T. Lee, MD
Associate Professor
Department of Head & Neck Surgery
UCLA David Geffen School of Medicine
Los Angeles, California, United States

John M. Lee, MD, FRCSC
Department of Otolaryngology—Head and Neck Surgery
University of Toronto
Toronto, Ontario, Canada

Randy Leung, MD, FRCSC
Clinical Lecturer
Otolaryngology—Head & Neck Surgery
University of Toronto
Toronto, Ontario, Canada

Brian C. Lobo, MD
Assistant Professor
Advanced Rhinology and Endoscopic Skull Base Surgery
Department of Otolaryngology
University of Florida
Gainesville, Florida, United States

Amber U. Luong, MD, PhD
Associate Professor
Department of Otorhinolaryngology—Head and Neck Surgery
McGovern Medical School
University of Texas
Health Science Center at Houston
Houston, Texas, United States

Michael Lupa, MD
Becker Nose and Sinus Center
Robbinsville, New Jersey, United States

Li-Xing Man, MSc, MD, MPA
Associate Professor and Program Director
Department of Otolaryngology Head and Neck Surgery
University of Rochester School of Medicine and Dentistry
Rochester, New York, United States

Avinash V. Mantravadi, MD
Assistant Professor
Department of Otolaryngology—Head and Neck Surgery
Indiana University School of Medicine
Indianapolis, Indiana, United States

Jose Mattos, MD, MPH
Assistant Professor
University of Virginia School of Medicine
Department of Otolaryngology—Head and Neck Surgery
Charlottesville, Virginia, United States

Marcel Menon Miyake, MD
Research Fellow
Otolaryngology
Massachusetts Eye and Ear Infirmary
Boston, Massachusetts, United States
Doctorate Student
Otolaryngology
Santa Casa de Sao Paulo School of Medical Sciences
Sao Paulo, Brazil

Yuresh Naidoo, BE (Hons), MBBS, FRACS, PhD
Associate Professor
Department of Otolaryngology
Macquarie University
Sydney, Australia

Jayakar V. Nayak, MD, PhD
Division of Rhinology and Endoscopic Skull Base Surgery
Department of Otolaryngology—Head and Neck Surgery
Stanford University School of Medicine
Stanford, California, United States

Bert W. O'Malley, Jr., MD
Gabriel Tucker Professor and Chairman
Department of Otorhinolaryngology—Head and Neck Surgery
University of Pennsylvania
Philadelphia, Pennsylvania, United States

Richard Orlandi, MD
Professor
Division of Otolaryngology—Head and Neck Surgery
University of Utah
Salt Lake City, Utah, United States

James N. Palmer, MD
Professor and Director, Division of Rhinology
Co-Director, Penn Center for Skull Base Surgery
Department of Otorhinolaryngology:HNS
Department of Neurosurgery
University of Pennsylvania
Philadelphia, Pennsylvania, United States

Arjun Parasher, MD, MPhil
Assistant Professor
Rhinology and Skull Base Surgery
Department of Otolaryngology—Head and Neck Surgery
University of South Florida
Tampa, Florida, United States

Aaron N. Pearlman, MD
Associate Professor of Clinical Otolaryngology
Weill Cornell Medical College
Associate Attending Otolaryngologist
New York—Presbyterian Hospital
New York, New York, United States

Shirley Shizue Nagata Pignatari, MD, PhD
Professor and Head
Division of Pediatric Otolaryngology
Federal University of Sao Paulo
Sao Paulo, Brazil

Vijay R. Ramakrishnan, MD
Associate Professor
Department of Otolaryngology
Department of Neurosurgery
University of Colorado, Denver School of Medicine
Aurora, Colorado, United States

Jeremy Reed, MD
Darnall Army Medical Center
Fort Hood, Texas, United States

Raymond Sacks, MBBCh, FCS (SA) ORL, FRACS
Professor and Chairman
Department of Otolaryngology
Macquarie University
Clinical Professor
The University of Sydney
Sydney, Australia

E. Ritter Sansoni, MD
Sydney Rhinology Fellow
Division of Rhinology & Skull Base Surgery
Department of Otolaryngology
St. Vincent's Hospital
Sydney, Australia

Rodney Schlosser, MD
Professor
Otolaryngology—Head and Neck Surgery
Medical University of South Carolina
Charleston, South Carolina, United States

Raj Sindwani, MD, FACS, FRCS
Section Head
Rhinology
Sinus and Skull Base Surgery
Head and Neck Institute
Cleveland Clinic
Cleveland, Ohio, United States

Rahuram Sivasubramaniam, FRACS (ORL-HNS), MS (ORL), MBBS (Hons), BSc(Med)
ENT Surgeon
Department of Otolaryngology, Head and Neck Surgery
Sydney Adventist Hospital
Wahroonga, Australia

Aldo Cassol Stamm, MD, PhD
Professor
Department of Otolaryngology and Head and Neck Surgery
Federal University of Sao Paulo
Director
ENT Center of Sao Paulo
Sao Paulo, Brazil

Jeffrey D. Suh, MD
Assistant Professor
Division of Head and Neck Surgery
University of California
Los Angeles, California, United States

Andrew Thamboo, MD
Division of Rhinology and Endoscopic Skull Base Surgery
Department of Otolaryngology—Head and Neck Surgery
Stanford University School of Medicine
Stanford, California, United States

Reza Vaezeafshar
Resident in Otolaryngology and Head and Neck Surgery
Stanford University
Palo Alto, California, United States

William A. Vandergrift III, MD
Assistant Professor
Division of Neurological Surgery
Department of Neurosciences
Medical University of South Carolina
Charleston, South Carolina, United States

Eric W. Wang, MD
Associate Professor
Department of Otolaryngology
University of Pittsburgh School of Medicine
Pittsburgh, Pennsylvania, United States

Calvin Wei, MD
Assistant Professor
Department of Otolaryngology—Head and Neck Surgery
Mount Sinai West Hospital
New York, New York, United States

Kevin C. Welch, MD
Associate Professor
Department of Otolaryngology—Head & Neck Surgery
Northwestern University, Feinberg School of Medicine
Chicago, Illinois, United States

Bradford A. Woodworth, MD
James J. Hicks Professor of Otolaryngology
Vice Chair, Department of Otolaryngology—Head and Neck Surgery
Associate Scientist
Gregory Fleming James Cystic Fibrosis Research Center
University of Alabama at Birmingham
Birmingham, Alabama, United States

P.J. Wormald, MD, FRACS, FRCS, MBChB
Professor
Department of Otolaryngology Head & Neck Surgery
Queen Elizabeth Hospital
Woodville South, South Australia, Australia

Jonathan Yip, MD
Department of Otolaryngology—Head & Neck Surgery
Toronto, Ontario, Canada

PREFACE

The field of sinus and skull base surgery continues to evolve in popularity, techniques, and practice. The way we think and learn has evolved as well. Podcasts, online videos, and the ability to access education at any time or place has become an expectation for many learners. On this edition of *Atlas of Endoscopic Sinus and Skull Base Surgery*, the editors and authors spent a great deal of time creating a multimedia experience to deliver educational content. Our learners can read, listen, and/or watch content. And the surgical videos are all narrated in stepwise fashion. We hope you enjoy the book and are on your way to becoming an expert in endoscopic sinus and skull base surgery!

CONTENTS

VIDEO CONTENTS

Nasal Surgery

Septoplasty

Michael Lupa, Marcelo Antunes, Samuel S. Becker, and
Daniel G. Becker

INTRODUCTION

- The nasal septum plays a key role in the form and function of the nose, nasal cavity, and paranasal sinuses.[1]
- Septal deformities are common and occur in nearly 77% to 90% of the general population worldwide.[2,3]
- Even small deviations in key areas have been shown to adversely affect nasal airflow, delivery of nasal medications, mucociliary clearance, and the external appearance of the nose.[4–6]
- Improving nasal airflow continues to be the primary goal of nasal septal surgery. Other indications include epistaxis, sinusitis, obstructive sleep apnea, and headaches.[5]
- This chapter focuses on three commonly used septoplasty techniques: traditional septoplasty performed with a headlight; septoplasty addressing caudal deformities; and endoscopic septoplasty, both for diffuse deflections and the directed endoscopic septoplasty approach, to address focal septal deviations (spurs).

ANATOMY[7–9]

- The nasal septum is a mucosa-covered bony and cartilaginous structure located in the rough midline of the nose, which separates the right nostril from the left nostril (Fig. 1.1).
- The nasal septum is situated in a sagittal plane extending from the skull base superiorly to the hard palate inferiorly and the nasal tip anteriorly to the sphenoid sinus and nasopharynx posteriorly.
- The bony portion of the septum includes the perpendicular plate of the ethmoid bone, the vomer, and the maxillary crest, which has contributions from the maxillary and palatine bones. The quadrangular cartilage forms the caudal portion of the septum.

- At the junction of the osseous and cartilaginous portions of the septum, the perichondrium and periosteum are not contiguous. Between the two layers are dense decussating fibers.
- The nasal septum forms the medial wall of each nasal cavity and contributes to the internal and external nasal valves.

PREOPERATIVE CONSIDERATIONS

- Patient history is important in establishing an operative plan. Preoperative history taking should elicit information regarding subjective nasal airway obstruction, prior trauma, epistaxis, nasal decongestant use, and drug use.
- Adequate mucosal decongestion and vasoconstriction are essential in reducing intraoperative bleeding and optimizing visualization during the procedure.
- Endoscopic examination prior to surgery is a valuable adjunct to anterior rhinoscopy to completely examine the nasal septum and allow accurate identification of the location and severity of a septal deviation.[10]
- Choice of septoplasty technique should be based on the nature and location of the deformity; patient history, including prior septoplasty; and surgeon skill and preference.[11]

RADIOGRAPHIC CONSIDERATIONS[4,12]

- Radiographic evaluation is not necessary to diagnose a septal deviation prior to surgery but is often available when septoplasty is performed in conjunction with other rhinologic procedures.[4]
- When available, coronal computed tomographic (CT) scan of the sinuses is the preferred study to evaluate the course of the nasal septum (Fig. 1.2).

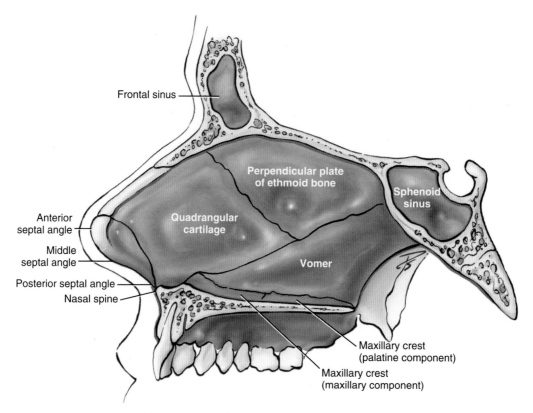

Fig. 1.1. Drawing of the nasal septum in the sagittal view.

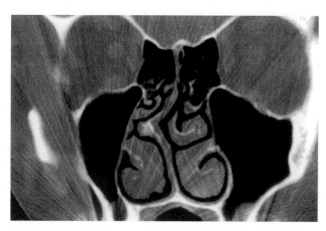

Fig. 1.2. Coronal computed tomographic scan of the sinuses demonstrating a large posterior septal deformity.

- The coronal CT scan may assist in identifying posterior deflections not visualized on anterior rhinoscopy or other sources of nasal obstruction, such as a concha bullosa.
- Despite its value, a CT scan may not accurately demonstrate the degree of septal deviation evident on physical examination.

INSTRUMENTATION (FIG. 1.3)

- Nasal specula of multiple lengths
- Bayonet forceps
- Scalpel with a No. 15 or No. 15C blade
- Small curved, sharp-pointed scissors
- Cottle elevator
- Freer elevator
- Takahashi forceps
- Open and closed double-action rongeur (Jansen-Middleton type)
- 0-degree endoscope with lens cleaner (endoscopic technique)
- Suction Freer elevator (endoscopic technique)

PEARLS AND POTENTIAL PITFALLS

- Establishing the proper subperichondrial plane before elevating the mucoperichondrial flap is essential to ensure a bloodless dissection and minimize the risk of tearing the mucosa.
- Bare cartilage is identified by its pearly white appearance and somewhat gritty feel.
- Septal perforations are an uncommon complication following septoplasty. The risk is increased when bilateral opposing mucosal tears occur during flap elevation[13–15]
- It is important to maintain a generous L-strut of at least 15 mm along the dorsal and caudal margins of the quadrangular cartilage to avoid long-term nasal tip and dorsal deformities (Fig. 1.4).[13–15]
- Care should be taken when addressing deviation of the ethmoid bone perpendicular plate, as aggressive

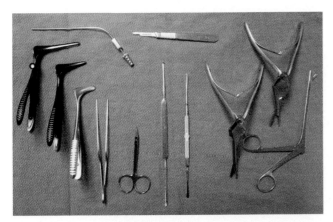

Fig. 1.3. Photograph of suggested instruments for septoplasty.

manipulation can violate the anterior skull base and cause a cerebrospinal fluid leak.[13–15]

SURGICAL PROCEDURES

Traditional Septoplasty[5,7,11]

- After adequate nasal decongestion is achieved using a topical agent, inject local anesthetic with a vasoconstrictor (1% lidocaine with 1:100,000 epinephrine) into the septal mucosa. Allow approximately 15 minutes for the anesthetic to take full effect.

Step 1: Initial Incision
- Retract the columella to the opposite side using a small nasal speculum, columellar retractor, or large two-prong hook and expose the caudal margin of the septum.
- Use a No. 15 blade or No. 15C blade to make a hemitransfixion incision along the caudal margin of the septum extending from the anterior septal angle to the posterior septal angle.
- A modified Killian incision may be used when more posterior deflections are being addressed or when less exposure is necessary (Fig. 1.5).

Step 2: Elevation of Mucoperichondrial Flaps
- Use a No. 15 blade, sharp-pointed scissors, or Cottle elevator to incise the perichondrium at or adjacent to the caudal septum.
- Perform a submucoperichondrial dissection along the inferior portion of the septum.
- Flap elevation should extend to encompass all areas of deflection, including bony spurs.
- A mucoperichondrial flap is then raised on the contralateral side of the septum beginning at the caudal margin if a hemitransfixion incision was used.

- If a modified Killian incision was used, gain access to the opposite side by incising the cartilage just anterior to the deflected portion.

Step 3: Removal of Offending Cartilage and Bone
- Using a No. 15 blade or sharp elevator, excise and remove the offending (deflected) portion of cartilage—again, maintaining a generous L-strut.
- A portion of the resected cartilage may be morselized or otherwise straightened and replaced into the septal pocket before the incision is closed.
- Any bony spurs can now be excised using controlled osteotomies.
- A double-action rongeur works well for areas of the perpendicular plate of the ethmoid or vomer.
- A septal chisel may be used for abnormalities of the maxillary crest.

Step 4: Closure of the Septal Pocket and Incision
- It is important to close the septal pocket to prevent the development of a septal hematoma postoperatively. Multiple methods have been described to accomplish this.
  - A running or interrupted quilting stitch can be placed using absorbable suture, such as 4-0 plain gut on a straight needle.
  - Internal silastic splints are often used in addition to further stabilize the septum and prevent fluid accumulation.
  - Additional nasal packing is often unnecessary.
- Close the hemitransfixion or Killian incision in a single layer using absorbable suture.

Caudal Septal Deformities[5,7,11,16]

Step 1: Initial Incision and Elevation of Mucoperichondrial Flaps
- Complete Steps 1 and 2 as described earlier for traditional septoplasty.

Step 2: Reduction of Cartilage Memory
- Use a No. 15 blade to score the deflected cartilage on the concave side.
- The direction of scoring should be vertical or along the axis of the deflection.

Step 3: Swinging Door/Doorstop Techniques
- Use a Cottle elevator to elevate the quadrangular cartilage out of the maxillary crest groove inferiorly.
- Using a knife, excise the inferior strip of cartilage that had been resting in the maxillary crest groove.
  - This should allow the remaining cartilage, attached only superiorly, to swing freely to the midline, where it can be secured caudally to the nasal spine with absorbable suture. Use a figure eight

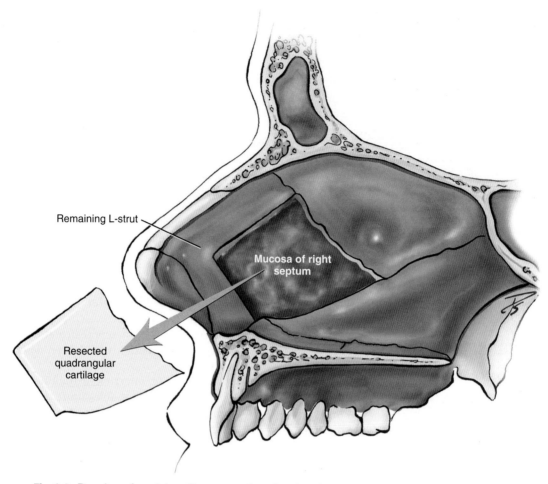

Fig. 1.4. Drawing of septal cartilage resection showing the remaining L-strut *(orange shading)*.

Labels in figure: Remaining L-strut; Mucosa of right septum; Resected quadrangular cartilage

of 3-0 polyglactin 910 (Vicryl) from septum to periosteum, overlying the anterior maxillary crest (Fig. 1.6).

■ A modification of this technique (doorstop method) eliminates the step of excising a strip of cartilage.

– After elevating the cartilage off of the maxillary crest, displace it to the side of the crest opposite the obstruction and suture it in place again.

Step 4: Closure of the Septal Pocket and Incision

■ Complete Step 4 as described for traditional septoplasty.

Endoscopic Septoplasty[9,7,11,17–19]

Step 1: Initial Incision and Initial Elevation of Mucoperichondrial Flaps

■ Complete Step 1 as described earlier for traditional septoplasty using a headlight and speculum.

Step 2: Elevation of the Mucoperichondrial Flap

■ Create a submucoperichondrial pocket with a Freer elevator or Cottle. Once a sufficient pocket is cre-

ated, continue the ipsilateral submucoperichondrial elevation using a suction Freer and 0-degree endoscope. Elevate past the bony cartilaginous junction.

■ Next, a septotomy is made just anterior to the area of greatest deviation and contralateral flaps are elevated.

Step 3: Removal of Offending Cartilage and Bone

■ Using a through-cutting instrument, a cut may be made above the deviated area of cartilage.

■ Any deviated cartilage may now be safely removed.

■ Any bony spurs can now be excised using controlled osteotomies, performed via the traditional approach.

■ There is no need to preserve bone of the posterior septum.

Step 4: Closure of the Septal Pocket and Incision

■ Closure is similar in technique to traditional septoplasty.

■ If suturing with endoscopic assistance, counterpressure is often required with the endoscope to allow the needle to pass from one nasal cavity to the other.

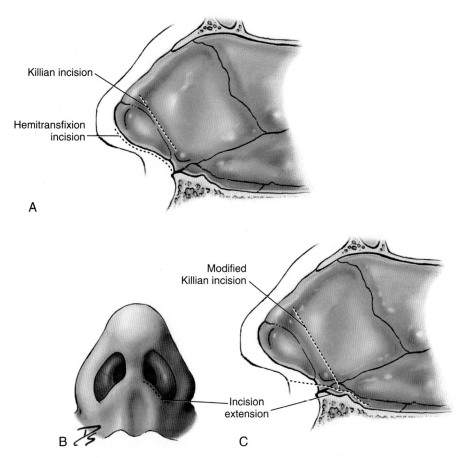

Fig. 1.5. **(A)** Drawing of standard hemitransfixion incision and Killian incision. **(B)** Inferior view modified Killian incision. **(C)** Sagittal view modified Killian incision.

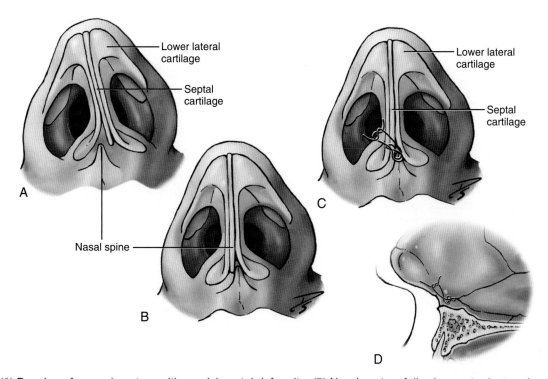

Fig. 1.6. **(A)** Drawing of a nasal septum with caudal septal deformity. **(B)** Nasal septum following septoplasty using the "doorstop technique." **(C)** and **(D)** Nasal septum following septoplasty with figure-eight suture.

- If no tear has occurred during the course of flap elevation, an incision should be made on the floor of one mucosal flap to prevent blood accumulation in the septum following surgery.

Directed Endoscopic Septoplasty[7,11,18,19]

- After adequate nasal decongestion is achieved using a topical agent, inject local anesthetic with a vasoconstrictor (1% lidocaine with 1:100,000 epinephrine) into the septal mucosa. Allow approximately 15 minutes for the anesthetic to take full effect.

Step 1: Incision and Elevation of Flaps
- Advance the 0-degree endoscope into the nasal cavity on the side of the deflection.
- Using a No. 15 blade or sharp elevator, make a horizontal incision directly over the apex of the spur or deflection.
- Raise mucosal flaps superiorly and inferiorly (Figs. 1.7 and 1.8).

Step 2: Removal of Offending Cartilage or Bone
- A bony spur may be excised simply using a microdébrider or through-cutting instrument.
- Alternatively, the septum may be incised anteriorly to the deflected cartilage or bony spur with a small flap raised on the opposite side.
- The deformed segment is then resected entirely as described for traditional septoplasty.

Step 3: Replacement of Flaps
- The flaps are simply redraped to their anatomic positions (Fig. 1.9).

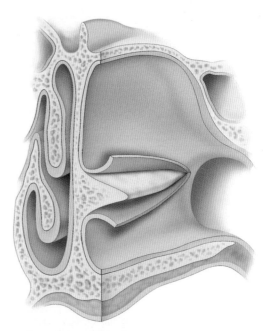

Fig. 1.8. Drawing showing the mucoperiosteal flaps raised superiorly and inferiorly. (From Friedman M, Schalch P. Endoscopic septoplasty. *Oper Tech Otolaryngol Head Neck Surg.* 2006;17[2]:139–142.)

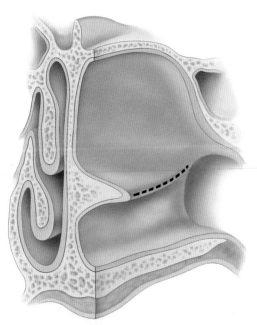

Fig. 1.7. Drawing depicting correct placement of the incision *(dashed line)* parallel to and directly over the apex of the spur. (From Friedman M, Schalch P. Endoscopic septoplasty. *Oper Tech Otolaryngol Head Neck Surg.* 2006;17[2]:139–142.)

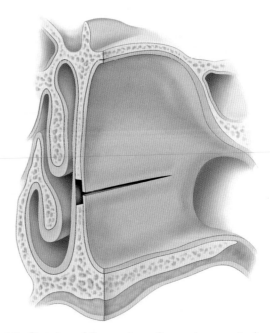

Fig. 1.9. Drawing of the septum after replacement of the flaps. (From Friedman M, Schalch P. Endoscopic septoplasty. *Oper Tech Otolaryngol Head Neck Surg.* 2006;17[2]:139–142.)

POSTOPERATIVE CONSIDERATIONS

- While nasal packing or splints are in place, the patient should receive an antibiotic with adequate coverage for *Staphylococcus aureus* to prevent toxic shock syndrome.[5]
- Splints are removed 2 to 7 days after surgery.[5]

SPECIAL CONSIDERATIONS

- An alternative approach to severe caudal deviation is ethmoid bone grafting, also referred to as ethmoid bone sandwich grafting.[20] The bony grafts are used as a buttress to provide rigidity to the caudal septum. Originally described via an open approach, a similar technique can be performed successfully via a closed endonasal approach using a unilateral bony graft.[21]

- An open approach via a columellar incision may be used when severe caudal deformities are encountered or when the septoplasty is performed in conjunction with a rhinoplasty.
- Open approach allows for extracorporeal septoplasty where the septum is completely resected and reconfigured into an L-shaped strut to address severe caudal deflections.
  - If the available cartilage is too damaged or is inadequate to create an L-shaped strut, then absorbable PDS foil may be used to augment the remaining cartilage.[22]

REFERENCES

Access the reference list online at ExpertConsult.com.

Middle and Inferior Turbinates

Richard Orlandi, Reza Vaezeafshar, and Peter H. Hwang

INTRODUCTION

- Turbinate surgery is performed most commonly to treat obstruction. Examples are nasal airway obstruction caused by oversized inferior turbinates and obstruction of sinus drainage by a lateralized middle turbinate or concha bullosa.
- The middle and inferior turbinates are dynamic functional structures within the nasal cavity and sinuses. Anatomic variations and/or dysfunction commonly lead to the need for turbinate reduction or resection.
- Total resection of an inferior turbinate is the extreme and is generally not recommended in most cases except for neoplasm resection (Fig. 2.1).

ANATOMY AND PHYSIOLOGY

- The turbinates comprise a set of three paired laminar structures that arise from the lateral wall and roof of the nasal cavity.
- The inferior turbinate is its own laminar structure; the middle and superior turbinates form part of the ethmoid bone.
- Each turbinate is composed of a bony base covered by respiratory epithelium with an intervening submucosal layer.
- Although the functions of the turbinates are not completely understood, it is known that they help to optimize oxygen exchange in the lungs by warming, humidifying, and filtering inspired air.
- The turbinates also assist in maintaining directional and laminar airflow in the nose and contribute to olfaction by directing air toward the olfactory cleft.
- The submucosa of the inferior turbinate contains a complex system of capacitance vessels that allow for selective engorgement or decongestion of the submucosal tissue. This change in turbinate thickness alters both the cross-sectional diameter of the nasal airway and the surface area of the turbinate.

- Fluctuations in vasomotor tone of the turbinates may be based on the temperature and humidity of inspired air and overall sympathetic tone of the individual.
- The cross-sectional area of the nasal cavity can also be altered by inflammatory swelling of turbinate soft tissue.

PREOPERATIVE CONSIDERATIONS

- When considering turbinate surgery, the surgeon should always remember that the turbinates are functional organs.
- Techniques should target the submucosal tissue, leaving the functional mucosa intact and undisturbed.

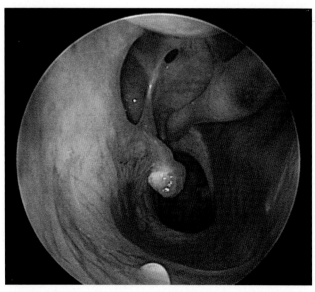

Fig. 2.1. Endoscopic view of the right nasal cavity after near total inferior turbinectomy. Patients with such extensive turbinate resection are at risk for atrophic rhinitis.

- Bleeding can be minimized by timely injection of 1:100,000 epinephrine (usually in combination with an anesthetic such as 1% lidocaine).
- Inferior turbinate outfracture does not address the vasoactive components of turbinate hypertrophy and is generally not sufficient as a standalone procedure.
- The surgeon should remember that the anterior-most 2 cm of the inferior turbinate account for the majority of its impact on patency of the nasal airway.
- Dissection posteriorly can injure larger vessels branching off the sphenopalatine artery as they enter the turbinates posteriorly.

Radiographic Considerations

- Radiologic imaging is not necessary to assess the inferior turbinates.
- For the middle turbinates, closely evaluate the axial and coronal computed tomographic scans.
- Identify the inferior and middle turbinates. Identify the nasolacrimal duct and take note of its location in relation to the inferior turbinate and inferior meatus.
- Identify the presence of any concha bullosa and note the anatomy of the middle turbinate as it inserts on the skull base. Prior surgical manipulation of the middle turbinate may predispose to middle turbinate lateralization, which may adversely affect drainage of the frontal or ethmoid sinuses.
- Assess the size and patency of the nasal cavity as well as the possible contributions of the inferior and middle turbinates, nasal septum, and other anatomic structures on nasal obstruction.

INSTRUMENTATION

- 0-degree and 30-degree endoscopes
- Boies-Goldman elevator
- Freer elevator
- Microdébrider with turbinate blade or pediatric cutting blade
- Monopolar or bipolar radiofrequency ablation device (optional)
- Monopolar needle electrocautery device (optional)
- Sickle knife or scalpel
- Straight and angled through-cutting forceps
- Endoscopic scissors

PEARLS AND POTENTIAL PITFALLS

- Care should be taken when operating on the turbinates, with the goal being to preserve or restore normal function.

- The most conservative procedure that can accomplish this goal is the best option. Techniques involving greater degrees of tissue resection or ablation should be reserved for treatment failures.
- Thermal injury caused by aggressive soft tissue reduction of the inferior turbinate can result in problematic complications such as mucosal sloughing and crusting.
- Surgery directed at the more posterior portions of the inferior or middle turbinate is generally less necessary to improve the nasal airway but can be associated with an increase in the risk of arterial bleeding.
- Overresection of the inferior turbinates may, in rare cases, lead to paradoxic nasal obstruction or empty nose syndrome (see Fig. 2.1). Therefore, a judicious approach to turbinate resection is indicated.

SURGICAL PROCEDURES
Surgery of the Inferior Turbinate

- Nasal obstruction is the primary indication for inferior turbinate surgery.
- Some evidence exists to support the use of inferior turbinate surgery to improve the symptoms of allergic rhinitis.
- Other indications include maxillary sinus hygiene, chronic rhinitis, and snoring.
- Surgery of the inferior turbinate can be classified into a sequence ranging from least invasive to most invasive: outfracture, soft tissue resection/reduction, resection of bone and soft tissue, and full-thickness resection of the anterior portion.

Inferior Turbinate Outfracture

- Outfracture is the simplest and least invasive of the inferior turbinate procedures because no tissue is removed.
- Because outfracture does not modify soft tissue, the vasoactive components of turbinate hypertrophy are not addressed by this technique.
- The inferior turbinate bone attaches to the lateral nasal wall at an angle, so that outfracture requires pressure on the bone in an inferior-lateral, not just lateral, direction.
- Gentle technique is necessary to avoid injury to the orifice of the nasolacrimal duct in the lateral wall of the inferior meatus.

Step 1

- Under direct visualization, place a Freer or similar elevator within the inferior meatus and fracture the turbinate upward and medially (Fig. 2.2A).

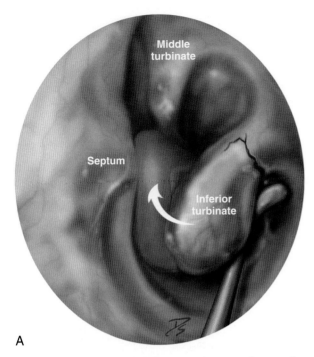
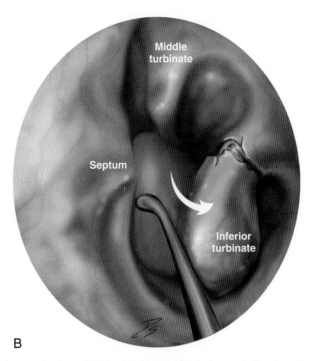

A   B

Fig. 2.2. Artist's depiction of inferior turbinate outfracture in endoscopic view. **(A)** The inferior turbinate is medialized so that the fracture point of the bone is at the attachment of the lateral nasal wall. **(B)** The inferior turbinate is lateralized with a Freer or Boies-Goldman elevator to create a larger inferior airway.

Step 2

- Place a Boies-Goldman or Freer elevator on the superior and medial surface of the turbinate and outfracture it laterally and inferiorly (Fig. 2.2B).

Inferior Turbinate Soft Tissue Reduction

- Many techniques can be used to address the soft tissue of the inferior turbinates, which have their own advantages and disadvantages (Table 2.1).
  - Thermal ablation: (1) Electrocautery, (2) Laser
  - Radiofrequency: (1) Bipolar, (2) Unipolar
  - Microdébrider
- Some devices that use thermal or radiofrequency energy remove tissue to some degree but work largely by causing wound contraction.
- Most, but not all, techniques target the submucosal tissue while leaving the functional mucosa intact.
- Submucosal needle electrocautery is, in many ways, the simplest of these techniques but is also very imprecise.
- Laser ablation essentially resurfaces the mucosa, with some ablation of the submucosa as well. The equipment costs can be substantial.
- Ablation and electrocautery both subject the overlying mucosa to thermal injury, which sometimes results in mucosal sloughing and crusting.[1]
- Radiofrequency devices for performing inferior turbinate reduction can be either unipolar or bipolar;

TABLE 2.1	Different Surgical Techniques for Inferior Turbinate Reduction With Advantages And Disadvantages for Each Technique	
Surgical Technique	**Advantages**	**Disadvantages**
Electrocautery/ diathermy	Minimally invasive	Unmeasured delivery of energy May necrose mucosa if not careful
Laser ablation	Minimally invasive May be performed in the office	Equipment costs Not mucosal sparing Long-term results vary
Radiofrequency (bipolar, unipolar)	Minimally invasive Minimal discomfort Mucosal sparing	Less control over degree of tissue reduction Equipment cost
Microdébrider	Can sculpt turbinate, especially for severe hypertrophy Can be performed in clinic or operating room Mucosa preserved	Risk of bleeding

no appreciable difference in outcomes is seen with the two methods.[2]

- The impact of soft tissue reduction on the nasal airway is largely due to alterations in the anterior portion of the inferior turbinate. Reduction posteriorly does not significantly improve the nasal airway and can significantly increase the risk of bleeding.

- Several careful analyses of outcomes following inferior turbinate surgery have been performed over the last few years.
- A large study comparing subtotal turbinectomy, laser cautery, electrocautery, cryotherapy, submucosal resection, and submucosal resection combined with outfracture found the best outcome at 6 years of follow-up in patients treated with submucosal resection combined with outfracture.[3]
- Bipolar radiofrequency has been proven safe and effective in both adult and pediatric populations.[4,5]
- Long-term (2-year) follow-up of radiofrequency (RF) turbinate reduction for allergic and nonallergic inferior turbinate hypertrophy has shown improvement in olfaction, decreased nasal resistance and subjective improvement in nasal obstruction.[6]
- Long-term (10-year) follow-up of microdébrider reduction has shown symptom improvement in 93% of cases. Endoscopy, mucociliary clearance time, and anterior rhinometry remained improved over the long term.[7]
- Comparisons between bipolar radiofrequency ablation and microdébrider submucosal resection have shown improvement in symptoms with both techniques, with the microdébrider technique yielding greater improvement over a longer period of time.[8,9]

Step 1

- Under direct visualization, either with a nasal speculum or 0-degree endoscope, inject the inferior turbinate with 1% lidocaine with 1:100,000 epinephrine.

Step 2

- Using a scalpel or similar leading edge of the microdébrider device, make a stab incision just posterior to the mucocutaneous junction of the inferior turbinate (Fig. 2.3).

Step 3

- Elevate soft tissue off of the underlying bone by subperiosteal dissection with a Freer or Cottle elevator or elevator portion of the microdébrider device (Fig. 2.4).

Step 4

- Once the tissue is elevated off of the bone, insert the oscillating microdébrider blade into the soft tissue pocket and engage the blade with soft tissue in a circular direction. Direct the active face of the microdébrider blade away from the turbinate bone.

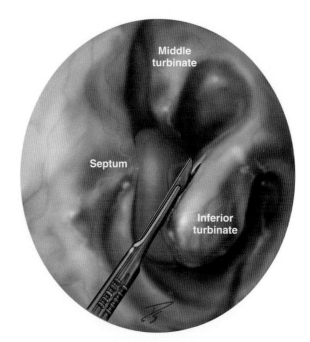

Fig. 2.3. Artist's depiction of the incision point into the left inferior turbinate submucosa in endoscopic view.

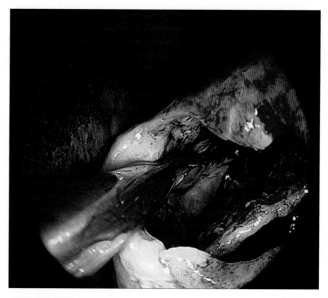

Fig. 2.4. Endoscopic view of the left inferior turbinate bone exposed by incising the anterior soft tissue.

- A slow oscillation speed facilitates controlled resection of the submucosal tissue without injuring the overlying mucosa.
- Direct soft tissue reduction toward the anterior two-thirds of the inferior turbinate.

Step 5

- Sculpt the soft tissue until adequate reduction is achieved.

- Preserve the overlying mucosa.
- Bleeding from the stab incision can be controlled, if necessary, using unipolar or bipolar electrocautery.

Other Methods

- Other techniques for soft tissue reduction, including electrocautery, radiofrequency ablation, and laser ablation, are implemented in accordance with the device manufacturer's instructions.
- In general, the device is inserted into the anterior surface of the turbinate, and multiple passes are made while the device is activated.
- The tip of the submucosal energy-delivering device should remain well below the surface to prevent mucosal injury.

Submucosal Resection of Bone and Soft Tissue of the Inferior Turbinate

- Submucosal resection of the inferior turbinate is indicated when the bone is significantly hypertrophic.
- This technique is often combined with other soft tissue procedures.

Step 1

- Develop a subperiosteal pocket of dissection, as outlined above in Steps 1 to 3 of the Inferior Turbinate Soft Tissue Reduction technique.

Step 2

- Remove the underlying bone with Blakesley forceps. The endoscope may be placed directly under the subperiosteal flap for enhanced visualization. The anterior one-half to two-thirds of the turbinate bone may be resected (Fig. 2.5).

Step 3

- Proceed with submucosal soft tissue resection with the microdébrider as described in Steps 4 and 5 of the Inferior Turbinate Soft Tissue Reduction technique.

Full-Thickness Resection of the Anterior Portion of the Inferior Turbinate

- Conservative resection of the anterior 1 to 2 cm of the inferior turbinate is usually well tolerated.
- The bone exposure resulting from this technique can sometimes lead to longer healing times and extensive crusting.
- Extensive removal of the inferior turbinate may lead to atrophic rhinitis, characterized by a paradoxical sense of obstruction due to loss of laminar airflow, and is therefore discouraged.
- Comparison between RF turbinate reduction and partial turbinectomy shows good clinical outcomes with improved nasal function with both techniques.

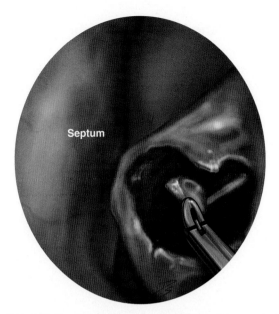

Fig. 2.5. Artist's depiction of the dissection of the pocket of the inferior turbinate bone in endoscopic view. Grasping with Blakesley forceps and using a twisting motion is a good method of removal.

However, histologic studies show that partial turbinectomy may be disruptive to the ciliated epithelium. Hence, compared to partial resection, RF turbinate reduction may be a preferable option to better preserve nasal physiology.[10]

Step 1

- Inject the anterior end of the inferior turbinate with 1% lidocaine with 1:100,000 epinephrine.

Step 2

- Under direct visualization with a 0-degree endoscope, place a Freer elevator into the inferior meatus and infracture the inferior turbinate medially and superiorly.

Step 3

- Remove the soft tissue overlying the lateral surface of the inferior turbinate either by using a microdébrider or by incising the mucosa and elevating it sharply off of the bone.

Step 4

- Remove the bone of the lateral and anterior surface of the inferior turbinate using through-cutting instruments and backbiters (Fig. 2.6).

Step 5

- Redrape the mucosa over the resected surface and lateral surface of the inferior turbinate and place packing, if necessary.

Surgery of the Middle Turbinate

Resection of a Concha Bullosa

- A concha bullosa is an enlargement of the middle turbinate caused by pneumatization of the turbinate bone.

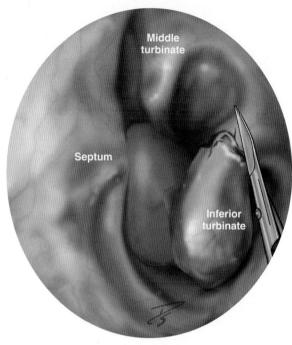

Fig. 2.6. Artist's depiction of an endoscopic view of resection of the anterior head of the left inferior turbinate using scissors.

- Concha bullosa of the middle turbinate is found more commonly in patients with chronic rhinosinusitis.[11]
- During the course of surgical treatment for chronic ethmoid sinusitis, it is typically necessary to partially resect this cell to ensure its drainage and facilitate access into the remainder of the ethmoid cavity.
- It is important to recognize that the concha bullosa represents a functioning ethmoid sinus cell. Surgical resection should consequently adhere to the same principles of mucosal preservation and promotion of physiologic drainage that are followed in other types of functional endoscopic sinus surgery.
- In nearly all cases, the medial aspect of the concha bullosa attaches to the cribriform plate, so that the lateral wall is typically removed during resection (Fig. 2.7).
- Crushing of a concha bullosa may provide only temporary reduction and may impair drainage of the mucus created within it.[12]

Step 1

- Under direct visualization of the middle turbinate with a 0-degree endoscope, infiltrate 1% lidocaine with 1:100,000 epinephrine into the turbinate and at its superior insertion before beginning the procedure.

Step 2

- Incise the anterior face of the concha bullosa vertically with a scalpel or sickle knife, making sure that the pneumatized cavity is entered.

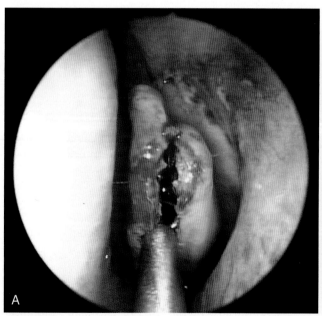
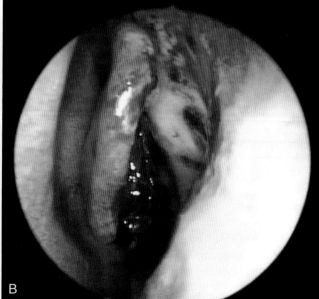

Fig. 2.7. **(A)** Endoscopic view of incision of a left concha bullosa to facilitate access to and drainage of the middle meatus. **(B)** Improved access following resection of the lateral lamella of the left concha bullosa [same nasal cavity as in **(A)**].

Step 3

- Spread the cavity open with a pair of straight or curved endoscopic scissors. Using the scissors, extend the incision to the posterior portion of the cell, usually at the basal lamella of the middle turbinate.

Step 4

- Extend the superior aspect of the vertical incision posteriorly and inferiorly until the entire lateral lamella of the concha bullosa is free.

Middle Turbinate Resection During Endoscopic Sinus Surgery

- Resection of the middle turbinate during endoscopic sinus surgery is controversial.
- Some surgeons advocate removal of the middle turbinate to facilitate access to the ethmoid sinus and prevent scarring of the turbinate to the lateral nasal wall.
- Others have stressed the importance of the middle turbinate as a landmark for revision sinus surgery and have argued for its preservation because of several potential complications associated with its removal.
- High resection or avulsion of the middle turbinate from the skull base carries the risk of cerebrospinal fluid leak.
- Removal of the highest part of the middle turbinate has the potential to result in olfactory disturbance, although conservative resection of the middle turbinate has not been shown to cause olfactory loss.[13]
- The remnant middle turbinate must be managed carefully, as it can lateralize and obstruct the frontal sinus, causing iatrogenic frontal sinusitis.
- There is some evidence to suggest that a select group of patients may actually benefit from middle turbinectomy.
- A lower rate of polyp recurrence has been demonstrated at 3-year follow-up in patients who underwent middle turbinate resection.[14]
- Other studies suggest that conservative middle turbinectomy does not negatively affect endoscopy scores or quality of life.[15,16]

Step 1

- Visualize the middle turbinate and its insertion on the skull base using a 0-degree endoscope.
- Inject the superior attachment of the turbinate with 1% lidocaine with 1:100,000 epinephrine.
- Perform a sphenopalatine injection as well, either through the greater palatine canal or transnasally.

Step 2

- Incise the superior attachment of the middle turbinate using straight or curved endoscopic scissors.

Minimize manipulation of the remnant turbinate to preserve its attachment to the skull base.

- In general, resecting the lower half of the middle turbinate can be performed safely without risk of disruption of the cribriform plate. Greater degrees of resection may be associated with higher risk of skull base disruption.

Step 3

- Incise the posterior attachment of the turbinate using either through-cutting forceps or endoscopic scissors until the turbinate is free.

Step 4

- Cauterize the posterior stump of the remnant middle turbinate as it may be a source of arterial bleeding, transmitting branches of the sphenopalatine artery.

Medialization Procedures and Other Alternatives to Middle Turbinate Resection

- As an alternative to middle turbinate resection, smaller instrumentation procedures can improve surgical access to narrow spaces.
- Endoscopic septoplasty can be easily integrated into an endoscopic sinus procedure when a deviation of the septum narrows access into the ethmoid sinuses. Such posterior deflections may not be aerodynamically relevant and may be difficult to appreciate on anterior rhinoscopy (Fig. 2.8).
- The inferior portion of the basal lamella should be preserved to avoid completely destabilizing the middle turbinate.
- Medialization can also be achieved by creating a small scar band between the middle turbinate and the nasal septum. Packing in the middle meatus is necessary to keep the surfaces in contact long enough to heal together and create an adhesion (usually 5–7 days).
- The middle turbinate can also be suture fixated to the nasal septum using a dissolving suture (Fig. 2.9). This technique can successfully secure a destabilized middle turbinate in most cases.[17] This is an effective method for preventing lateralization of the middle turbinate.[18]
- Knot-free suture medialization of the middle turbinate has been described as well.[19]

POSTOPERATIVE CONSIDERATIONS

- Most turbinate procedures can be performed on an outpatient basis or as in-office procedures.
- Postoperative pain is usually minimal and can be treated with acetaminophen alone. Patients should maintain a moist environment around the surgical site via the use of nasal saline.

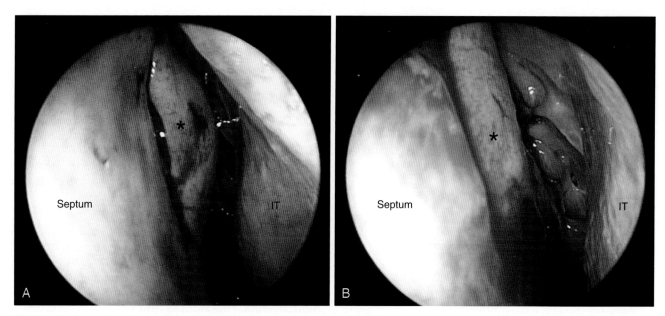

Fig. 2.8. Endoscopic views before and after septoplasty to allow medialization of the middle turbinate. **(A)** Left nasal cavity with poor access to the middle meatus caused by a posterior septal deviation *(asterisk).* An incision has been made in anticipation of an endoscopic septoplasty. **(B)** After endoscopic septoplasty, the middle meatus has opened access without the need for surgery on the middle turbinate. *IT,* Inferior turbinate.

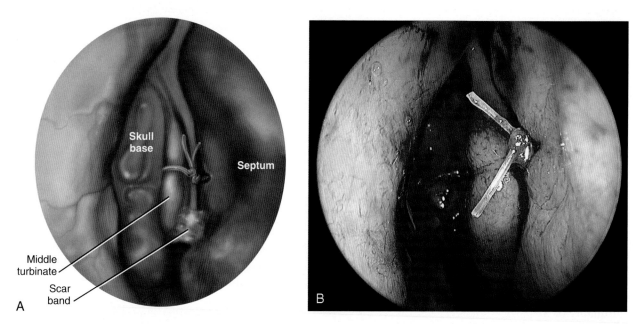

Fig. 2.9. (A) Artist's depiction of suture medialization of the right middle turbinate in endoscopic view. The suture can be tied more anteriorly in the nasal septum as well. **(B)** Endoscopic image illustrating how suture medialization can be combined with controlled scar creation between the middle turbinate head and septum.

- After some more aggressive inferior turbinate procedures, nasal packing may be helpful in keeping mucosal flaps in place but is not required.
- Patients should be evaluated postoperatively to assess healing and to débride any crusts or synechiae.
- Synechiae formation after middle turbinate procedures can be prevented by medializing the turbinate at the conclusion of the case.

REFERENCES

Access the reference list online at ExpertConsult.com.

Sphenopalatine/Internal Maxillary Artery Ligation

Li-Xing Man, Samer Fakhri, Amber U. Luong, and Martin J. Citardi

INTRODUCTION

- Epistaxis is one of the most common otolaryngologic emergencies.
- Minor epistaxis usually originates from the anterior nasal septum and is often satisfactorily treated with direct pressure or anterior nasal packing.
- Epistaxis that is not controlled by adequate anterior nasal packing can be pragmatically defined as posterior epistaxis.[1] Refractory posterior epistaxis is continued hemorrhage that occurs despite placement of anteroposterior nasal packing or shortly after its removal.
- Traditionally, the initial management of posterior epistaxis involved placement of anteroposterior nasal packing and inpatient observation. This procedure, however, is associated with significant morbidity. This has led to earlier intervention with a variety of means, including transarterial embolization, internal maxillary artery ligation, anterior ethmoid artery ligation, and endoscopic sphenopalatine artery (SPA) ligation.
- Embolization is a nonsurgical option to controlling epistaxis. It may not be available in many institutions and is typically more costly than endoscopic surgical control.[2]
- Transantral internal maxillary artery ligation through a Caldwell-Luc antrostomy is relatively straightforward but is now rarely performed since there is decreased morbidity and increased effectiveness with surgical ligation of the SPA and the anterior ethmoid artery.[3]
- Anterior ethmoid artery ligation via an external (or even an endoscopic) approach can be performed as an adjunct to SPA ligation. Vascular supply to the nasal mucosa from this branch of the internal carotid artery is usually of secondary importance.

- Endoscopic SPA ligation was first described in 1992.[4] As rigid endoscopes have become increasingly available, this technique has been refined to require minimal dissection. Because the endoscopic technique provides excellent visualization and is associated with low morbidity, it is now the first-line surgical treatment for refractory posterior epistaxis.
- SPA ligation is not intended for the treatment of epistaxis associated with the use of anticoagulants and antiplatelet drugs. Patients with this type of epistaxis are better treated with limited cauterization and placement of resorbable hemostatic packing materials.
- SPA ligation is also unlikely to provide long-term improvement in epistaxis associated with hereditary hemorrhagic telangiectasia.

ANATOMY

- The lateral nasal wall is supplied by the SPA as well as the anterior and posterior ethmoid arteries (Fig. 3.1A and Fig. 3.1B).
- The SPA, a terminal branch of the internal maxillary artery (IMA) from the external carotid artery, supplies blood to up to 90% of the nasal mucosa.[5]
- The anterior and posterior ethmoid arteries, branches of the ophthalmic artery from the internal carotid artery, also contribute significantly to nasal blood flow.
- The anterior ethmoid artery is larger than the posterior ethmoid artery and is more clinically significant. It is the major blood supply to the anterior third of both the septum and lateral nasal wall.

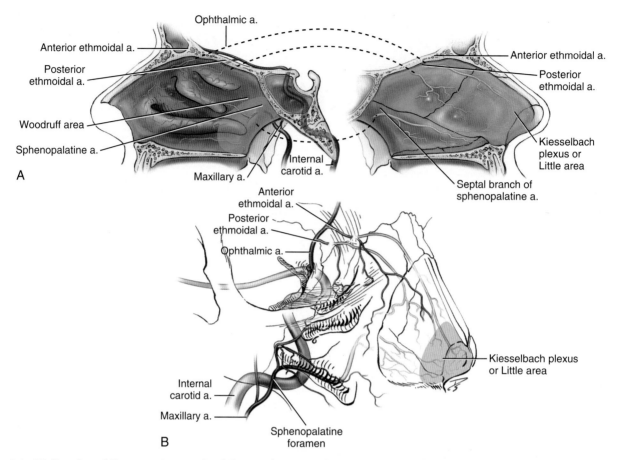

Fig. 3.1. (A) Drawing of the vascular supply of the nasal septum. Note that the sagittal cuts are as if the patient's right nose had been opened like a book. The anterior and posterior ethmoid arteries arise from the ophthalmic artery and perfuse the superior septum and lateral nasal wall. The sphenopalatine artery, which comes off the internal maxillary artery, perfuses most of the lateral nasal wall and septal mucosa. The septal branch of the sphenopalatine artery crosses from the lateral nasal wall to the septum just under the sphenoid sinus ostium. **(B)** Drawing showing three-quarter view of the blood supply of the nose. The contents of the orbit are treated as if transparent. The ophthalmic artery enters through the optic canal and sends branches of the posterior and anterior ethmoid arteries to supply the superior portions of the nasal cavity. *a.,* Artery.

- The posterior ethmoid artery supplies a small area on the superior concha and adjacent septum.
- The labial artery, a branch of the facial artery, also supplies the nasal vestibule. In addition, branches of the greater palatine artery supply the inferior anterior septum.
- The SPA, a terminal branch of the IMA from the external carotid artery, supplies blood to up to 90% of the nasal mucosa.[5]
- The network of vessels found in the Little area on the anterior septum is known as the Kiesselbach plexus (Fig. 3.2A and Fig. 3.2B). It has a rich blood supply from the anterior ethmoid artery and the SPA.
- The Woodruff plexus is located at the posterior 1 cm of the nasal floor, inferior meatus, inferior turbinate, and middle meatus (Fig. 3.3). It is predominantly supplied by the SPA.

Anatomy of the Sphenopalatine Artery

- The SPA branches from the IMA in the pterygomaxillary fossa and enters the nose through the sphenopalatine foramen.
- The sphenopalatine foramen is located on the lateral nasal wall at the superior aspect of the vertical plate of the palatine bone. It can be found where the inferior portion of the middle turbinate basal lamella meets the medial orbital wall.
- The SPA divides into the lateral nasal artery and the posterior septal nasal artery, which supply the lateral nasal wall and posterior septum, respectively. The posterior septal nasal branch is often termed the posterior nasal artery and runs across the inferior aspect of the sphenoid rostrum.

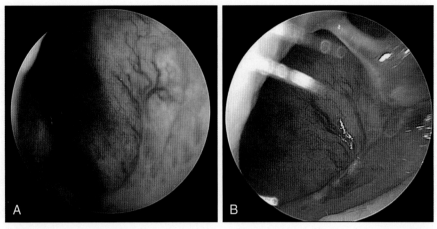

Fig. 3.2. (A) and **(B)** Endoscopic views of the Kiesselbach plexus in the Little area.

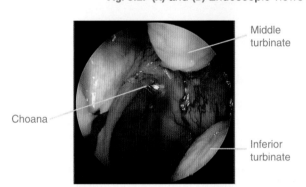

Middle turbinate

Choana

Inferior turbinate

Fig. 3.3. Endoscopic view of the Woodruff plexus in the left nasal cavity.

- The branching of the SPA occurs prior to exiting the sphenopalatine foramen in 42% of cadaveric specimens and results in separate bony foramina.[6]
- The SPA has 2+ branches immediately medial to the crista ethmoidalis in 97%, 3+ branches in 67%, and 4+ branches in 35% of individuals.[7]

Anatomy of the Crista Ethmoidalis

- During surgery, the most consistent landmark for the sphenopalatine foramen is the crista ethmoidalis of the palatine bone.
- The crista ethmoidalis is a small, raised bony crest just anterior or anterior-inferior to the sphenopalatine foramen.
- The crista ethmoidalis is located within 1 mm of the sphenopalatine foramen in 95% of cadaveric specimens.[8]
- Careful dissection posterior or posterior-superior to the crista ethmoidalis will typically reveal the sphenopalatine neurovascular bundle.
- Posterior-superior nasal branches of the maxillary nerve, including the nasopalatine nerve, emerge from the sphenopalatine foramen with the SPA. Neurologic deficits from injury to these structures have not

been described, but it is often possible to dissect free the nasopalatine nerve prior to SPA ligation.
- Removal of the crista ethmoidalis, as opposed to not removing the bone, has been associated with a lower rate of rebleeding after SPA ligation.[9]

PREOPERATIVE CONSIDERATIONS

- Preoperative evaluation includes a careful history to identify risk factors for epistaxis, including coagulopathy, hypertension, nasal trauma, and the use of anticoagulant or antiplatelet medications. Patients may not realize that a number of complementary and alternative medicines (such as fish oils and vitamin E, among many others) have antiplatelet effects.
- Symptoms such as nasal obstruction, facial hypoesthesia, or diplopia may indicate epistaxis secondary to an undiagnosed sinonasal neoplasm.
- Hematologic laboratory tests are unnecessary unless the patient has a history of recurrent bleeding or easy bruising.
- Although preoperative imaging is usually not essential, an unusual history or an abnormal physical examination may prompt a computed tomographic (CT) scan of the sinuses. A CT scan with image guidance may be helpful for intraoperative localization of anatomic structures.
- Patients may be consented for possible concurrent anterior ethmoid artery ligation.
- General anesthesia is utilized for patient comfort and to prevent aspiration.

INSTRUMENTATION (FIG. 3.4A AND FIG. 3.4B)

- 0-degree and 30-degree endoscopes
- Ball-tip, maxillary probe/seeker (Fig. 3.4A)
- Cottle elevator

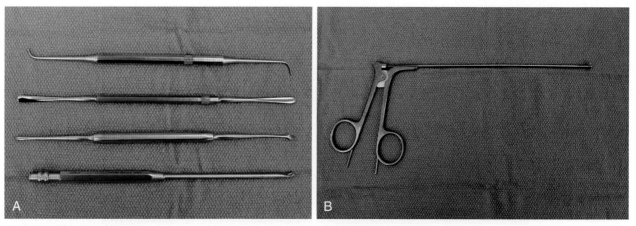

Fig. 3.4. Photographs of instruments used in sphenopalatine artery ligation. **(A)** Ball-tip seeker, Freer elevator, Cottle elevators, and suction Freer elevator. **(B)** Bipolar forceps.

- Freer elevator
- Bipolar cautery and/or hemoclip appliers (Fig. 3.4B)
- Suction Freer (optional)
- 1-mm Kerrison rongeur (optional)

PEARLS AND POTENTIAL PITFALLS

- The sphenopalatine foramen is located just posterior or posterior-superior to the crista ethmoidalis.
- It is not uncommon for the SPA to branch proximal to the foramen.
- Almost all individuals have at least two major SPA branches and two-thirds have at least three. Careful dissection is required to identify all SPA branches for ligation.
- Profuse bleeding at the time of the procedure will prevent adequate visualization. A transpalatal block of the sphenopalatine neurovascular bundle via a transpalatal injection of 1% lidocaine with 1:100,000 epinephrine through the greater palatine foramen of the hard palate may provide adequate vasoconstriction of the SPA trunk so that the bleeding slows sufficiently (Fig. 3.5). Mucosal bleeding also may be temporarily controlled using oxymetazoline-soaked pledgets, irrigation with hot water (50° C),[10] or bipolar cauterization.
- To create more space to address the sphenopalatine artery, the middle turbinate is gently moved medially using a Freer elevator and an oxymetazoline-soaked pledget is placed in the middle meatus. In addition, the uncinate may be removed, especially when it is large.
- If SPA localization is difficult, performing a maxillary antrostomy will provide the additional anatomic landmark of the posterior maxillary wall. Once this is performed, raise a flap posteriorly and inferiorly off the lateral nasal wall mucosa—this mucosa is contiguous with the mucosa over the crista ethmoidalis.

SURGICAL PROCEDURE

Step 1 (Fig. 3.6)
- Identify the middle turbinate basal lamella attachment to the palatine bone (Fig. 3.6).
- Make a vertical incision through the mucosa and periosteum approximately 1 cm anterior to the middle turbinate basal lamella attachment site.
- The demarcation between the maxillary sinus antrum and the palatine bone can be palpated using a ball-tip probe or Cottle elevator.
- If access is limited, removal of the uncinate may be helpful.

Step 2 (Fig. 3.7)
- A mucoperiosteal flap is elevated posteriorly by sweeping a Cottle, Freer, or Freer suction elevator in an inferior-to-superior direction (Fig. 3.7).

Step 3 (Fig. 3.8)
- A small crest of bone, the crista ethmoidalis, is observed just anterior or anterior-inferior to the tented SPA (Fig. 3.8) at the sphenopalatine foramen.
- Optionally, the crista ethmoidalis and bone of the foramen superficial to the SPA may be removed using a 1-mm Kerrison rongeur to expose the SPA prior to its branching point.
- Whether or not the crista is removed, perform gentle dissection 360 degrees around the SPA pedicle. A ball-tip probe is ideal for this maneuver.

Step 4 (Fig. 3.9)
- Place individual hemoclips on the main trunk and each terminal branch of the SPA. Perform bipolar cautery on the terminal branches distally (Fig. 3.9).

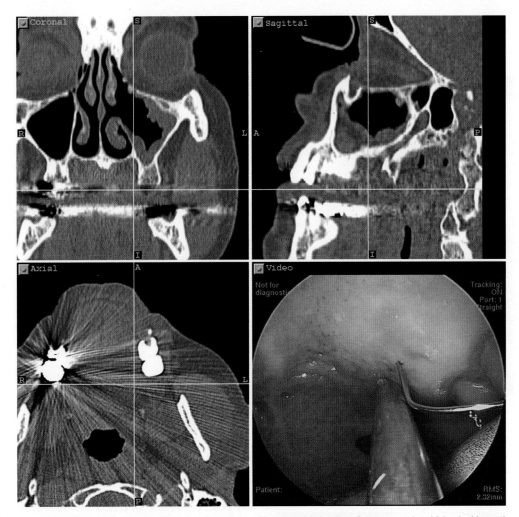

Fig. 3.5. CT scans and endoscopic image showing location of intraoral injection for transpalatal block. Note the greater palatine foramen and canal on the sagittal view.

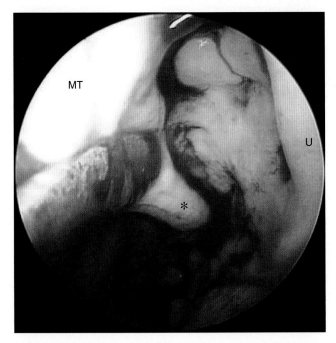

Fig. 3.6. Endoscopic view of the anatomy of the left lateral nasal wall. The asterisk is at the middle turbinate attachment. If difficulty is encountered in identifying the sphenopalatine artery (SPA), remember that the SPA is the major blood supply of the middle turbinate (MT) and follow that attachment to identify the SPA. *U,* Uncinate.

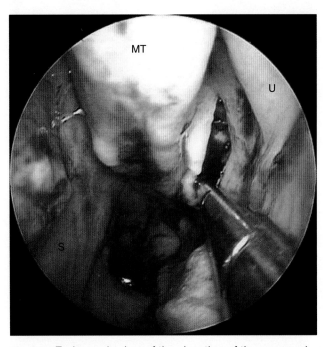

Fig. 3.7. Endoscopic view of the elevation of the mucoperiosteal flap. *MT,* Middle turbinate; *S,* septum; *U,* uncinate.

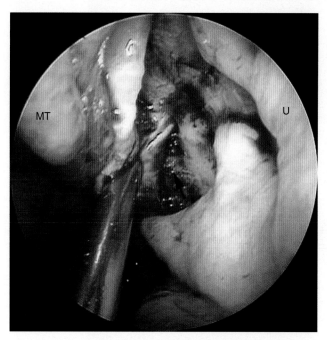

Fig. 3.8. Endoscopic view of the sphenopalatine artery. The arrow points to the sphenopalatine artery. *MT,* Middle turbinate; *U,* uncinate.

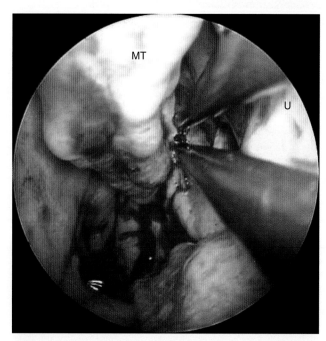

Fig. 3.9. Endoscopic view of bipolar cautery of the sphenopalatine artery. The artery may also be clipped. *MT,* Middle turbinate; *U,* uncinate.

- Alternatively, perform bipolar cautery without placing hemoclips.
- At the end of the procedure, redrape the mucoperiosteal flap laterally over the exposed palatine bone.
- An absorbable hemostatic spacer may be placed in the middle meatus to lateralize the mucoperiosteal flap and to keep the middle turbinate medialized.

POSTOPERATIVE CONSIDERATIONS

- Avoid synechiae formation between the middle turbinate and lateral nasal wall by medializing the middle turbinate at the end of the case.
- If diffuse anterior nasal mucosal trauma has occurred from prior nasal packing or cautery, the placement of resorbable dressing materials will minimize the risk of bleeding from the mucosal edges and help prevent adhesion formation.
- Postoperatively, patients can usually be discharged after observing for 12 hours.
- The main complication of endoscopic sphenopalatine artery ligation is failure to control epistaxis. This is usually due to the surgeon's failure to clip or coagulate all branches of the SPA or to bleeding from mucosa supplied by the anterior ethmoid artery.

SPA LIGATION CARE PATHWAYS

- Early SPA ligation has been associated with shorter hospitalizations, lower costs, and lower risks.[11,12]
- SPA ligation may be integrated into an epistaxis treatment algorithm such that this procedure is offered to all patients with posterior epistaxis as a means to an early, definitive intervention. This approach results in better outcomes, including greater patient safety and reduced costs.[13]

CONCLUSIONS

- Endoscopic SPA ligation has emerged as a mainstay in the management of severe epistaxis.
- Endoscopic SPA is a low-morbidity procedure with a high likelihood of success.
- Endoscopic SPA ligation may obviate the need for traditional anteroposterior nasal packing.

REFERENCES

Access the reference list online at ExpertConsult.com.

Endoscopic and Open Anterior/ Posterior Ethmoid Artery Ligation

Yuresh Naidoo and P.J. Wormald

INTRODUCTION

- The anterior ethmoid artery (AEA) and the posterior ethmoid artery (PEA) are major vessels supplying the ethmoid sinus, septum, and anterior skull base.
- Control of these vessels is a key step in performing extended sinus and skull base procedures.
- The critical location of these vessels, which traverse the orbit and roof of the ethmoid sinus, makes iatrogenic damage to these vessels potentially dangerous during endoscopic sinus and skull base surgery (Fig. 4.1).
- Retraction of the AEA into the orbit can lead to permanent vision loss if not managed appropriately.
- Elective ligation of the AEA and PEA is indicated for extended endonasal procedures when control of these vascular structures is an essential component of the procedure, such as in endoscopic craniofacial resections.
- Rarely, intractable or traumatic epistaxis requires ligation of these arteries, but this is probably best managed externally with endoscopic assistance.
- This chapter explains how to reliably perform an endoscopic endonasal ligation of the AEA and PEA before surgery of the anterior skull base as well as to perform open arterial ligation for epistaxis.

ANATOMY—ENDOSCOPIC PERSPECTIVE

- The AEA and PEA are branches of the ophthalmic artery.
- The PEA is smaller than the AEA and is found at the junction of the roof of the sphenoid and posterior ethmoid sinuses.

- The AEA lies between the second and third lamella of the lateral nasal wall (ethmoid bulla and middle turbinate, respectively). This is posterior to the anterior face of the ethmoid bulla unless a suprabullar recess exists. In general, it is found one cell behind the frontal ostium along the skull base (Fig. 4.2).
- The AEA passes between the superior oblique and medial rectus muscles before leaving the orbit at the anterior ethmoid foramen, together with the anterior ethmoid nerve, to enter the roof of the ethmoid sinus. It crosses the cribriform plate and enters the nose through a tiny slit adjacent to the crista galli to become the dorsal nasal artery.
- Depending on the pneumatization of the ethmoid sinuses and the height of the lateral lamella of the cribriform plate, the AEA may lie on a mesentery below the skull base within the ethmoid sinus (seen in 36% of cases; Fig. 4.3).[1,2]
- Sixteen percent of AEAs are found to be in a mesentery *and* dehiscent and therefore at significant risk of traumatic injury in endoscopic sinus surgery.[2]
- These arteries also supply the meninges of the anterior cranial fossa and can be considerably enlarged in the presence of meningiomas and other tumors arising in this region.[3]
- The crucial *external* landmark is the frontoethmoid suture line[4]:
  - The AEA is approximately 24 mm posterior to the anterior lacrimal crest along the frontoethmoid suture line.
  - The PEA lies approximately 12 mm farther posterior to the AEA along the frontoethmoid suture line.
  - The optic nerve is approximately 6 mm posterior to the PEA.

20–40% BELOW SKULL BASE

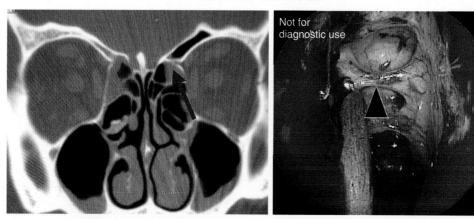

Fig. 4.1. Coronal computed tomographic scan *(left)* and endoscopic image *(right)* with the left anterior ethmoid artery indicated *(left, arrow; right, arrowhead).*

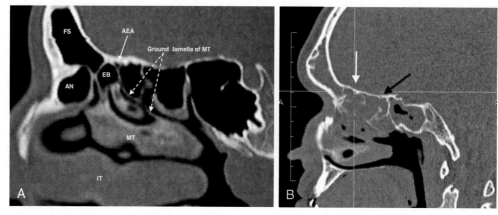

Fig. 4.2. **(A)** Parasagittal computed tomographic (CT) scan showing the location of the anterior ethmoid artery (AEA), which is usually found between the second and third basal lamellae of the lateral nasal wall. The anterior ethmoid foramen is seen on the skull base between these two structures. **(B)** Parasagittal CT scan showing the anterior *(white arrow)* and posterior *(black arrow)* ethmoid arteries on the skull base. *AN,* Agger nasi; *EB,* ethmoid bulla; *FS,* frontal sinus; *IT,* inferior turbinate; *MT,* middle turbinate.

PREOPERATIVE CONSIDERATIONS

■ Complete exposure of the skull base is required for identification and endoscopic endonasal ligation. Tumor debulking and a complete sphenoethmoidectomy are required to achieve this exposure. The exposure is further aided by an endoscopic modified Lothrop procedure.

■ For epistaxis, use of an endoscopic approach, which requires significant sinus dissection for exposure and places the skull base at risk, seems unnecessary purely to avoid the small external scar associated with an external incision.

Radiographic Considerations

■ Examine the coronal, parasagittal, and axial computed tomographic scans.

■ Identify the first coronal scan in which the globe is no longer seen. Look for the protuberance on the lamina papyracea between the superior oblique and medial rectus muscles. This is the anterior ethmoid foramen.

■ Follow the artery anteriorly to ascertain whether it lies above the skull base in its entirety or whether it descends into the nasal cavity.

■ Determine whether a suprabullar recess exists. If so, determine whether the AEA lies in front of the anterior face of the ethmoid bulla.

■ In expanded endonasal procedures, computer-aided surgery is helpful. The images should be reviewed preoperatively to identify the AEA or PEA in each plane and its relationship to the tumor.

INSTRUMENTATION

■ 0-degree and 30-degree endoscopes

■ Lens washer (e.g., Endo-Scrub 2 [Medtronic ENT], Jacksonville, Florida)

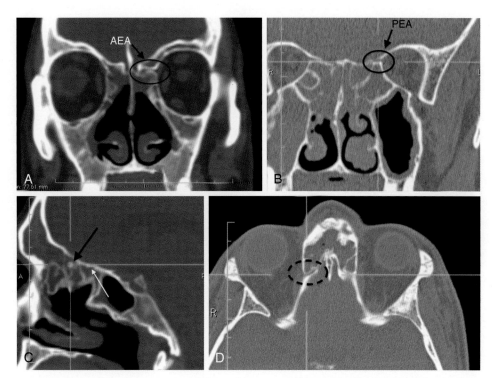

Fig. 4.3. (A) Computed tomographic (CT) scan of a patient with an anterior ethmoid artery (AEA) lying below the skull base. This coronal CT shows the left AEA on a mesentery, leaving the orbit between the medial rectus and superior oblique muscles. **(B)** Coronal CT scan showing the posterior ethmoid artery (PEA) on the skull base at the level of the posterior ethmoids. **(C)** Parasagittal CT showing the AEA lying well below the skull base in the ethmoid sinus *(black arrow).* The PEA is not as clearly seen *(white arrow),* but it is lying in its usual position at the junction of the posterior ethmoids and front face of the sphenoid. **(D)** Axial CT showing the AEA as it exits the orbit.

- Routine functional endoscopic sinus surgery instruments (ball-tip probe, microdébrider, straight and angled cutting and grasping instruments)
- 3.2-mm diamond bur or dacrocystorhinostomy (DCR) bur (Medtronic ENT)
- Wormald Suction Bipolar Forceps (Medtronic ENT)
- Malleable suction curette (Wormald Malleable Frontal Sinus Surgery Instrument Set [Medtronic ENT])
- Vascular clips
- For open AEA and PEA ligation, additional instruments include the following:
  - Scalpel with a No. 15 blade
  - Freer elevator
  - Thin, malleable retractors
  - Standard head and neck bipolar forceps

PEARLS AND POTENTIAL PITFALLS

Pearls

- Endoscopically, the key to finding the AEA and PEA is to define the level of the skull base. This is reliably and safely achieved by identifying the roof of the sphenoid sinus.
- Dissect between ethmoid septations that extend from the skull base.

  - Move the débrider or malleable suction curette in and out between the septations rather than across bony septations from posterior to anterior.
  - This will clear disease and/or debulk tumor without transecting the AEA or PEA, which might be present in the septation.
- The AEA is usually found one cell posterior to the frontal ostium on the skull base.
- When performing an ethmoid bullectomy, look for the characteristic posterolateral to anteromedial slant of the AEA in the roof of the ethmoid bulla.
- The PEA is identified in the roof of the posterior ethmoid adjacent to the sphenoid.
- Even if the artery is in a mesentery, it can be difficult to apply a vascular clip, because the artery is often still encased in bone.[2,5] The artery therefore must be freed from its bony confines so that a clip can be applied. Alternatively, bipolar forceps can be applied to the exposed component of the artery.

Potential Pitfalls

- The PEA usually causes minimal problems if accidentally transected, but it can be abnormally large when tumors of the anterior skull base are present or

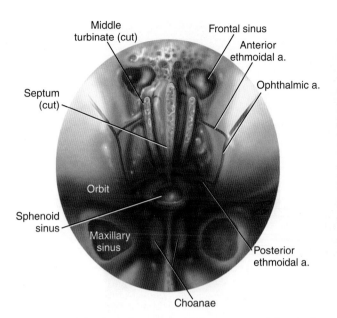

Fig. 4.4. Artist's depiction of required exposure of the skull base in endoscopic view. A complete sphenoethmoidectomy and bilateral frontal sinusotomy has been performed. Often a Draf 3 (frontal sinus) drill-out procedure is added. The septum has been released from the skull base. The anterior and posterior ethmoid arteries are identified before bipolar cautery is used. *a.*, Artery.

when prior sphenopalatine artery (SPA) ligation has been performed.[3,4]

- Retraction of the AEA behind the orbit can occur if the AEA is accidentally severed, with resultant orbital hematoma. This requires emergency decompression of the orbit.
- Refrain from using monopolar cautery to control bleeding from the AEA or PEA. This can result in a bony fracture of the adjacent skull base leading to cerebrospinal fluid leak.
- For an open procedure, careful exposure is necessary before cauterization or vascular ligation because the optic nerve lies directly posterior to vessels.

SURGICAL PROCEDURES

- For tumors of the anterior skull base, such as an anterior cranial fossa meningioma, the surgical steps are as described below.

Endoscopic Ligation

Step 1: Identify Critical Landmarks and Fully Expose the Skull Base (Fig. 4.4)

- Open the sinuses and identify the skull base.
- Perform an uncinectomy with identification of the maxillary ostium. This is a landmark for the floor of the orbit and also guides the surgeon to the approximate height of the sphenoid ostium.

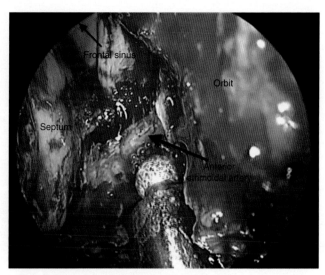

Fig. 4.5. Endoscopic view of the left anterior ethmoid artery *(arrow)*. After the artery is identified, the drill is used to remove its bony covering.

- Clear the frontal recess and identify the frontal ostium.
- Remove the lower half of the ethmoid bulla and enter the posterior ethmoids.
- Identify the superior turbinate and remove the inferior third to identify the sphenoid ostium.
- Enlarge the sphenoid to identify the skull base.
- Continue the dissection along the skull base, completely removing all cells from the sphenoid roof posteriorly to the frontal ostium anteriorly.
- If indicated because of the need for an entire skull base resection, an endoscopic modified Lothrop procedure may aid in exposing the anterior skull base and AEA.

Step 2: Identify and Confirm the AEA and PEA With Image Guidance

- After completing this step, proceed to the next step.

Step 3: Use a Diamond Bur to Thin the Bone Overlying the AEA/PEA

- Remove bone over a broad front over the artery to reduce the risk of transecting the artery (Fig. 4.5).
- Do not approach the orbit because the bur may transect the artery. If this happens directly adjacent to the orbit, retraction of the artery into the orbit with subsequent hematoma can occur.

Step 4: Expose the Artery So That Bipolar Forceps Can Be Applied

- See Fig. 4.6.

Step 5. Ligate the PEA in the Same Fashion (Fig. 4.7)

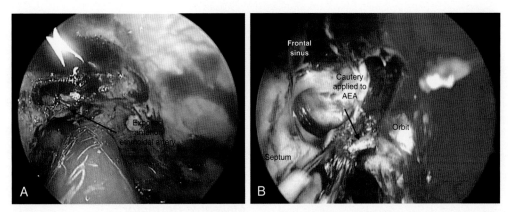

Fig. 4.6. Endoscopic views of ligation of the anterior ethmoid artery (AEA). **(A)** The left AEA is exposed in its midportion *(arrow)* and is ready for application of the bipolar forceps. **(B)** Cauterization of the exposed artery is performed with the bipolar forceps *(arrow; Wormald style shown)*.

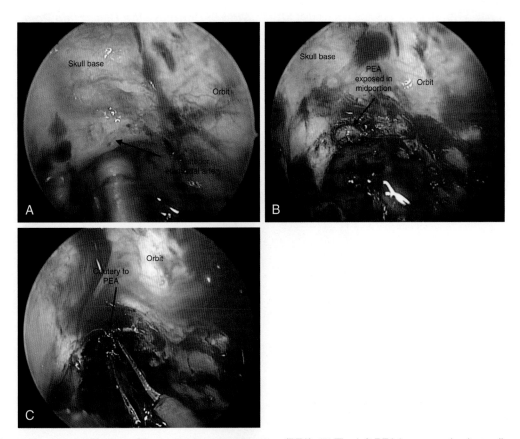

Fig. 4.7. Endoscopic views of ligation of the posterior ethmoid artery (PEA). **(A)** The left PEA is exposed using a diamond bur in the midportion of the artery along its course on the roof of the ethmoid cavity *(arrow)*. **(B)** The bony covering of the PEA has been exposed at the midportion of the artery *(arrow)*. **(C)** Bipolar cauterization of the PEA is performed after bone removal *(arrow)*.

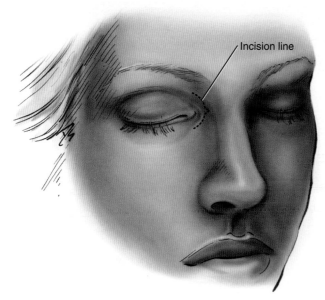

Fig. 4.8. Drawing of the incision for external ligation. The incision is made with a No. 15 blade held perpendicular to the skin. A notch at the level of the medial canthus helps prevent webbing after surgery. The incision is taken down to bone and the tissue elevated at the subperiosteal plane.

External Ligation

Step 1: Make the Incision

- After injecting a local vasoconstrictive agent, make a semicircular incision (Lynch incision) as shown in Fig. 4.8. Note the notch made to minimize scar retraction.

Step 2: Dissect Soft Tissue Down to Bone

- Diploic veins are often identified here, and bipolar cautery can be used for hemostasis.

Step 3: Retract Soft Tissue With a Thin, Malleable Retractor

- After completing this step, proceed to the next step.

Step 4: Continue the Dissection Posteriorly Until the Nasolacrimal Sac Is Identified

- This step can be done either with loupes or with a 0-degree endoscope (Fig. 4.9).

Step 5: Continue the Dissection Posteriorly Until the AEA and PEA Are Identified

- The 24/12/6 rule as described previously is useful to identify the arteries (Fig. 4.10).

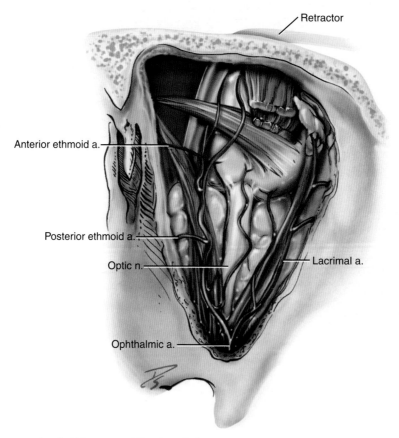

Fig. 4.9. Drawing of the operative field in external ligation. Soft tissues of the orbit are retracted laterally. Dissection is continued in the subperiosteal plane and extended until the anterior and subsequent posterior ethmoid arteries are identified. Typically, the superior oblique muscle will not be identified because the vessels are inferior, and the superior oblique is held in the fascial planes of the orbital contents above the dissection plane. *a.,* Artery; *n.,* nerve.

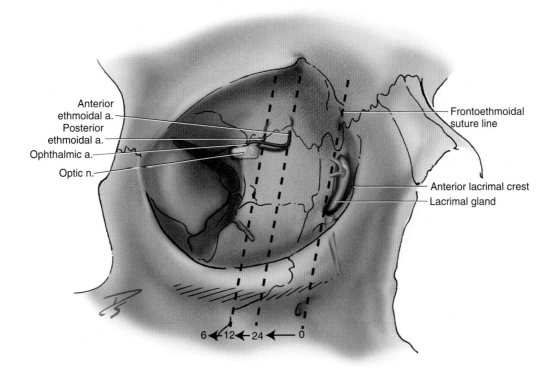

Fig. 4.10. As illustrated in the drawing, once the lacrimal sac is identified, the anterior ethmoid artery, posterior ethmoid artery, and optic nerve typically follow the "24/12/6" rule from the anterior lacrimal crest. *a.,* Artery; *n.,* nerve.

Step 6: Ligate the Vessels With Endoscopic Clip Appliers or Bipolar Cautery

■ After completing this step, proceed to the next step.

Step 7: Close Soft Tissue and Skin Using a Standard Facial Closure

■ Take great care to close the deep layers in perfect apposition to minimize scarring.

Transcaruncular Approach

■ Another open approach to AEA and PEA ligation is similar to a Lynch incision. However, the incision is made across the caruncle and is taken down to the subperiosteal/bony plane. The surgery then proceeds as described earlier in Steps 3 through 7.

POSTOPERATIVE CONSIDERATIONS

■ Check the patient's visual acuity and range of motion hourly for 6 hours postoperatively.
■ The optic nerve and superior oblique muscle are at risk of thermal injury from the bipolar diathermy in the external approach.[6-8]
■ A small amount of periorbital bruising can be expected.

SPECIAL CONSIDERATIONS

■ Endonasal ligation of the AEA and PEA as they exit the orbit has been described in small case series and cadaver studies.[9,10] A small amount of the lamina papyracea surrounding the artery is removed to expose the artery sufficiently to apply a vascular clip. However, this technique has the potential to expose orbital fat and medial rectus muscles with potentially devastating consequences if they are subsequently caught in the débrider.
  – Loss of control of the AEA at this point is more likely to cause retraction of the AEA within the orbit and subsequent hematoma.
  – Fat prolapse from this exposure may hinder dissection of an intracranial tumor once it is accessed (Fig. 4.11).
■ The recommended protocol is to achieve control of the AEA and PEA as they cross the midpoint of the ethmoid roof when performing skull base surgery because the fovea ethmoidalis needs to be exposed and removed as part of this surgery. An external endoscopically assisted approach for ligating the artery is preferred when the procedure is performed for epistaxis.

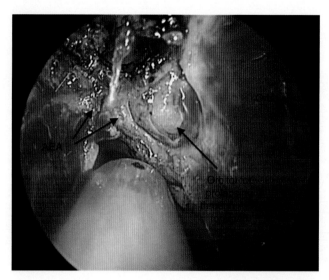

Fig. 4.11. Endoscopic view of prolapse of orbital fat as the anterior ethmoid artery (AEA) exits the AEA foramen *(arrow).* The periorbita is relatively weak where the AEA exits the orbit to enter the AEA foramen *(arrow).* Hence, ligation is most safely achieved in the midportion of the anterior or posterior ethmoid artery as it traverses the skull base.

Orbital Hematoma

- An expanding orbital hematoma can occur if the AEA is severed and retracts within the orbit.
- This requires immediate action:
  - Endoscopic orbital decompression if it occurs intraoperatively
  - Lateral canthotomy and cantholysis if vision is at risk

REFERENCES

Access the reference list online at ExpertConsult.com.

Endoscopic Repair of Choanal Atresia

Aldo Cassol Stamm, Shirley Shizue Nagata Pignatari, and Leonardo Balsalobre

INTRODUCTION

The opening of choanal atretic plates can be obtained by various techniques. Despite the substantial available published literature on the treatment modalities of choanal atresia, the optimum technique is not fully established. The choice many times depends on the surgeon's preference.[1] This chapter describes the cross-over flap technique, which can be employed in unilateral or bilateral choanal atresia.[2]

Surgical endoscopic techniques incorporating mucosal flaps have been shown to minimize the healing reaction, reduce subsequent scarring, and may present less chance of restenosis.[2–5] Knowledge of the anatomy, good visualization (0-degree endoscope), and utilization of very delicate surgical instruments facilitate an easier, faster, and safer procedure.

ANATOMY

- The choanal atretic plate may consist of a mucosal membrane or of bone covered by mucosa. The bony part is usually an extension of the medial pterygoid plate laterally and the vomer medially.
- The nasal cavity itself is usually preserved anatomically.

PREOPERATIVE CONSIDERATIONS

- Choana atresia patients are usually children, often newborns, who present with narrow and small nasal cavities. Every initial step should be directed to preventing unnecessary mucosal trauma and bleeding and to create more operating exposure. Preoperative mucosal topical decongestion is recommended. At least 5 minutes should elapse to allow the vasoconstrictive pledgets to decongest the mucosa.

- To create more space to address the posterior part of the nasal cavity, cover the inferior turbinate with a piece of cotton and, with a delicate Freer elevator, gently move and outfracture it against the nasal lateral wall.
- In order to facilitate tailoring while displacing the posterior septal mucosa and the mucosa of the posterior floor of the nasal cavity, infiltration elevation can be accomplished by using a saline solution.

Preoperative Considerations— Radiographic Considerations

- Review in detail the axial and coronal computed tomography (CT) scans.
- Identify the atretic plate verifying the presence or absence of bone. Not uncommonly, septal deviations coexist, further narrowing the operating field exposure (Fig. 5.1).

INSTRUMENTATION

- 0-degree scope
- Suction elevator
- Ball-tip probe
- Backbiter
- Downbiter
- Delicate scissors
- Micro Kerrison punch
- Curette
- Drill

PEARLS

- Adequately delicate instruments are essential to shorten the surgical procedure. In some cases, particularly

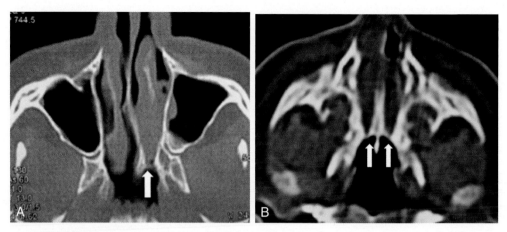

Fig. 5.1. **(A)** Axial computed tomographic (CT) scan showing unilateral choanal atresia *(white arrow)*. **(B)** Axial CT scan showing bilateral choanal atresia *(white arrows)*.

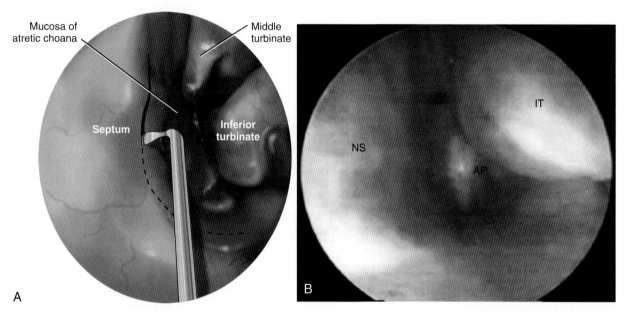

Fig. 5.2. **(A)** Artist's depiction of the L-shaped incision *(dashed line)* made in left-sided choanal atresia (endoscopic view). **(B)** Endoscopic view of an atretic plate *(AP)* of the left nasal cavity. *IT,* Inferior turbinate; *NS,* nasal septum.

in newborns, otologic microinstruments may be employed.

- After infiltration, before proceeding to displacing and elevating the mucosa, one may take advantage of the support of the osteocartilaginous septum to make linear incisions on the mucosa, creating the desired shape for the flaps.

SURGICAL STEPS

- The entire surgical procedure can be accomplished with a 0-degree endoscope. If bilateral, choose the side with more space, thus with more operating exposure. If unilateral, begin by making an L-shaped (left side; Fig. 5.2) or J-shaped (right side) incision at the posterior part of the nasal septum, vertically on

the septum mucosa and obliquely toward the end of the inferior turbinate on the floor of the nasal cavity.

- Before displacing the mucosa toward the atretic plate and removing the osteocartilaginous septum, it may prove helpful to incise the mucosa, creating the shape of the flaps. Incisions can be accomplished with a delicate horizontal knife (similar to the otologic horizontal knife).

Step 1: Incise the Mucosa, Drawing the Flaps

- Creation of Flaps for Unilateral Left-Side Atresia: After proper infiltration, make a transfixing vertical incision on the nasal septum, about 1 cm ahead of the atretic plate. On the atretic side, this incision will start at the level of the inferior edge of the middle turbinate, continuing vertically down and reaching

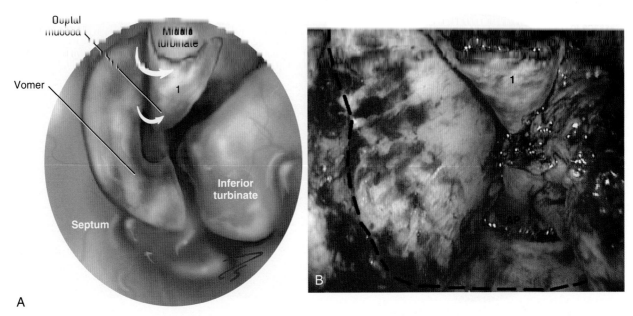

Fig. 5.3. Artist's depiction **(A)** and endoscopic photograph **(B)** of the flap *(1)* harvested from the initial L-shaped incision (*dashed line* in B) left-sided choanal atresia. *AP,* Atretic plate.

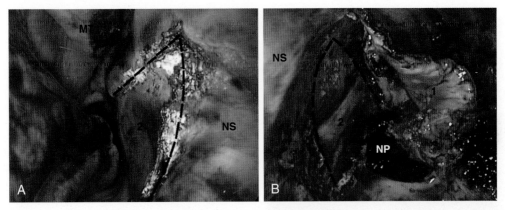

Fig. 5.4. (A) Endoscopic view through the right nasal cavity showing the creation of the shape of the contralateral flap (2). **(B)** Endoscopic view though the left nasal cavity showing the shape of the right flap (2). *1,* Left flap; *IT,* inferior turbinate; *MT,* middle turbinate; *NP,* nasopharynx; *NS,* nasal septum.

the nasal floor mucosa in an L-shaped fashion on the mucosa of the floor toward the end of the inferior turbinate (Figs. 5.3A and 5.3B).

■ On the other side, the upper part of this vertical incision will turn posteriorly toward the superior edge of the choana following the level of the free border of the middle turbinate, reaching the end of the septum, opening the mucosa vertically, and creating a communication with the nasopharynx (Figs. 5.4A and 5.4B).

■ The mucosal flaps can now be displaced bilaterally and preserved. The flap of the atretic side will be elevated to the upper part of the nasal cavity, and the opposite flap will be preserved. The pharyngeal mucosa of the atretic plate can be removed along with the atretic bone.

Step 2: Remove the Posterior Nasal Septum

■ The posterior nasal septum (bony-cartilaginous) is now removed, along with the atretic plate (Fig. 5.5). Different instruments may be necessary for this step. The atretic plate can be removed with a micro Kerrison punch, diamond drill, or even a microdébrider. The posterior nasal septum can be removed with a micro Kerrison punch, backbiting and downbiting forceps, or a strong through-cutting forceps.

■ The superior limit of septum removal is the inferior edge of the middle turbinate. At this point, one may realize that the mucosal flaps are redundant and some will need to be tailored with a delicate pair of scissors.

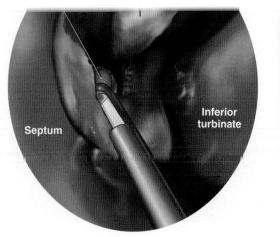

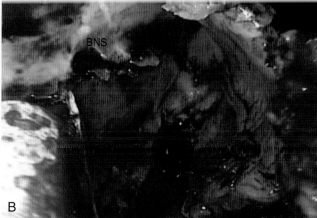

Fig. 5.5. Artist's depiction **(A)** and endoscopic photograph **(B)** of removal of the posterior nasal septum using a micro Kerrison punch. *1,* Left mucosal flap; *2,* right septal mucosa from which the contralateral flap will originate; *BNS,* bony nasal septum.

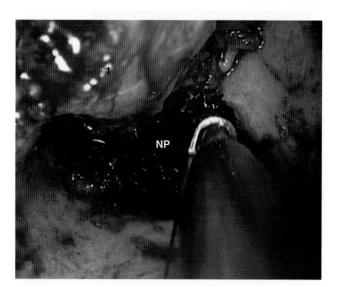

Fig. 5.6. Endoscopic view of removal of the pterygoid lamina using a micro Kerrison punch. *1,* Left flap; *NP,* posterior wall of the nasopharynx after removal of the atretic plate.

Step 3: Remove the Thickened Extension of the Pterygoid Lamina Laterally

- Use a horizontal knife or elevator (45- or 90-degree lamina) to carefully displace and separate the pharyngeal from the nasal mucosa of the lateral edge of the new choana, exposing the bony border (extension of the medial pterygoid lamina). The bone can then be removed with a micro Kerrison punch, drill, or curette (Fig. 5.6).

Step 4: Positioning the Flaps

- The flaps are positioned, covering the entire denuded exposed area of the neochoana (floor and roof) by using a seeker probe or Freer elevator (Figs. 5.7A and 5.7B).

Step 5: Attaching the Flaps

- In order to keep the flaps in position (Figs. 5.8A and 5.8B), fibrin glue or a soft anchored packing (with a suture guide attached on the external part of the nose with a bandage) is kept in place for 1 to 2 days. Fig. 5.9 shows the final aspect of the new choana after 1 week postoperatively.

POSTOPERATIVE CONSIDERATIONS

- Nasal wash with saline solution using a syringe (1 mL for newborns) is recommended for at least 3 times a day during the first month. Steroid eye drops are also prescribed in decreasing doses in the first 3 weeks.
- Nasal aspiration probes should be avoided during the first weeks because of the risk of displacement of the flaps.
- Nasal endoscopy is recommended after 10 days and periodically for the first year.

FINAL CONSIDERATIONS

In the past 8 years, the authors have operated exclusively by this surgical technique on more than 25 patients from

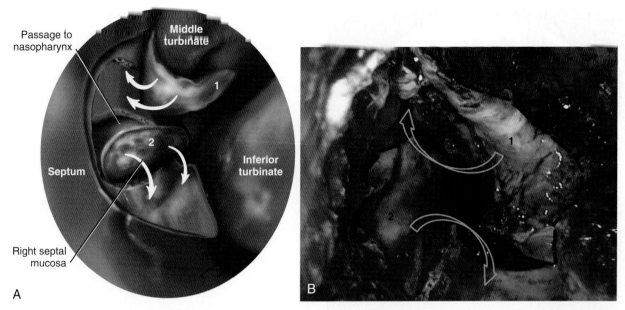

Fig. 5.7. Artist's depiction **(A)** and endoscopic photography **(B)** of the view after removal of the posterior bony septum and creation of the left *(1)* and right *(2)* flaps. The arrows indicate the position of the flaps. The dashed lines outline both left and right flaps.

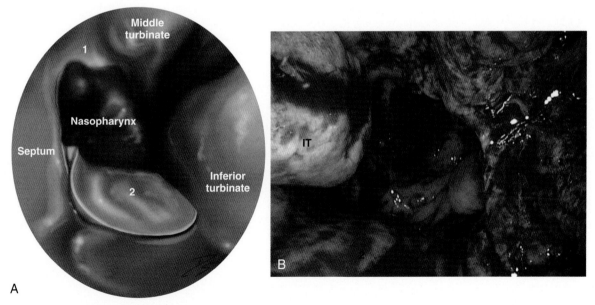

Fig. 5.8. Artist's depiction **(A)** and endoscopic photography **(B)** of the final aspect of the neochoana after the flaps are attached with fibrin glue. *1,* Left flap; *2,* right flap; *IT,* inferior turbinate.

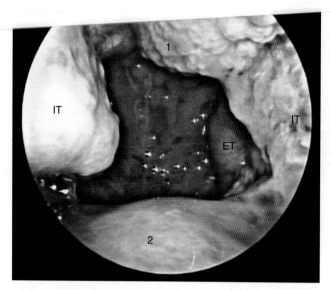

Fig. 5.9. Endoscopic view of the neochoana on the eighth postoperative day. *1,* Left flap; *2,* right flap; *ET,* eustachian tube torus; *IT,* inferior turbinate.

...served in this series of patients.

- In some cases with more than 5 years of follow-up, we have observed a worsening of breathing due to the inferior turbinate's posterior aspect hypertrophy at the level of the posterior nasal septum defect. In selected cases, partial turbinectomy may be useful.

REFERENCES

Access the reference list online at ExpertConsult.com.

Basics of Primary Endoscopic Sinus Surgery

Maxillary Antrostomy

Alexander G. Chiu and James N. Palmer

INTRODUCTION

- The maxillary antrostomy is the first step in performing functional endoscopic sinus surgery.
- Based on a good working knowledge of the anatomy and using proper visualization and mucosa-sparing techniques, a well-performed maxillary antrostomy will not only address maxillary sinus disease but properly set up the remaining portions of the sinus surgery.

ANATOMY (FIGS. 6.1, 6.2, AND 6.3)

- The uncinate process is composed of thin bone covered by mucosa. It has attachments superiorly to the agger nasi cell or skull base.
- The uncinate process covers the infundibulum—the functional area where the maxillary sinus, anterior ethmoids, and frontal sinus drain.
- The uncinate process attaches anteriorly to the lacrimal bone and is in the shape of a quarter moon. The posterior-inferior portion of the uncinate runs in a horizontal plane toward the posterior fontanelle.
- The maxillary line is the attachment of the uncinate process to the lacrimal bone. The natural *os* of the maxillary sinus can be visualized at the junction of the lower ⅓ and upper ⅔ on the maxillary line (Fig. 6.4). The ostiomeatal complex is a functional area not an anatomic area. Opening the ostiomeatal complex involves removing the uncinate process and ethmoid bulla as well as enlarging the natural maxillary ostium.
- The middle turbinate serves to humidify inspired air. Care should be taken to preserve the middle turbinate if possible when performing a maxillary antrostomy. If removal is necessary, consider amputating only the anterior inferior quadrant of the turbinate.

Radiographic Considerations

- Look at the axial and coronal computed tomographic (CT) scans
- Identify the uncinate process and its relation to the medial orbital wall.
  - Beware of an uncinate process that is lateralized against the medial orbital wall (Fig. 6.5). If identified, make sure to take great caution in using a sickle knife or microdébrider against the uncinate to prevent inadvertent orbital entry.
- Identify the presence of any Haller cells, also called *infraorbital ethmoid cells,* that may be contributing to the obstruction of the middle meatus.
- Identify the presence of any pathologic process along the floor and/or anterolateral walls of the maxillary sinus. If a retention cyst or polyp is present, make preparations to have angled instruments and endoscopes available to address these hard-to-reach locations.

INSTRUMENTATION (FIG. 6.6)

- 0-degree and 30-degree endoscopes
  - 45-degree or 70-degree endoscopes if lesions must be removed along the floor or anterior wall
- Ball-tip probe
- Backbiter
- Downbiter
- Angled microdébrider
- Straight through-cutter
- 120-degree giraffe
  - Used for removal of retention cysts along the anterior and/or floor of the maxillary sinus

PREOPERATIVE CONSIDERATIONS

- The first 15 minutes after anesthesia induction is often a time when the patient's heart rate and blood pressure

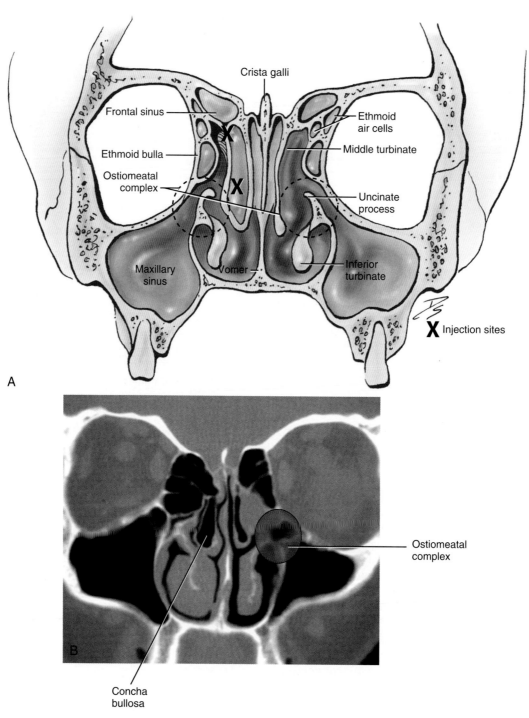

Fig. 6.1. **(A)** Drawing in coronal view of the middle turbinate, uncinate, and ostiomeatal complex. Dashed circles represent the ostiomeatal complexes. Local anesthetic should be infiltrated at both Xs, which correspond to the axilla of the middle turbinate as it attaches to the lateral nasal wall, and injected into the anterior face of the middle turbinate itself. **(B)** Coronal CT scan showing bilateral conchae bullosae, which are air cells inside the middle turbinate.

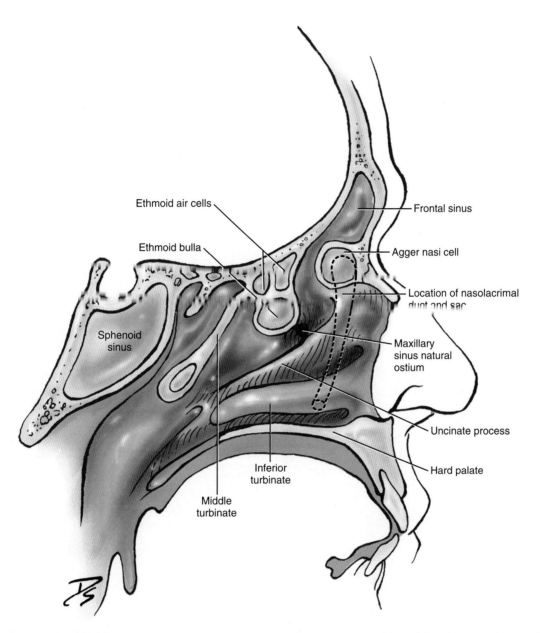

Fig. 6.2. Drawing in sagittal view showing the curvature of the uncinate process, location of the natural ostium, and nasolacrimal duct and sac *(dashed line)*.

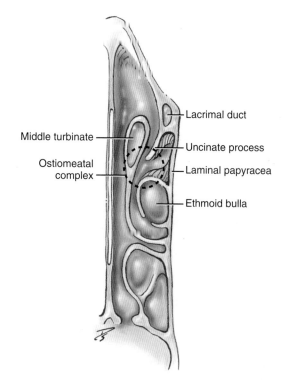

Middle turbinate

Ostiomeatal complex

Lacrimal duct

Uncinate process

Laminal papyracea

Ethmoid bulla

Fig. 6.3. Drawing in axial view showing the relationship between the uncinate process, ethmoid bulla, and middle turbinate. *Dashed circle* represents the ostiomeatal complex.

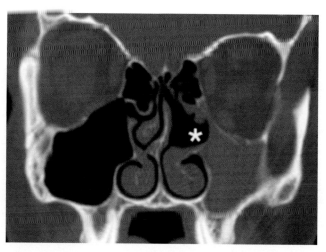

Fig. 6.5. Coronal CT scan showing a lateralized left uncinate process *(asterisk).* With the decreased maxillary volume and low orbital floor, this CT scan is consistent with maxillary atelectasis or silent sinus syndrome.

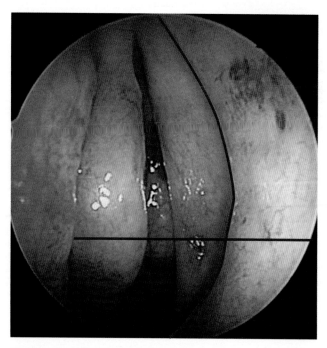

Fig. 6.4. Endoscopic photograph illustrating how to locate the maxillary os.

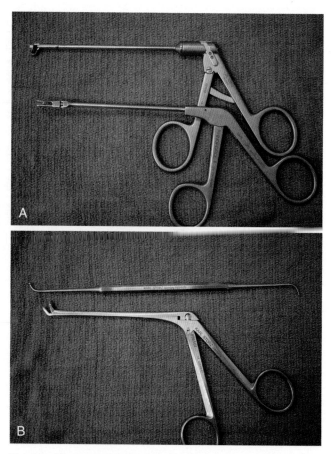

Fig. 6.6. Photographs of instruments used in maxillary antrostomy. **(A)** Downbiter and backbiter forceps. **(B)** Ball-tip probe and 45-degree Blakesley forceps.

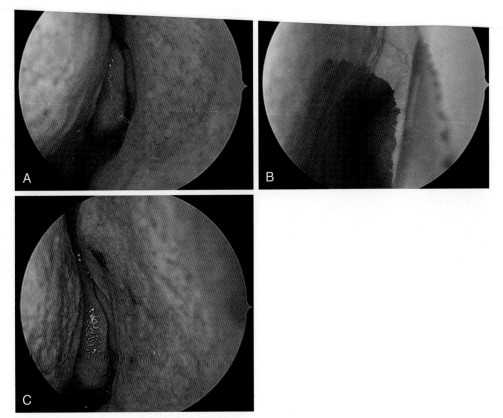

Fig. 6.7. (A–C) Accurate placement of decongestive pledgets will allow better visualization of the middle meatus. Here, endoscopic placement of the pledgets superiorly will allow for adequate decongestion of the nasal swell body, thus improving visualization of the superior attachment of the middle turbinate and the superior middle meatus.

are at their highest. Starting to operate before proper mucosal decongestion and local injection have been accomplished will often result in mucosal trauma and excess mucosal bleeding, especially in the areas of the anterior septum, anterior middle turbinate, and lateral nasal wall. Trauma to these areas will add to the difficulty of the remainder of the procedure.

- Take at least 5 minutes to allow the vasoconstrictive pledgets to decongest the mucosa and local injections to take effect.
- It is important to accurately place the nasal pledgets to optimize the visual field. A common mistake is to place the pledgets low in the nose, failing to decongest the nasal swell bodies, which can obscure endoscopic visualization of the middle meatus and frontal recess (Fig. 6.7).
- To avoid unnecessary trauma and clouding of the operative field, be careful in manipulation of the middle turbinate. To create more space to address the uncinate process, gently move the middle turbinate medially with a Freer elevator and slide an oxymetazoline-soaked pledget into the middle meatus for 5 minutes.

- When in doubt, perform a septoplasty if a septal deflection is preventing access to the middle meatus. A septal deflection will not only make intraoperative access difficult but will also create problems for effective postoperative débridement.

PEARLS AND POTENTIAL PITFALLS

Pearls

- Removal of the uncinate process will often enlarge the middle meatus, making what appears to be a narrow space adequate for maneuvering endoscopic instruments.
- The uncinate process is in the shape of a crescent moon that vanishes in the superior plane.
- The key to a proper antrostomy is to find the natural ostium and enlarge it by removing the fontanelle posteriorly and the uncinate process anteriorly.
- When the uncinate process is intact, the height of the lower $\frac{1}{3}$ of the middle turbinate approximates the location of the natural ostium.

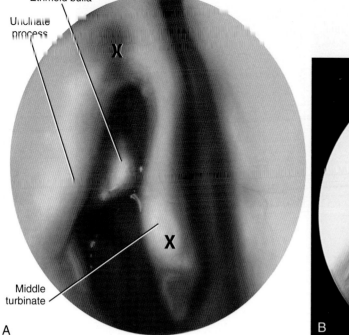

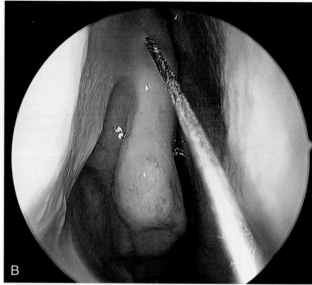

Ethmoid bulla

Uncinate process

Middle turbinate

X

X

A

B

Fig. 6.8. Injection of local anesthesia. **(A)** Artist's depiction of endoscopic view. Local anesthetic should be infiltrated at the points marked with an *X*. **(B)** Endoscopic photograph demonstrating infiltration of lidocaine with epinephrine. On slow injection, the mucosal lining of the middle turbinate and uncinate process should blanch.

- The antrostomy may be started with a 0-degree scope, but use of a 30-degree scope makes it much easier to identify the natural ostium.
- A 45-degree or 70-degree scope is useful to visualize the anterior wall and floor of the sinus after an antrostomy has been performed. It is especially useful in removing a retention cyst along the floor or anterior wall.

Potential Pitfalls

- Beware of an uncinate process that is atelectatic and pressed against the lamina. Incision of the uncinate with a sickle knife or microdébrider can result in orbitotomy and damage to the orbital contents.
- Remove the uncinate process from posterior to anterior, starting from the free edge, with backbiting forceps. The bone of the uncinate process is thin. Bite anteriorly until the hard lacrimal bone is encountered. "Bite to the hard bone, not through the hard bone." Biting through the lacrimal bone may result in an injury to the lacrimal duct system.
- Be careful in manipulation of the middle turbinate. Take care to gently move the middle turbinate medially with the smooth back end of the instruments while using the working end to remove the uncinate. Trauma to the lateral surface of the middle turbinate will cloud the operative field with blood and make visualization and instrumentation difficult.
- When using the microdébrider, "tap" the pedal to use in short bursts. This will prevent a prolonged

débridement and damage to orbital contents if the orbit is entered.

SURGICAL PROCEDURE

- You may elect to begin with a 0-degree endoscope for the removal of the uncinate process, but as you gain experience, you will find that a 30-degree endoscope allows much better visualization of the natural ostium.
- Inject 1 mL of 1% lidocaine with epinephrine at the superior attachment of the middle turbinate to the lateral nasal wall (Fig. 6.8).
- Inject 1 mL of local anesthetic into the anterior head of the middle turbinate. This will limit bleeding, which will cloud the operative field if the lateral surface of the middle turbinate is roughened.
- While looking in the nose with a 0-degree endoscope, identify the curve and free edge of the uncinate process, the anterior bulge of the agger nasi cell, and the superior attachment of the inferior turbinate.

Step 1: Medialize the Middle Tubinate

- A vertical relaxing incision starting inferiorly at the junction of the horizontal and vertical portion of the basal lamella and extending superiorly can help to medialize the middle turbinate.

Step 2: Outfracture the Inferior Turbinate to Better Visualize the Middle Meatus

- After completing this step, proceed to the next step.

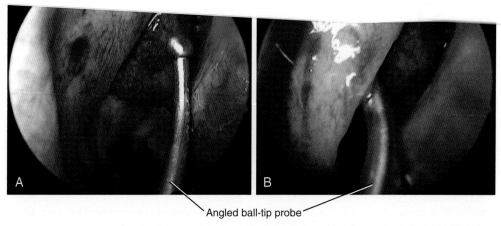

Angled ball-tip probe

Fig. 6.9. **(A)** and **(B)** Endoscopic photographs showing use of an angled ball-tip probe to identify and medialize the uncinate process.

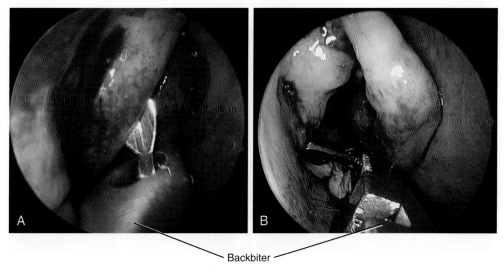

Backbiter

Fig. 6.10. **(A)** and **(B)** Views through a 30-degree endoscope used to visualize the right maxillary sinus. A backbiter is used to palpate behind the uncinate process and cut it in a posterior to anterior direction initially.

Step 3: Remove the Uncinate Process and Identify the Natural Ostium

- Use a ball-tip probe to reflect anteriorly the free edge of the uncinate process (Fig. 6.9).
- Use the backbiter to remove the uncinate process from posterior to anterior to its attachment to the lacrimal bone (Fig. 6.10).
- When first using the backbiter, place and open the blade at the 12 o'clock position in the middle meatus, then pronate your wrist to slide behind the free edge of the uncinate process.
- Stray mucosal edges of the uncinate process can be removed with a straight or angled microdébrider.

Step 4: Reflect and Remove the Superior Uncinate Process (Fig. 6.11)

- Remove the superior attachment of the uncinate process by first reflecting the uncinate anteriorly with a ball-tip probe and then excising it with a 45-degree or 90-degree through-cutting forceps or angled microdébrider.

Step 5: Remove the Inferior Uncinate Process (Fig. 6.12)

- Use the downbiter angled microdébrider or ball-tip probe to take down the inferior uncinate process to the superior border of the inferior turbinate.

Step 6: Enlarge the Antrostomy by Removing the Posterior Fontanelle (Fig. 6.13)

- Use a 30-degree endoscope to visualize the natural ostium.
- To make a larger antrostomy, use a straight through-cutter to excise the fontanelle posterior to the natural ostium.

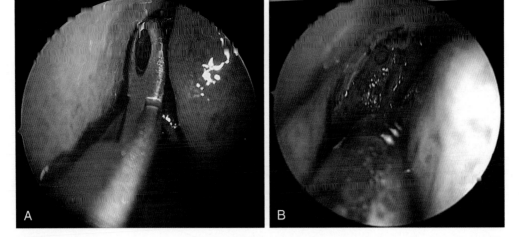

Fig. 6.11. **(A)** Endoscopic photograph showing use of upbiting forceps to remove the superior uncinate. **(B)** Endoscopic photograph showing use of a microdébrider to remove the uncinate using a "tap, tap" technique.

Downbiter

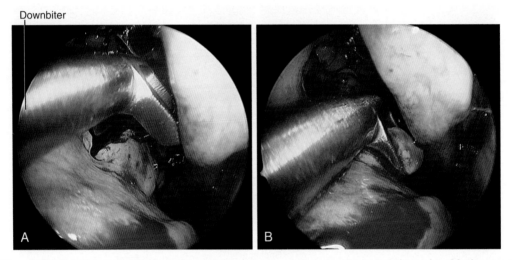

Fig. 6.12. **(A)** and **(B)** Use of a downbiter to enlarge the antrostomy inferiorly. Views are through a 30-degree endoscope.

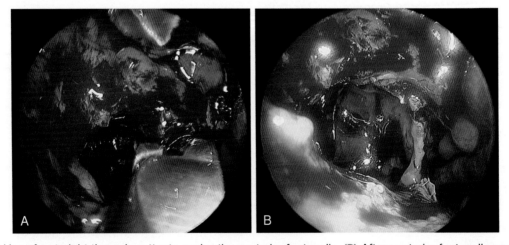

Fig. 6.13. **(A)** Use of a straight through-cutter to excise the posterior fontanelle. **(B)** After posterior fontanelle removal. Views are through a 30-degree endoscope.

recurrent, acute rhinosinusitis with hyperplastic mucosa.

- Larger antrostomy with complete removal of the uncinate process and posterior fontanelle to the palatine bone for significant nasal polyposis, hyperplastic mucosa, or revision surgery.

Step 7: Débride Polyps Within the Maxillary Sinus (If Present; Fig. 6.14)

- Using an angled endoscope and débrider, débride polypoid tissue from the sinus.

POSTOPERATIVE CONSIDERATIONS

- Avoid formation of synechiae between the middle turbinate and lateral nasal wall.
- Prevent synechiae formation by medializing the middle turbinate at the end of the case.
  - This can be done in multiple ways, either by suture or controlled scarring
- Before finishing, make sure to look one last time with a 30 degree or 70-degree endoscope at the natural ostium. Use a ball-tip probe to feel the lacrimal bone anteriorly and ensure that the uncinate process has been completely removed. This will help prevent postoperative mucus recirculation.

sinus, and saline irrigations can be used to flush the mucin out of the sinus.

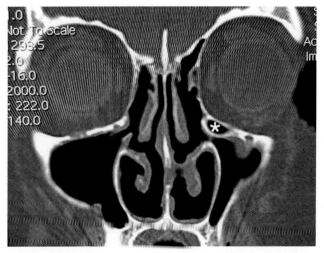

Fig. 6.15. Coronal CT scan showing a left Haller cell *(asterisk)*. The cell may narrow the natural ostium or may be a source of chronic inflammation.

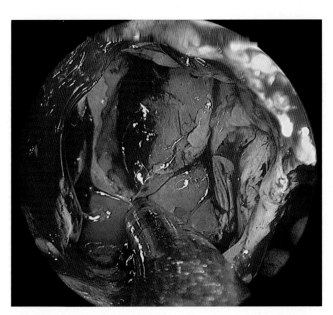

Fig. 6.14. Removal of polyps from the lateral sinus using a 40-degree microdébrider. View is through a 30-degree endoscope.

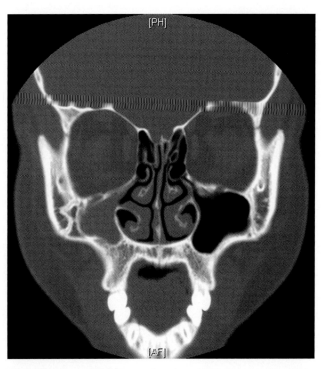

Fig. 6.16. Coronal CT scan showing silent sinus syndrome of the right maxillary sinus. Note the atelectatic uncinate and retracted orbital floor.

SPECIAL CONSIDERATIONS

- An intraorbital ethmoid cell (Haller cell) will crowd the middle meatus, may be difficult to reach, and may harbor disease (Fig. 6.15).
  - Angled endoscopes, 90-degree forceps, and giraffe forceps are needed to remove the cell.

- Silent sinus syndrome is from an atelectatic uncinate process that results in negative pressure producing a downward retraction of the floor of the orbit (Fig. 6.16).

Partial and Complete Ethmoidectomy

Nithin D. Adappa, James N. Palmer, and Alexander G. Chiu

INTRODUCTION

- The terms *partial* and *complete ethmoidectomy* refer to the removal of the anterior and posterior ethmoids (Figs. 7.1 and 7.2, respectively).
- A *partial ethmoidectomy* is the removal of the ethmoid bulla and any cells against the medial orbital wall anterior to the basal lamellae.
- A partial ethmoidectomy is often combined with a maxillary antrostomy and termed *mini–FESS*. The most common indication is recurrent acute rhinosinusitis or nonpolypoid chronic rhinosinusitis involving mainly the maxillary and anterior ethmoids.
- A *complete ethmoidectomy* is the removal of the anterior and posterior ethmoid air cells.
- A complete ethmoidectomy follows a maxillary antrostomy and is one component of complete functional endoscopic sinus surgery.
- Complete removal of all ethmoid cells entails the "skeletonizing" of the medial orbital wall and skull base of all ethmoid bony partitions.
- The safest method of performing a complete ethmoidectomy is to remove the inferior anterior and posterior ethmoid cells until the sphenoid face is reached, then identify the skull base at the posterior ethmoid or sphenoid sinus roof and dissect along the skull base from a posterior to anterior direction.
- Indications for a complete ethmoidectomy include the following:
  - Chronic rhinosinusitis with polyps
  - Revision surgery for chronic rhinosinusitis
  - Disease in the posterior ethmoids and sphenoid sinus

ANATOMY
Anterior Ethmoids

- The anterior ethmoids are those cells that lie anterior to the basal lamella (portion of the middle turbinate that attaches to the lateral nasal wall).
- The anterior ethmoid air cells consist of the ethmoid bulla, agger nasi cell, and those cells that lie against the medial orbital wall.
- The space just posterior to the ethmoid bulla and anterior to the basal lamellae is termed the *retrobullar space*.

Posterior Ethmoids

- The posterior ethmoid air cells are those that lie posterior to the basal lamellae and anterior to the sphenoid sinus.
- The posterior ethmoid cells can consist of anything from a single cell to multiple layers of cells. They are bordered laterally by the orbital apex and superiorly by the skull base.

Basal Lamellae

- Anatomically, the basal lamella is the portion of the middle turbinate that attaches to the lateral nasal wall.
- Functionally, the basal lamella is the bony-mucosal junction between the anterior and posterior ethmoid air cells.
- There are two components of the basal lamellae (Fig. 7.3):
  - Vertical portion
  - Horizontal portion

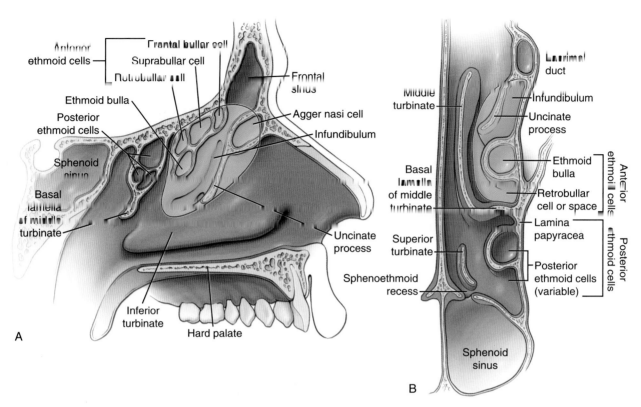

Fig. 7.1. Schematic drawings of the ethmoid sinuses showing sagittal (A) and axial (B) views of the structures involved in a partial ethmoidectomy *(shaded area).*

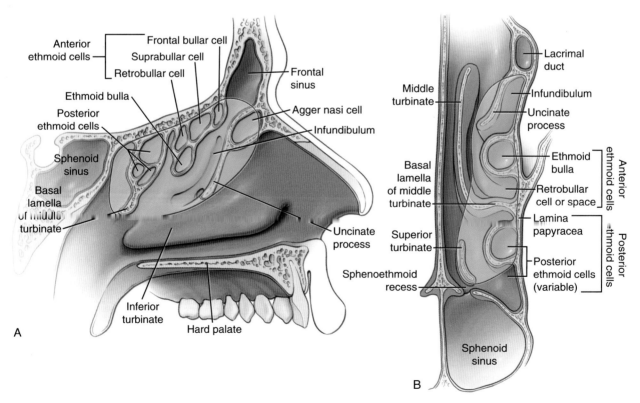

Fig. 7.2. Schematic drawings of the ethmoid sinuses showing sagittal (A) and axial (B) views of the structures involved in a complete ethmoidectomy *(shaded area).*

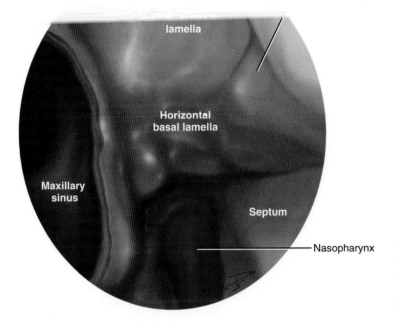

Labels on image:
lamella
Horizontal basal lamella
Maxillary sinus
Septum
Nasopharynx

Fig. 7.3. Artist's depiction of a 0-degree endoscopic view of the right basal lamellae. The ethmoid bulla has been removed; the vertical and horizontal segments of the basal lamellae are shown. The posterior ethmoids are entered at the junction between the vertical and horizontal segments.

■ Handling of the basal lamellae is extremely important. Excessive resection of the horizontal portion of the basal lamellae can result in destabilization of the middle turbinate. Destabilization can lead to lateralization of the middle turbinate and postoperative obstruction of the middle meatus and frontal recess. However, if the surgeon is too conservative and the vertical portion of the basal lamella is not dissected inferiorly enough, surgeons can often dissect too far superiorly in the posterior ethmoid cavities as they are working toward the sphenoid sinus. Optimally, the vertical portion of the basal lamella is fully removed and the horizontal portion is preserved.

Onodi Cell

■ An Onodi cell is a posterior ethmoid cell that lies superior and/or lateral to the sphenoid.
■ Onodi cells are important to identify preoperatively because the optic nerve traverses the roof of these cells.

PREOPERATIVE CONSIDERATIONS

■ When a complete ethmoidectomy is performed, a greater palatine or sphenopalatine artery injection

of 1% lidocaine with 1:100,000 epinephrine can be helpful in controlling intraoperative bleeding.
■ A sphenopalatine artery injection is performed transnasally. Identify the inferior attachment of the middle turbinate to the lateral nasal wall and inject roughly 1 cm above the inferior border (Fig. 7.4) with 1 to 2 mL of 1% lidocaine with 1:100,000 epinephrine. Often, a curved tonsil needle or spiral needle is needed to reach the appropriate position.
■ A greater palatine artery injection is performed through the mouth. The greater palatine canal is in the hard palate, usually medial and posterior to the second molar. Bend a 27-gauge needle at 1.5 to 2 cm from the tip, identify the foramen, aspirate, and then inject with 1 mL of 1% lidocaine with 1:100,000 epinephrine.

Radiographic Considerations

■ The axial, coronal, and sagittal computed tomographic scans are helpful to understand the anatomy.
■ Identify the ethmoid bulla and get a general idea of the number of ethmoid cells (Fig. 7.5).
■ While looking at the sagittal view, identify the slope of the skull base.
■ Look at the height of the roof of the maxillary sinus in relation to the height of the skull base.

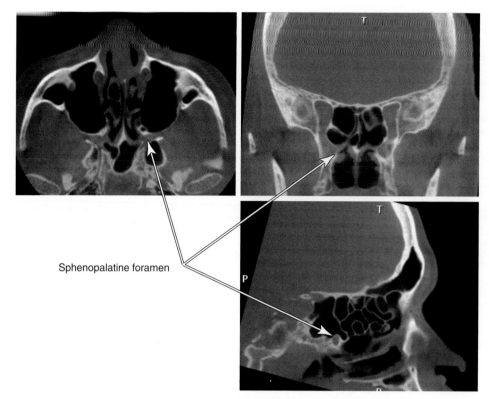

Fig. 7.4. Computed tomographic scans of the sphenopalatine foramen in three planes. Note the location anterior to the sphenoid, posterior and superior to the middle turbinate.

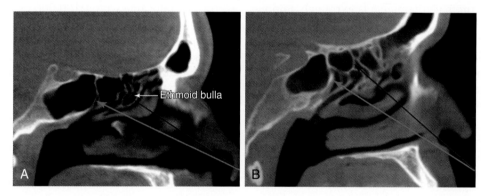

Fig. 7.5. (A,B) Sagittal computed tomographic scans showing the ethmoid air cells. Note the lower-sloping skull base in scan **(B)** that predisposes surgeons to a higher cerebrospinal fluid (CSF) leak risk during dissection of the posterior ethmoid air cells if the trajectory of dissection is not accurate. *Green arrows* indicate the correct level at which to cross the basal lamella into the posterior ethmoid. *Red arrows* denote too high an entry into the basal lamella, which encourages the surgeon to dissect into the skull base and create a CSF leak.

- Count the number of ethmoid cells above the height of the roof of the maxillary sinus. The roof of the maxillary sinus is a critical landmark surgically as one dissects anteriorly to posteriorly through the ethmoid cavity.
- Identify the presence of any Onodi cells.

Cribriform Plate and Skull Base
- Note the hard bone of ethmoid roof compared with the thin bone of lateral lamellae of cribriform plate (Fig. 7.6).

INSTRUMENTATION (FIG. 7.7)

- J-curette
- Straight mushroom punch
- 2- and 4-mm Kerrison rongeurs—especially useful for removing ethmoid cell partitions off the medial orbital wall laterally
- Straight and upbiting through-cutting forceps and Blakesley forceps

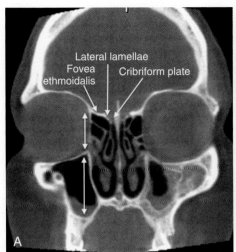
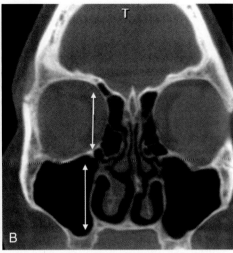

Fig. 7.6. Coronal computed tomographic scans showing a short and tall ethmoid roof. **(A)** Note the large maxillary height associated with a short ethmoid roof height. This configuration, when viewed in the sagittal plane (see Fig. 7.5A), can be seen to put the surgeon at risk of crossing the basal lamella too far superior and therefore entering the cranial base in the posterior ethmoid and causing a cerebrospinal fluid (CSF) leak. **(B)** A smaller maxillary sinus height translates into a higher ethmoid roof and therefore carries less chance of intracranial injury, as can be seen in Fig. 7.5B.

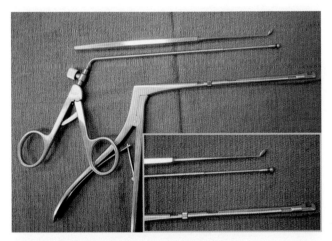

Fig. 7.7. Photograph showing specialized instrumentation for ethmoidectomy. *Top to bottom:* J-curette, straight mushroom punch, Kerrison rongeur. Inset displays instrument tips.

PEARLS AND POTENTIAL PITFALLS

Pearls

- When removing ethmoid bony partitions, dissect from "known to unknown." Identify air spaces around the bony partitions and remove the ethmoid partitions at each air space.
- When dissecting anteriorly to posteriorly through the ethmoid cavity, stay low in the cavity to avoid inadvertent injury to the skull base as it slopes down posteriorly.
- Dissecting anteriorly to posteriorly through the ethmoid air cells at the level of the height of the roof of the maxillary sinus will assist in staying low and avoiding the skull base in the posterior ethmoid sinus.
- Learn to medialize the middle turbinate with an instrument while placing the endoscope in the ethmoid cavity. This will create more space for the endoscope and avoid blood clouding of the endoscope tip.
- The inferior ethmoidectomy is performed with a 0-degree scope as one dissects anteriorly to posteriorly through the ethmoid cavity. Once the face of the sphenoid sinus is reached, begin to dissect posteriorly to anteriorly along the skull base, removing ethmoid bony attachments from the skull base.
- Use a 30-degree scope and angled suction tools to dissect along the skull base. A reverse or offset 30-degree scope is extremely helpful to prevent physical interference between hand instruments and the camera head's light cord attachment.
- Use mucosa-sparing techniques. Through-cutting instruments are used to remove ethmoid bony partitions. Blakesley forceps should be used only to remove loose bony fragments.
- Limit the use of the microdébrider along the skull base and medial orbital wall. Use it to clean mucosal fragments but never to dissect bone off the skull base.

Potential Pitfalls

- Always keep the height of the roof of the maxillary sinus in mind when dissecting anteriorly to posteriorly through the ethmoid cavity.

- Learn to "zoom out." To avoid getting lost in the ethmoid cavity, intermittently bring the endoscope out of the ethmoid cavity anterior to the middle turbinate to get an overall picture of where dissection is occurring.
- Avoid cutting though the horizontal portion of the basal lamellae. This will destabilize the middle turbinate, which often results in postoperative lateralization.
- When performing an anterior ethmoidectomy, avoid cutting the mucosa of the posterior agger nasi and superior ethmoid bulla at the same vertical level. This decreases the chance for the two raw surfaces to scar together and result in postoperative frontal sinus disease.
- Identify the presence of an Onodi cell preoperatively as well as intraoperatively. Mistaking the anterior surface of an Onodi cell for the sphenoid face can result in inadvertent injury to the orbital apex.
- Be aware of the branches of the sphenopalatine artery as it exits the sphenopalatine foramen. Resection of the inferior portion of the basal lamellae may injure a branch of the sphenopalatine artery. Bleeding in this area can be addressed with a suction Bovie cautery.
- Avoid stripping mucosa off the skull base or medial orbital wall. This will often lead to prolonged localized postoperative mucosal edema and long-term neo-osteogenesis.

SURGICAL PROCEDURE

Step 1

- With a 0-degree endoscope, identify the medial border of the ethmoid bulla. This will often require medializing the middle turbinate with the back end of a J-curette or a Freer elevator (Fig. 7.8).

Step 2

- Starting from the space medial to the bulla and posterior to the bulla (retrobullar space), use the J-curette to fracture the bulla in an anterolateral direction (Fig. 7.9).

Step 3

- Once the bulla has been fractured, remove all bony fragments with Blakesley forceps or a straight microdébrider (Fig. 7.10). Dissect along the medial orbital wall with Kerrison rongeurs to remove the lateral partitions of the ethmoid bulla. Angled through-cutting instruments are helpful.

Step 4

- Identify the roof of the maxillary sinus and keep the height of the roof in mind. This will serve as a vertical landmark for dissection as you progress from anterior to posterior through the ethmoid cavity. At the height of the roof of the maxillary sinus, perforate the medial-inferior basal lamellae with a J-curette (Fig. 7.11).

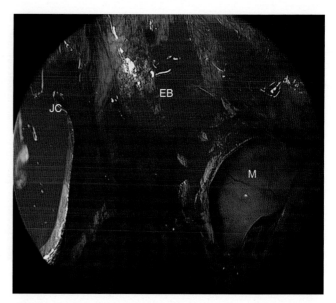

Fig. 7.8. Endoscopic view of a left maxillary antrostomy *(M)* with the ethmoid bulla *(EB)* superiorly. Note the J-curette *(JC)* medializing the middle turbinate.

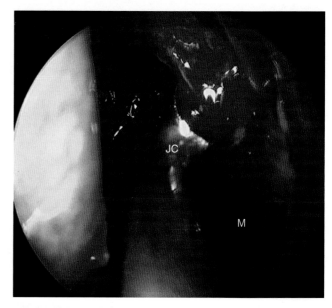

Fig. 7.9. Endoscopic view of a J-curette *(JC)* entering the retrobullar space and fracturing the ethmoid bulla in an anterolateral direction. Note the left-sided maxillary antrostomy *(M)* in the background.

Step 5

- Use the straight microdébrider and through-cutting instruments to dissect the basal lamella inferiorly to the horizontal portion and superiorly to the height of the roof of the maxillary sinus (Fig. 7.12). Use angled through-cutting instruments and a rotating Kerrison rongeur to remove ethmoid bony partitions laterally attached to the medial orbital wall.

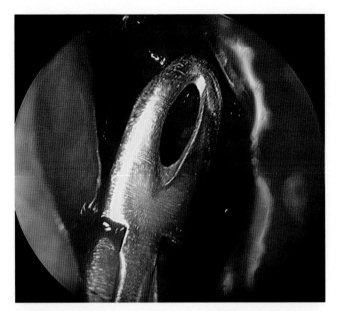

Fig. 7.10. Left-side endoscopic view of Blakesley forceps removing the previously outfractured ethmoid bulla.

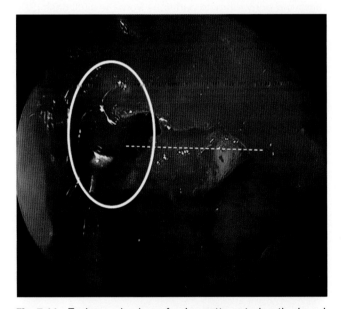

Fig. 7.11. Endoscopic view of a J-curette entering the basal lamellae *(oval)* at the height of the maxillary sinus roof *(dashed line).*

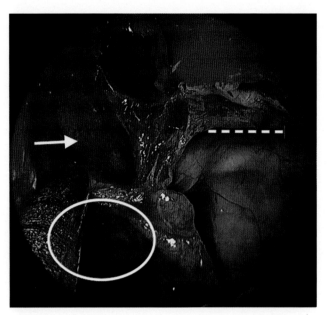

Fig. 7.12. Endoscopic view of a left superior turbinate *(arrow)* after removal and microdébridement of the basal lamellae. Note the height of the maxillary roof *(dashed line)* in relation to the superior turbinate. The horizontal portion of the basal lamellae remains inferiorly *(oval)* to prevent destabilization.

Step 6

■ Dissect the posterior ethmoids until the anterior face of the sphenoid sinus is reached. At this point, identify the skull base superiorly and begin to dissect posteriorly to anteriorly along the skull base. Use an angled 30-degree endoscope to begin removing the superior ethmoid bony fragments off of the skull base (Fig. 7.13).

Step 7

■ Use curved suction tools, image guidance if available, and angled endoscopes to visualize around the bony partitions that are attached to the skull base. Use upbiting through-cutters to remove bony partitions attached to the skull base (Fig. 7.14). As a general principle, if you can see in front of a bony partition and feel behind it, then it is safe to cut with a through-cutting instrument.

Step 8

■ Dissect along the skull base in a posterior to anterior direction until the roof of the ethmoid bulla and roof of the suprabullar recess are reached. This marks the area of the anterior ethmoid artery and the beginning of the frontal recess dissection (see Chapter 9).
  – Finished partial and complete ethmoidectomies are shown in Fig. 7.15.

POSTOPERATIVE CONSIDERATIONS

■ Preventing postoperative synechiae between the middle turbinate and lateral nasal wall is critical for long-term success. This can be accomplished by medializing the middle turbinate at the end of the case. Techniques for medializing the middle turbinate include suturing or controlled scarring of the middle turbinate to the nasal septum (see Chapter 2).
■ Meticulous postoperative care will also prevent lateralization and synechia (see Chapter 12).

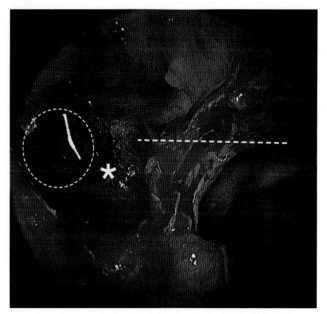

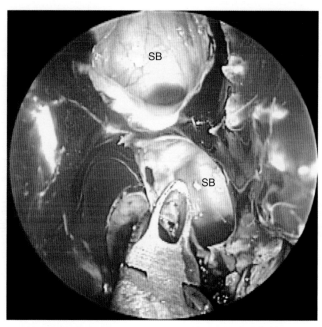

Fig. 7.13. Endoscopic view of the anterior sphenoid face *(circle)* with the horizontal lamellae of the superior turbinate removed *(asterisk* denotes the remnant of the superior turbinate). Note the location of the maxillary sinus roof *(dashed line)* and the superior turbinate.

Fig. 7.14. Endoscopic view of a straight through-biter removing bony ethmoid partitions from the skull base *(SB)*.

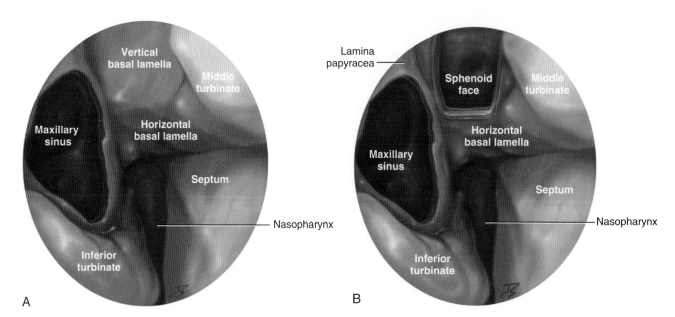

Fig. 7.15. Artist's depiction of a partial **(A)** and complete **(B)** ethmoidectomy in endoscopic view.

Sphenoidotomy

Alexander G. Chiu and Jeremy Reed

INTRODUCTION

- There are two ways to approach and perform a sphenoidotomy: transnasal and transethmoid.
- In the *transnasal* approach, the sphenoidotomy is performed while sparing the ethmoid cavity. Dissection proceeds medial to the middle turbinate. Common indications for this approach are isolated pathologic processes within the sphenoid sinus (e.g., fungal ball, isolated sphenoid sinusitis). This approach may also be combined with a posterior septectomy for an endoscopic transnasal approach to the pituitary sella (see Chapter 28).
- In the *transethmoid* approach, the uncinate process and inferior ethmoid air cells are removed to access the anterior face of the sphenoid sinus. This technique may be used in cases of isolated sphenoid disease, but most commonly is performed as a component of a complete functional endoscopic sinus surgery.

ANATOMY

Sphenoid

- The sphenoid sinus has the following borders (Fig. 8.1):
  - Anterior: superior turbinate and posterior ethmoid cells
  - Medial: intersinus septum and nasal septum
  - Posterior: pituitary sella superiorly, clival recess inferiorly
  - Lateral: cavernous sinus, optic nerve, and infratemporal fossae
  - Superior: planum sphenoidale, anterior skull base
- The natural os of the sphenoid sinus lies in the medial and inferior portion of the sphenoid face, nearly always medial and posterior to the superior turbinate (Fig. 8.2).

Onodi Cell

- An Onodi cell is a posterior ethmoid cell that lies superior or lateral to the sphenoid sinus.
- When a sphenoidotomy is performed, it is crucial not to confuse the posterior wall of an Onodi cell with the anterior face of the sphenoid.
- A common cause of optic nerve or orbital apex injury in the early days of functional endoscopic sinus surgery was dissection through the posterior wall of an Onodi cell because it was mistaken for the anterior face of the sphenoid sinus (Fig. 8.3).

Vasculature

- The septal branch of the sphenopalatine artery runs horizontally along the inferior and anterior face of the sphenoid sinus.

PREOPERATIVE CONSIDERATIONS

- When a sphenoidotomy is performed, a greater palatine or sphenopalatine artery injection can be helpful in controlling intraoperative bleeding.
- A greater palatine artery injection is performed through the mouth. The greater palatine canal is in the hard palate, opposite the second molar. Bend the needle at 1.5 to 2 cm from the tip at a 45-degree angle, aspirate, and then inject 1 to 2 mL of 1% lidocaine with 1:100,000 epinephrine.
- A sphenopalatine artery injection can be performed transnasally. Identify the inferior attachment of the middle turbinate to the lateral nasal wall and inject roughly 1 mL of 1% lidocaine with 1:100,000 epinephrine 1 cm above the inferior border.

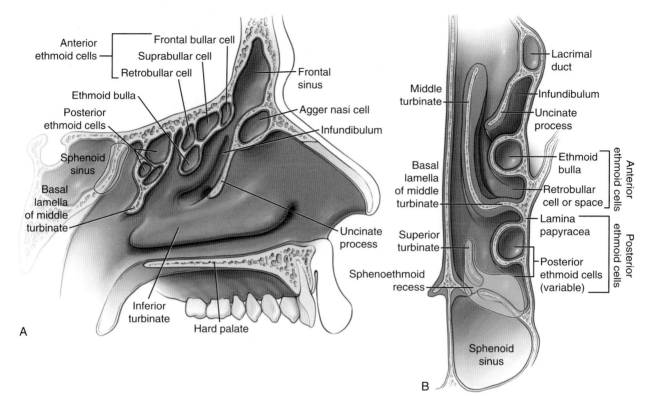

Fig. 8.1. Schematic drawings of the sphenoid sinus showing sagittal **(A)** and axial **(B)** views of the structures involved in a sphenoidotomy *(shaded area).*

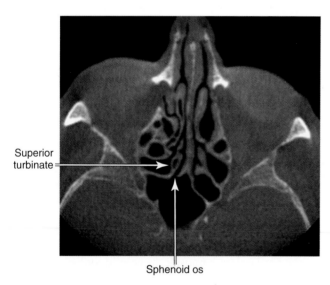

Fig. 8.2. Axial CT scan showing the position of the natural sphenoid os medial, posterior, and inferior to the superior turbinate.

Radiographic Considerations

- The axial, coronal, and sagittal computed tomography (CT) scans are helpful to understand the anatomy.
- Identify the size and pneumatization of the sphenoid sinus.

- Look at the nature of the bone of the sphenoid walls. Fungal balls or long-standing inflammatory disease often results in thickened bone of the anterior face (sometimes requiring a drill for sphenoidotomy enlargement).
- Identify the presence of any Onodi cells.
- Identify the intersinus septum and track its path back to the posterior wall. Beware of any attachments to the internal carotid artery. If such an attachment is identified, it is advisable to avoid aggressive manipulation of the intersinus septum for fear of injuring the artery (Fig. 8.4).

INSTRUMENTATION

- 30- or 70-degree endoscope if the lateral or inferior portion of the sinus must be examined
- Straight microdébrider
- Straight sphenoid punch
- 45-degree through-cutting instrument
- J-curette
- 2- and 4-mm Kerrison rongeurs

PEARLS AND POTENTIAL PITFALLS

- Avoid operating in a narrow space when entering the sphenoid. Visualization is significantly improved by removing superior ethmoid air cells, which allows greater access to light from the endoscope.

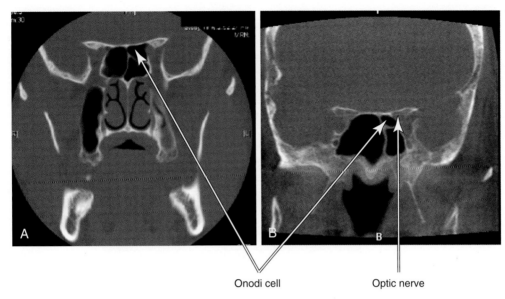

Onodi cell   Optic nerve

Fig. 8.3. Coronal CT scans (**A** and **B**) revealing left Onodi cells. Note the location of the optic nerve in the roof of these cells.

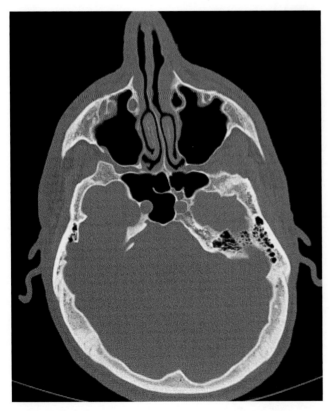

Fig. 8.4. Axial CT scan showing a left intersinus septum leading to the carotid artery.

- A reliable method to identify the natural os of the sphenoid is to truncate the lower half of the superior turbinate. Avoid excising too much of the superior turbinate, because olfactory fibers are located in its most superior portion.
- Dissect from "known to unknown." Identify the natural os first and then expand the antrostomy laterally.

- If image guidance is available, estimate the height of the septal branch of the sphenopalatine artery. This can be done by looking at the axial computed tomography (CT) sections and noting the location of the sphenopalatine foramen.
- Identify the presence of an Onodi cell preoperatively as well as intraoperatively. Mistaking the anterior surface of an Onodi cell for the sphenoid face can result in inadvertent injury to the orbital apex (Fig. 8.5).
- Avoid stripping mucosa off the skull base or medial orbital wall. This will often lead to prolonged localized postoperative mucosal edema and long-term neo-osteogenesis.

SURGICAL PROCEDURES

Transnasal Sphenoidotomy

Step 1

- With a 0-degree endoscope, gently lateralize the middle turbinate to identify the lower half of the superior turbinate.
- Use a straight through-cutter to excise the lower half of the superior turbinate. This is done to identify the natural os of the sphenoid sinus (Fig. 8.6).

Step 2

- Enter the natural os with a J-curette and then dilate the os by fracturing the anterior sphenoid face in a lateral direction. Remove bony fragments.
- The sphenoid antrostomy can be enlarged with a Kerrison punch or straight mushroom punch.

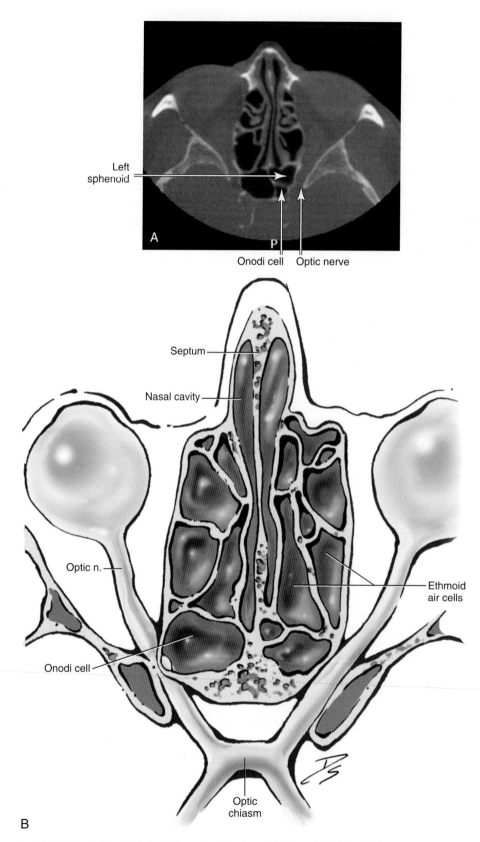

Fig. 8.5. Computed CT **(A)** and **(B)** artist depiction showing the right Onodi cell in relation to the optic nerve. *n.,* Nerve.

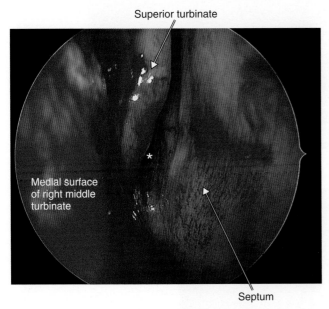

Fig. 8.6. Endoscopic view of the right sphenoethmoid recess. In a direction medial to the right middle turbinate, the natural os of the sphenoid sinus *(asterisk)* is visible posterior and medial to the superior turbinate.

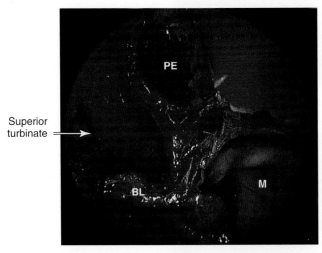

Fig. 8.7. Endoscopic view of the left superior turbinate (identified with the suction device) after the basal lamellae have been removed and a posterior ethmoidectomy has been performed. *BL,* Basal lamella; *M,* maxillary sinus; *PE,* posterior ethmoid.

Transethmoid Sphenoidotomy

Dilation of the Natural Os

- After a posterior ethmoidectomy has been performed, identify the superior turbinate and its horizontal lamellae (Fig. 8.7).

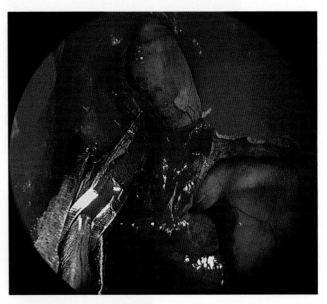

Fig. 8.8. Endoscopic view of resection of the left superior turbinate with straight through-cutter forceps to allow visualization of the anterior sphenoid face.

- Remove the lower half of the superior turbinate to identify and then enlarge the natural os (Fig. 8.8). It is safest to find the os in its medial location and then, using a J-curette, fracture the anterior sphenoid face in a lateral direction.
- Enlarge the antrostomy by using an upbiting through-cutting instrument, Kerrison rongeur, or straight mushroom punch (Fig. 8.9).
- The final antrostomy is shown in Fig. 8.10.

Bolger Box Method

- The "Bolger box" method is a technique for performing a sphenoidotomy without finding or resecting the superior turbinate.
- Draw a rectangular box with the borders being the superior turbinate medially, superior turbinate lamellae inferiorly, skull base superiorly, and orbit laterally. Draw a diagonal line through the box and enter the sphenoid face medial and inferior to the line (Fig. 8.11).

SPECIAL CONSIDERATIONS—ONODI CELL

- An Onodi cell lies superior to the natural os of the sphenoid sinus. Continued dissection through the posterior wall of an Onodi cell results in intracranial or orbital apex injury.
- The floor of an Onodi cell may be removed to create one continuous sphenoid cavity (Fig. 8.12).

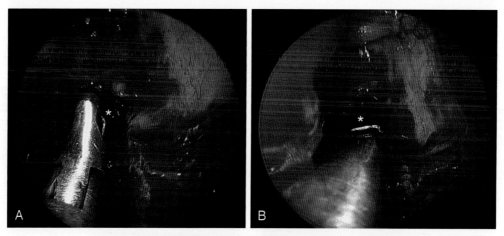

Fig. 8.9. Endoscopic view (**A** and **B**) of the widening of the antrostomy *(asterisk).*

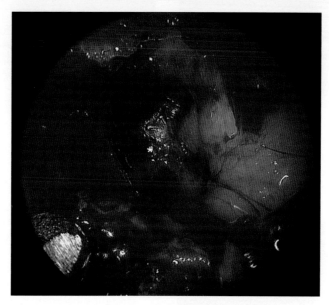

Fig. 8.10. Endoscopic view of the final antrostomy.

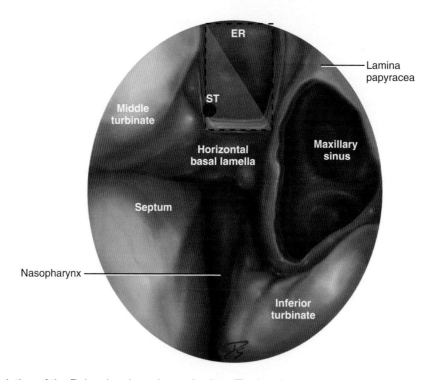

Fig. 8.11. Artist's depiction of the Bolger box in endoscopic view. The box is a parallelogram bounded by the medial orbital wall laterally, basal lamella of the superior turbinate inferiorly, superior turbinate (ST) medially, and ethmoid roof (ER) superiorly. The natural sphenoid os is indicated by the red dot.

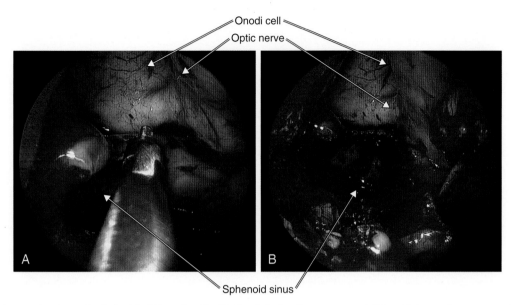

Fig. 8.12. Endoscopic view of a left-sided Onodi cell with the inferior floor removed **(A)**, which creates one continuous sphenoid cavity **(B)**.

Frontal Sinusotomy—Draf I and IIa

Alexander G. Chiu and James N. Palmer

INTRODUCTION

- Dissection of the frontal recess is the most difficult of the basic endoscopic dissections.
- Care must be taken to preserve the mucosa surrounding the frontal recess. Stripping of mucosa can result in postoperative stenosis and neo-osteogenesis.
- The frontal recess is difficult for another reason: the variable anatomy that can present an obstruction within the frontal recess. Frontal recess cells, posteriorly located frontal bullar cells, and intersinus septal cells all vary in presence and location from patient to patient but must be dissected for a complete frontal recess dissection (Fig. 9.1).
- Although a frontal recess dissection can be performed without removing the ethmoid bulla, a more complete and thorough surgery is possible only after the skull base has been cleared of all superior ethmoid bony partitions.
- When performed as part of complete functional endoscopic sinus surgery, the frontal recess dissection follows the completion of the maxillary antrostomy, sphenoidotomy, and complete ethmoidectomy.
- Proper postoperative care and débridements are critical for long-term patency of the frontal recess.
- Other keys to success are the following:
  - Proper instrumentation
  - Use of angled through-cutting instruments and probes specially designed for the frontal recess
  - Good visualization with a minimum of a 45-degree and preferably a 70-degree endoscope
  - Maintenance of a well-mucosalized frontal recess
- Endoscopic frontal procedures can be described by the following classification, based on Wolfgang Draf's initial work in 1991 using the microscope for endonasal frontal recess dissections:
  - Draf I: Removal of the superior uncinate with preservation of the agger nasi (Fig. 9.2)

  - Draf IIa: Removal of all cells within the frontal recess (Fig. 9.3)
  - Draf IIb: Draf IIa dissection plus removal of the ipsilateral floor of the frontal recess (Fig. 9.4)
  - Draf III: Bilateral Draf IIb dissection plus removal of the intersinus septum and the superior nasal septum to create a single common opening (Fig. 9.5)
- Nearly all primary cases and a substantial number of revision cases can be adequately treated using a Draf IIa procedure. This chapter discusses the technique

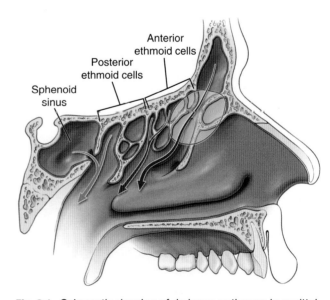

Fig. 9.1. Schematic drawing of drainage pathways in sagittal view. The frontal sinus drainage pathway is shown in *red*. The posterior ethmoid and sphenoid sinus drainage pathways through the sphenoethmoid recess are indicated in *green*. The drainage pathways from the anterior ethmoid are shown in *purple*. The *green-shaded* portion should be removed in frontal recess dissection.

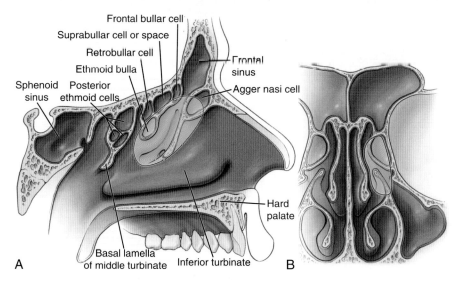

Fig. 9.2. Schematic drawings in sagittal (A) and coronal (B) views showing the portions of cells and bones removed in a Draf I dissection. The frontal recess cells, anterior ethmoid, uncinate process, and infundibulum are cleared, but the internal frontal sinus ostium (or thinnest part of the frontal recess drainage pathway) is not manipulated.

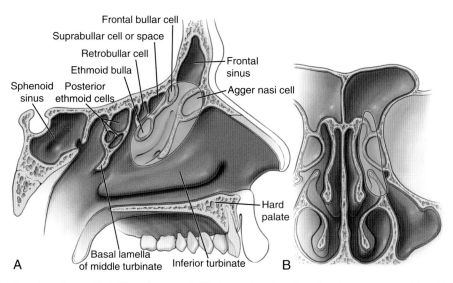

Fig. 9.3. Schematic drawings in sagittal (A) and coronal (B) views showing the structures removed in a Draf IIa frontal recess procedure. A Draf IIa dissection removes the cells excised in a Draf I procedure; in addition, it removes all cells lateral to the middle turbinate attachment and opens the internal frontal ostium.

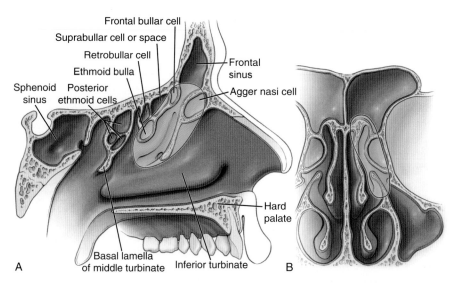

Fig. 9.4. Schematic drawings in sagittal (A) and coronal (B) views showing the structures removed in a Draf IIb dissection. The Draf IIb procedure includes the dissection of the Draf IIa procedure with the addition of the ipsilateral middle turbinate attachment to the floor of the frontal sinus; it, therefore, removes all the ipsilateral frontal sinus floor from septum to orbital wall.

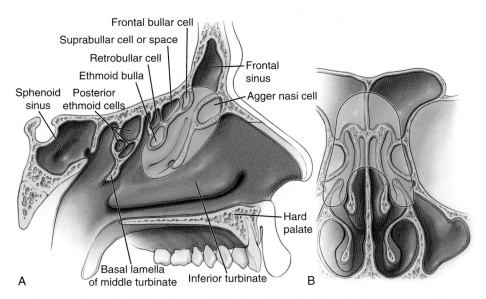

Fig. 9.5. Schematic drawings in sagittal (**A**) and coronal (**B**) views showing the structures removed in a median frontal sinus drainage, or Draf III, procedure, also called a *frontal sinus drill-out* or *endoscopic modified Lothrop procedure.* The procedure includes removal of the midline septum, both middle turbinate attachments to the floor of the frontal sinus, and all of the frontal sinus floor from orbital wall to orbital wall.

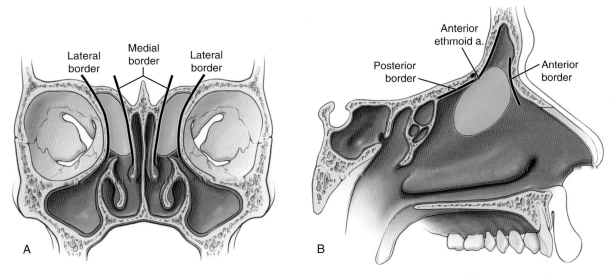

Fig. 9.6. Schematic drawings showing the boundaries of the frontal recess. (**A**) In the coronal plane, the medial boundary is the attachment of the middle turbinate. The lateral boundary is the orbit. (**B**) In the sagittal plane, the anterior border is the anterior wall of the agger nasi cell, which is continuous with the anterior buttress of the nasal spine, also called the *nasal beak.* The posterior-superior border is the attachment of the ethmoid bulla and/or the suprabullar cell.

for a Draf IIa dissection; the following chapters are devoted to the Draf IIb and Draf III procedures.

ANATOMY

■ The anatomic shape of the frontal sinus and frontal recess can be visualized as an hourglass, with the narrowest point corresponding to the frontal sinus ostium.

■ For the purpose of dissection, the frontal recess can be thought of as a box with four borders (Fig. 9.6). Enlarging the recess requires dissection of each wall of the box:
  – Anterior: the superior uncinate process and agger nasi cell
  – Medial: the lateral lamellae of the skull base and intersinus septum, and the attachment of the middle turbinate

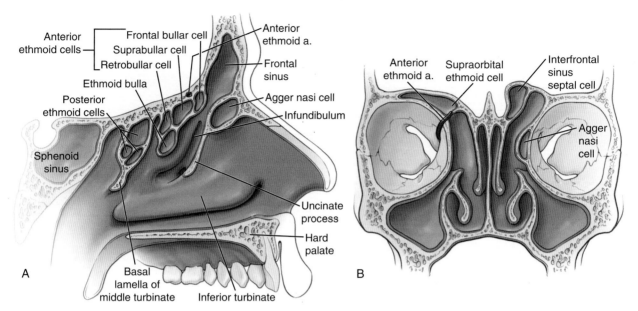

Fig. 9.7. **(A)** Schematic drawing showing an agger nasi cell, suprabullar cell, and frontal bullar cell, which are best appreciated on a sagittal section (as depicted here). **(B)** Schematic drawing in coronal view of a supraorbital cell, which pneumatizes up and over the orbit. One should be aware of its orientation just superior and anterior to the anterior ethmoid artery.

– Posterior: the supraorbital ethmoid cell and the anterior border of the ethmoid bulla
– Lateral: the medial wall of the orbit

Cells of the Frontal Recess

Agger Nasi Cell

■ The most anterior of the ethmoid air cells, the agger nasi cell often has the appearance of a bulge in the superior uncinate process. The cap of the agger nasi cell often makes the floor of the frontal recess (Fig. 9.7A).

Interfrontal Sinus Septal Cell

■ An interfrontal sinus septal cell is a cell that arises along the midline septum of the frontal sinus. As it pneumatizes, it narrows the frontal recess from medial to lateral (see Fig. 9.7B).

Supraorbital Ethmoid Cell

■ A supraorbital ethmoid cell pneumatizes into the frontal bone over the orbit and behind the frontal recess. It may extend lateral to the frontal recess (see Fig. 9.7B).

Suprabullar Cell

■ A suprabullar cell arises above the ethmoid bulla and pneumatizes up to the attachment of the bulla to the skull base. It is best seen in sagittal view (see Fig. 9.7A).

Frontal Bullar Cell

■ A frontal bullar cell arises anterior and superior to the bulla and pneumatizes toward the frontal recess but does not enter the frontal sinus proper. If a cell is pneumatized into the frontal sinus, it is classified as a type 3 frontal cell. Because this cell travels along the skull base, it is extremely difficult to identify on endoscopy alone without the aid of image guidance. It is seen best on sagittal section (see Fig. 9.7A).

Frontal Recess Cell

■ Frontal recess cells are located superior to the agger nasi cell. Variable in their presentation and seen in anywhere from 25% to 40% of frontal recess dissections, these cells make up the floor of the frontal recess.
– Type 1: One cell above the agger nasi (Fig. 9.8).
– Type 2: Two separate cells above the agger nasi or a tier of separate cells. They do not enter the frontal sinus proper (see Fig. 9.8).
– Type 3: One large cell that pneumatizes into the frontal sinus proper and can have a wall in common with either the anterior or posterior wall of the frontal sinus (Fig. 9.9).
– Type 4: Isolated cell within the frontal sinus (Fig. 9.10). This cell is seen rarely, if ever, and looks like a balloon blown up from the ethmoid into the frontal sinus with walls completely distinct from the sinus itself.

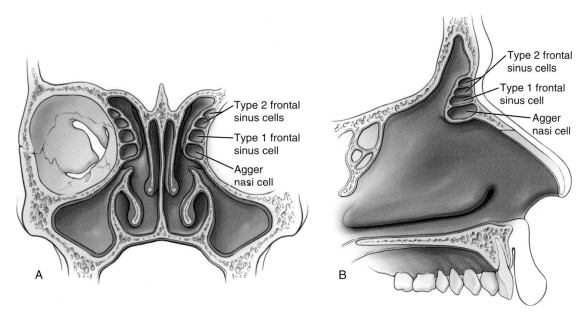

Fig. 9.8. Schematic drawings in coronal (A) and sagittal (B) views showing agger nasi and frontal sinus cells in a tier above the agger nasi cell. Note that one cell above the agger nasi cell is a type 1 cell, whereas multiple cells above a type 1 cell are all classified as type 2 frontal sinus cells until they enter the frontal sinus. At that point, they are type 3 cells.

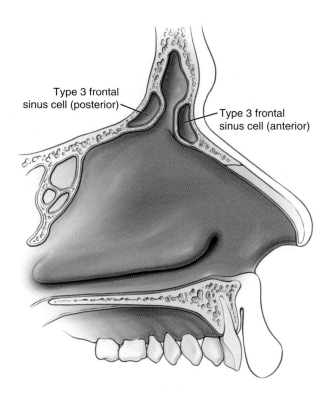

Fig. 9.9. Schematic drawing in sagittal view showing type 3 frontal sinus cells. These cells can pneumatize into the frontal sinus from anterior or posterior, and they have a common wall with either the anterior or posterior frontal sinus wall. These are frontal recess cells that pneumatize into the frontal sinus itself.

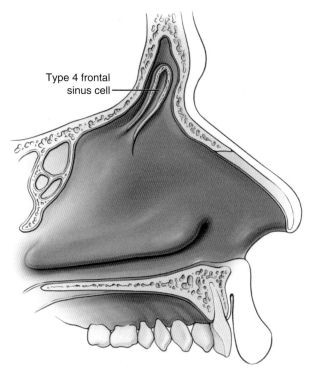

Fig. 9.10. Schematic drawing in sagittal view showing a type 4 frontal sinus cell. It arises entirely from the ethmoid and pneumatizes into the frontal sinus without a common wall, as if a balloon were blown up into the sinus.

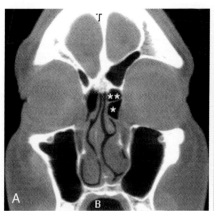 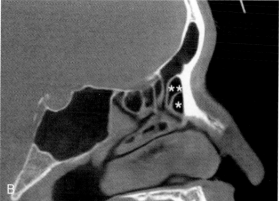

Fig. 9.11. Coronal **(A)** and sagittal **(B)** CT scans showing agger nasi cells *(single asterisk)* and type 1 frontal cells *(double asterisks)*.

PREOPERATIVE CONSIDERATIONS

- Limit bleeding to improve visualization by taking the following measures:
  - Elevate the head of the bed to 30 degrees.
  - Take the time to inject at least 2 mL of lidocaine with epinephrine at the most superior attachment of the middle turbinate to the lateral nasal wall.
  - Take time in the dissection and be prepared to use pledgets to dry the operative field if it gets too bloody.
  - Use 1:1000 epinephrine pledgets for improved hemostasis and local visualization.

Radiographic Considerations

- Axial, coronal, and sagittal computed tomographic (CT) scans are helpful to understand the anatomy (Figs. 9.11 to 9.15 and 9.17).
- Special attention should be paid to the sagittal views of the frontal recess. These will provide an idea of the anterior-posterior dimension of the frontal recess (Fig. 9.16).
- More than any other measurement, the anterior-posterior diameter is the indicator of the ease of the upcoming frontal recess dissection. The larger the diameter, the easier the dissection. Recesses with small anterior-posterior diameters must be treated with extreme care, because any stripping of the mucosa within the recess will likely result in postoperative stenosis (Fig. 9.18). In these cases, it may be advantageous to use a balloon dilation tool to start the dissection of the recess. Once the recess has been dilated, hand instruments can be used to remove the agger nasi cell and supraorbital ethmoid bony partitions.

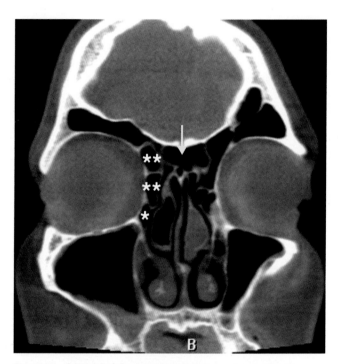

Fig. 9.12. Coronal CT scan showing an agger nasi cell *(single asterisk),* type 2 frontal cells *(double asterisks),* and interfrontal sinus septal cell *(arrow).*

INSTRUMENTATION

- 45-degree mushroom punch (Fig. 9.19)
- Bachert forceps (see Fig. 9.19)
- Through-cutting giraffe forceps (Fig. 9.20)
- Hosemann punch and larger-sized Bachert forceps (Figs. 9.19 and 9.21)
- Bolger-Kuhn probes (Fig. 9.22)

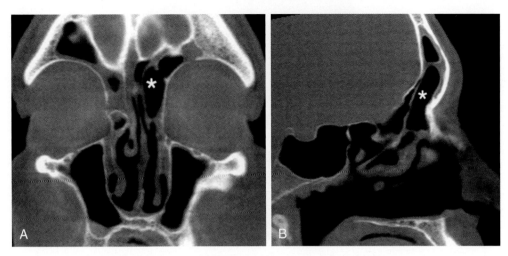

Fig. 9.13. Coronal **(A)** and sagittal **(B)** CT scans showing a type 3 frontal cell *(asterisk)*.

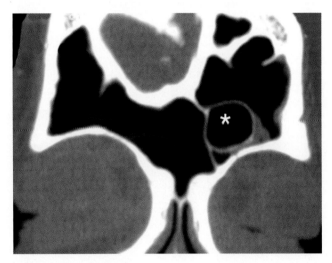

Fig. 9.14. Coronal CT scan showing a type 4 cell *(asterisk)*. Note that these cells are rarely seen. Most are actually type 3 cells.

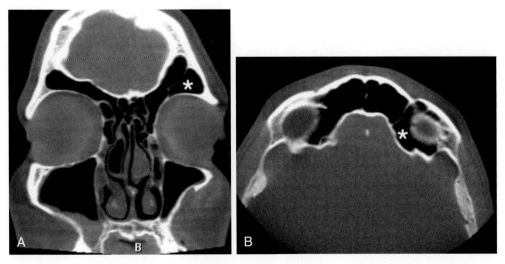

Fig. 9.15. Coronal **(A)** and axial **(B)** CT scans of a supraorbital ethmoid cell *(asterisk)*.

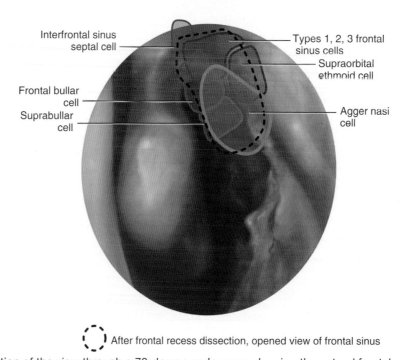

Interfrontal sinus septal cell

Types 1, 2, 3 frontal sinus cells

Supraorbital ethmoid cell

Frontal bullar cell

Suprabullar cell

Agger nasi cell

After frontal recess dissection, opened view of frontal sinus

Fig. 9.16. Artist's depiction of the view through a 70-degree endoscope showing the natural frontal recess pathway and the influence of surrounding cells.

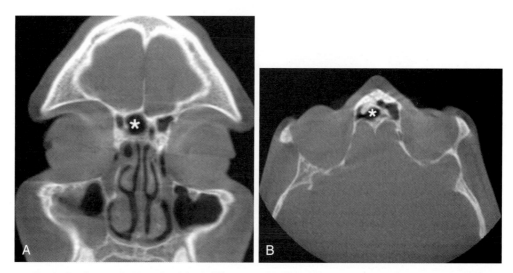

Fig. 9.17. Coronal **(A)** and axial **(B)** CT scans of an interfrontal sinus septal cell *(asterisk)*.

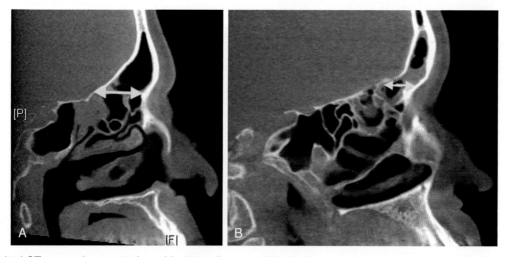

Fig. 9.18. Sagittal CT scans demonstrating wide **(A)** and narrow **(B)** anterior-posterior frontal diameters (indicated by *arrows*).

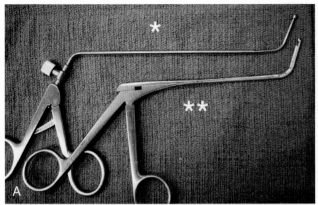

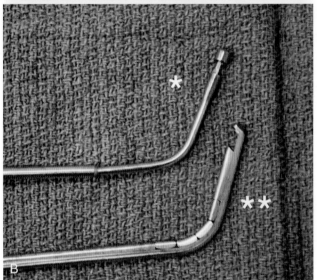

Fig. 9.19. (A) Photograph of a 45-degree Hosemann mushroom punch *(single asterisk)* and Bachert forceps *(double asterisks),* affectionately referred to as the "cobra" at the University of Pennsylvania. The latter instrument is the workhorse in frontal recess dissections. Essentially a 45-degree Kerrison punch that punches back to front, this instrument is used for the removal of agger nasi cell caps and frontal recess cells. **(B)** Zoomed-in view of instrument tips.

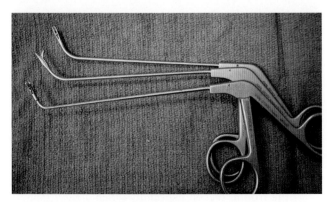

Fig. 9.20. Photograph of through-cutting giraffe forceps. They come in side-to-side and front-to-back versions at both 45- and 90-degree angles.

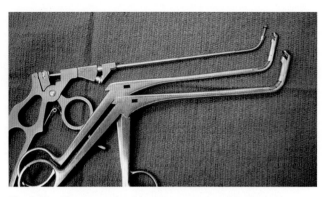

Fig. 9.21. Photograph of instruments used in frontal sinusotomy. Top instrument is a Hosemann punch. It is a 45-degree mushroom punch with greater cutting strength than a traditional mushroom punch. This instrument is best used for removal of osteitic bone of the frontal floor of the recess. The bottom two instruments are larger-sized Kerrison punches made for the frontal recess.

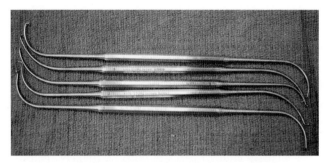

Fig. 9.22. Photograph of Bolger-Kuhn probes. They are sleek, ball-tipped instruments that have an extended length. They are very useful in the dissection of frontal recess cells that are located high in the frontal sinus.

- Image guidance systems
  - Even for the most experienced frontal sinus surgeons, image guidance is an extremely helpful tool in performing a *complete* frontal recess dissection.
  - The surgeon should learn to use the image guidance system planning station preoperatively to anticipate the anatomic variants and then intraoperatively to help guide the dissection.

PEARLS AND POTENTIAL PITFALLS

Pearls

- Even when one is first learning to perform frontal recess dissections, it is a good idea to use the 70-degree endoscope. The first attempts should focus only on visualization. The point cannot be stressed enough

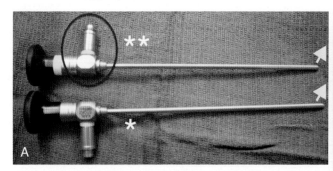

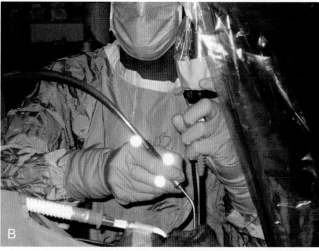

Fig. 9.23. (A) Photograph of a traditional endoscope *(single asterisk),* in which the light post is located down while the light is shining up, and a reverse endoscope *(double asterisks),* in which the light post is situated at the top of the scope. *Yellow arrows* represent the field of view; the *red circle* highlights the difference in the light post on the reverse endoscope. (B) The reverse endoscope allows for easier use of curved frontal sinus instruments without interference from the standard endoscope light post.

that *the key to good frontal recess surgery is proper visualization.*

- Reverse or offset 70-degree scopes are extremely helpful (Fig. 9.23). Getting the light post out of the way helps in instrument maneuvering, especially with the heavily angled giraffe-style instruments that are designed for the frontal recess.
  - These endoscopes are also extremely helpful when line-of-sight image guidance systems are used. The light cord will be out of the way so as not to block the tracking systems of the image guidance system.
- The goal of surgery is to identify the natural os of the frontal recess and expand "from known to unknown." This means finding the natural drainage pathway of the frontal recess and expanding the natural recess.
- Viewed endoscopically, natural drainage pathways will look like shadowed or dark recesses. These are often called *transition zones* and will guide the surgeon around the bony ethmoid walls to the frontal recess (Fig. 9.24).

Potential Pitfalls

- Through-cutting instruments should be used as much as possible to avoid stripping of mucosa within the frontal recess.
- Microdébrider use should be limited to cleaning up loose mucosal edges. The microdébrider lacks the tactile feedback for delicate dissection of subcentimeter structures.

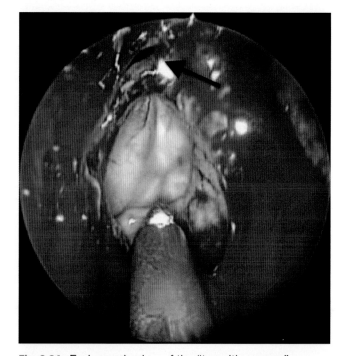

Fig. 9.24. Endoscopic view of the "transition zone," a shadowed area *(arrow)* that represents the natural drainage pathway. Bone and skull base always appear white, and mucosa appears red. Air pathways appear black; this is what one looks for when dissecting out the frontal recess.

- Move the light post around to improve visualization of the frontal recess. Especially when a *right* frontal recess dissection is performed by a right-handed surgeon, the natural tendency is to dissect in a medial

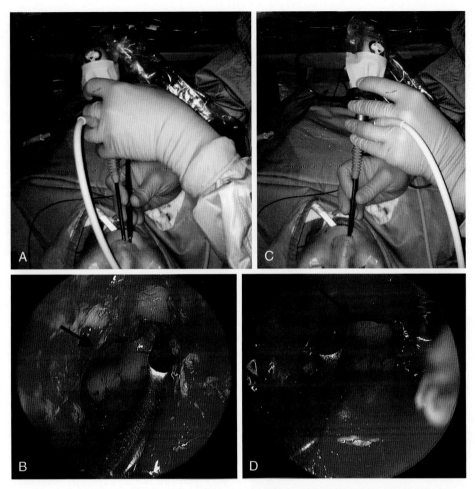

Fig. 9.25. (A) Photograph of a surgeon performing an endoscopic right frontal dissection using a 70-degree reverse endoscope with the light post at the 12 o'clock position. **(B)** Intranasal view with the light post at the 12 o'clock position. Note how the lateral true frontal recess *(arrow)* appears. **(C)** Photograph of the same right frontal dissection, now with the endoscope light post at the 10 o'clock position. **(D)** Intranasal view with the light post at the 10 o'clock position. Note that the frontal recess *(arrow)* is now centered in the view, which allows for better visualization.

direction toward the cribriform plate. Turning the light cord to "lateralize" the view will correct the angle of dissection (Fig. 9.25).

SURGICAL PROCEDURE

Step 1: Identifying the Anterior Ethmoid Artery

- Start with a 30-degree reverse endoscope. The anterior ethmoid artery is often identified at the beginning of the frontal recess as one moves posterior to anterior (Fig. 9.26). This signals the beginning of the frontal dissection. At this point, place a 70-degree reverse endoscope for better visualization. When the frontal recess is viewed, the most common arrangement is the agger nasi cell anteriorly and the supraorbital ethmoid and ethmoid bulla posteriorly.

Step 2: Identifying the Natural Drainage Pathway

- Identify the natural drainage pathway by the appearance of a transition zone (Fig. 9.27). In nearly all cases, the pathway is medial-posterior to the posterior wall of the agger nasi cell.
- Using a curved suction or frontal sinus curette, direct dissection toward this area to identify a transition zone. Once the transition zone is identified, work to dilate this space and remove the bone surrounding it. In this case, the bony walls to be removed are the agger nasi cell anteriorly and the ethmoid bulla posteriorly.

Step 3: Removing the Posterior Wall of the Agger Nasi Cell

- Use 45-degree front-to-back through-cutting giraffe forceps to remove the posterior wall of the agger nasi cell (Fig. 9.28).

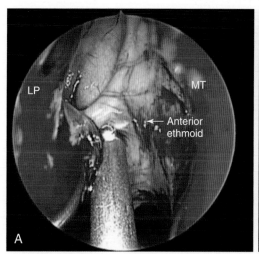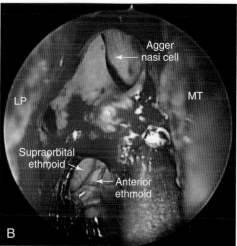

Fig. 9.26. (A) View of the anterior ethmoid artery through a 30-degree reverse endoscope. (B) View of the frontal recess after changing to a 70-degree reverse endoscope. *LP,* Lamina papyracea (medial orbital wall); *MT,* middle turbinate.

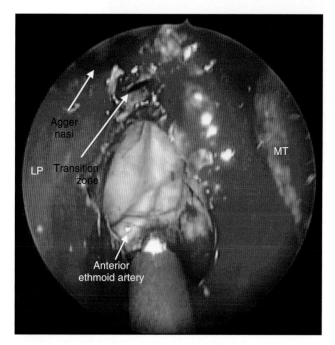

Fig. 9.27. Endoscopic view of the transition zone that identifies the natural drainage pathway. In nearly all cases, the frontal recess pathway is medial-posterior to the posterior wall of the agger nasi cell. *LP,* Lamina papyracea; *MT,* middle turbinate.

- This move alone already exposes the frontal recess, and the skull bone can be identified based on its characteristic appearance.

Step 4: "Enlarging the Box"—Remove Surrounding Bony Partitions to Widen the Frontal Recess

- With the posterior wall of the agger nasi cell removed, remove the medial wall of the agger nasi cell. The skull base is located posterior to the dissection (Fig. 9.29).

- Use a combination of front-to-back and side-to-side through-cutting giraffe forceps to cut the medial wall of the agger nasi cell (Fig. 9.30).

Step 5: Removing the Cap of the Agger Nasi Cell

- As the next step, remove the cap of the agger nasi cell (Fig. 9.31). This is best accomplished with a frontal sinus Kerrison punch (Bachert). A 45-degree mushroom punch can also be used.
- Open the Bachert forceps wide and then remove the cap in a posterior to anterior direction. Remove the cap of the agger nasi cell all the way anteriorly to the hard shelf of the nasofrontal bone.
- Removing the cap of the agger nasi cell has the greatest effect in widening the frontal recess.

Step 6: Expanding the Posterior Frontal Recess

- Remove the bony wall separating the supraorbital ethmoid and frontal recess. Removing the ledge back to the skull base will allow expansion of the frontal recess into the supraorbital ethmoid recess, which will greatly enlarge the dissection (Fig. 9.32).
- Remove the posterior bone with either a 45-degree mushroom punch or through-cutting giraffe forceps. Identifying the anterior ethmoid artery more posteriorly before this move will provide greater confidence in working in the posterior frontal recess.

Step 7: Performing the Finishing Touches

- Perform finishing touches to maximize the opening into the frontal sinus. Use a 45-degree mushroom or Hosemann punch to remove some of the medial floor of the frontal recess.
- After a properly performed frontal recess dissection, the roof and posterior skull base should be clearly visualized with a 70-degree endoscope (Fig. 9.33).

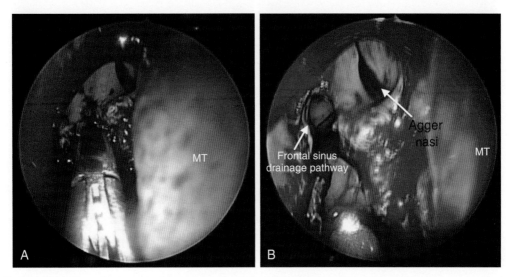

Fig. 9.28. (A) Endoscopic view of removal of the posterior wall of the agger nasi cell using 45-degree front-to-back through-cutting giraffe forceps. **(B)** Endoscopic view demonstrating that the frontal recess has been exposed by this move. *MT,* Middle turbinate.

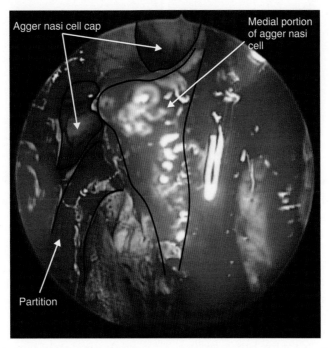

Fig. 9.29. Endoscopic view of the agger nasi cell. With the posterior wall of the agger nasi cell removed, the next step is to remove the medial wall of the cell. The skull base is located posterior to the dissection.

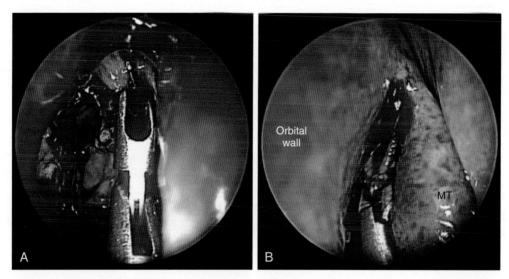

Fig. 9.30. Endoscopic images of dissection of the medial wall of the agger nasi cell using a combination of front-to-back **(A)** and side-to-side **(B)** through-cutting giraffe instruments. *MT*, Middle turbinate.

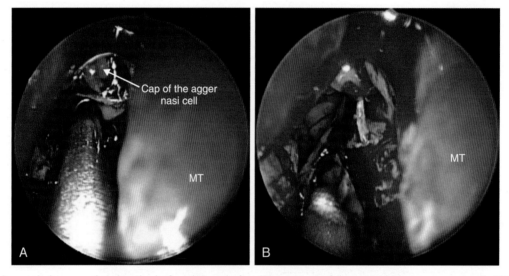

Fig. 9.31. Endoscopic images showing the before **(A)** and after **(B)** removal of the cap of the agger nasi cell. *MT*, Middle turbinate.

Step 8: Placing a Frontal Sinus Stent (Optional)

- Cut the frontal sinus stent from a 0.25-mm silicone sheet (Fig. 9.34A). To place the stent, roll the base and hold with pediatric side-to-side giraffe forceps.
- Fig. 9.34B shows the frontal sinus stent in position. The stent is generally left in place for 1 to 2 weeks.
- Alternatively, there are now steroid-eluting stents that are made to dissolve in 4 weeks and designed to fit the frontal recess. An advantage of this stent is the decreased need for postoperative débridements and local application of steroids to the surrounding mucosa. A disadvantage for use is the cost of the stent and a potential for infection, necessitating early removal. Use of either the silastic stent or steroid-eluting stent is based on surgeon preference.

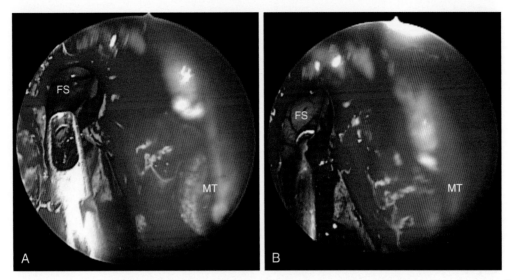

Fig. 9.32. **(A)** Endoscopic view of removal of the bony wall separating the supraorbital ethmoid and frontal recess. **(B)** Endoscopic view of removal of the posterior bone. *FS,* Frontal sinus; *MT,* middle turbinate.

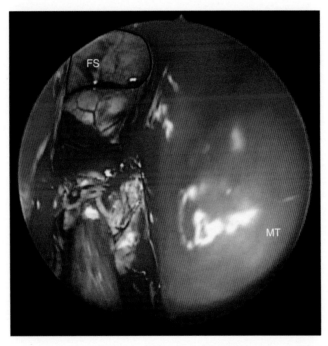

Fig. 9.33. Endoscopic view of a completed frontal recess dissection. *FS,* Frontal sinus; *MT,* middle turbinate.

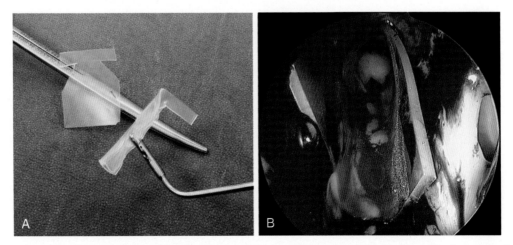

Fig. 9.34. **(A)** Photograph of a frontal sinus stent cut from a 0.5-mm silicone sheet. **(B)** Endoscopic view of the frontal sinus stent in place.

Frontal Sinusotomy—Draf IIb

Henry P. Barham and Vijay R. Ramakrishnan

INTRODUCTION

- Endoscopic sinus and skull base surgery has become an effective part of the management of chronic rhinosinusitis (CRS) and tumors of the sinuses and anterior skull base. Technologic advances have been critical in advancing endoscopic surgical procedures, with the introduction of improved optics and lighting, advanced instrumentation, and image-guided surgical navigation. Hemostatic materials and devices have similarly evolved to assist in the management of the surgical field and postoperative cavity.

- The vast majority of inflammatory frontal disease can be treated with a well-performed Draf I or Draf IIa dissection. Common causes of continued disease after a complete Draf IIa dissection include membranous stenosis, middle turbinate lateralization, osteitis, neoosteogenesis, and prominence of the nasofrontal beak.

- Extended endoscopic approaches offer improved exposure of the frontal sinus and may be preferred over external approaches in some cases. Table 10.1 describes the advantages of such endoscopic approaches. Extended frontal sinus approaches are also useful for the resection of benign and malignant tumors of the frontal sinus. The procedure has helped to expand endoscopic techniques to include recalcitrant frontal sinus disease, frontal sinus mucoceles, cerebrospinal fluid (CSF) leaks, frontoethmoid fractures, frontal sinus tumors, and endoscopic skull base surgery. The procedure also improves the postoperative delivery of topical irrigation and tumor surveillance.

- The Draf IIb procedure is an extension of the Draf IIa dissection in the medial direction, with partial removal of the anterior-superior middle turbinate and frontal sinus floor. As in basic frontal sinus surgery, it is critical to preserve mucosa and avoid exposed bone wherever possible. Ideally, complete Draf IIa dissection is performed before progressing to Draf IIb dissection.

- Patients undergoing extended frontal approach procedures often have challenging anatomy; the use of image guidance is preferred in these cases. The progression to Draf IIb dissection commits both the patient and the surgeon to more meticulous and prolonged postoperative care.

ANATOMY

Frontal Sinus

- The reader is referred to Chapter 9 for discussion and illustration of the anatomy of the frontal recess, anterior ethmoid region, and accessory frontal cells. Given the high degree of variability in pneumatization of the sinus, certain basic relationships are important to understand. The frontal sinus is a pyramidal, funnel-shaped structure. It is divided in the midline by an intersinus septum and may contain an intersinus cell. The intersinus septum separates the paired sinuses and is a surgical target for maximal expansion of outflow.

- Extended frontal sinus approaches seek to remove the floor of the frontal sinus for maximal enlargement of the outflow pathway. Fig. 10.1 shows the dissection boundaries for the Draf classification of extended frontal sinus approaches. The nasofrontal beak is the variably thick bony projection at the junction of the

TABLE 10.1 Advantages of Extended Endoscopic Approaches Over External Approaches
■ Decreased pain
■ Shorter hospital stay
■ No risk of dysesthesia
■ Improved cosmesis
■ Ability to perform subsequent endoscopic surveillance

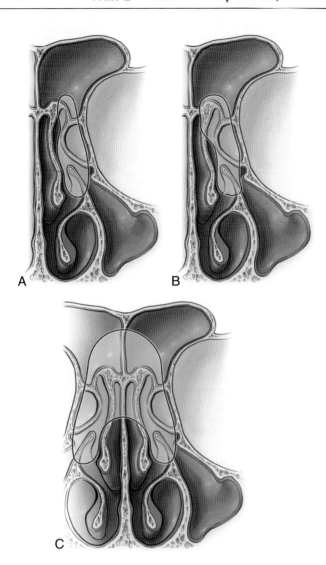

Fig. 10.1. Drawings showing areas of dissection in Draf extended frontal sinus approaches. **(A)** Boundaries of dissection for the Draf IIa procedure. **(B)** Boundaries of dissection for the Draf IIb procedure. The middle turbinate attachment at the floor of the frontal sinus is removed, as is the entire ipsilateral floor of the frontal sinus. The remainder of the middle turbinate is preserved. **(C)** The Draf III procedure is bilateral Draf IIb procedures combined with removal of the superior nasal septum and frontal intersinus septum.

nasal and frontal bones. If this structure is prominent, it may narrow frontal sinus outflow. The anterior limit of dissection is the periosteal layer of the superficial glabellar cutaneous tissue. Lateral boundaries of the frontal sinus floor consist of the medial orbital wall and orbital roof. These structures are generally left undisturbed during extended frontal sinus approaches.

Anterior Fossa and Cribriform Plate

- The olfactory fossa is the lowest point in the floor of the anterior cranial base. The skull base slopes

downward in a lateral to medial direction in the coronal plane and in an anterior to posterior direction in the sagittal plane. The degree of slope is highly variable and should be studied on preoperative images. The olfactory fossa contains an anterior projection into the frontal sinus that is most easily seen in axial view (Fig. 10.2). The distance from this projection to the anterior table of the frontal sinus is referred to as the anterior-posterior (A-P) diameter.
- The cribriform plate of the ethmoid bone may vary in depth and slope and is often asymmetric.

Middle Turbinate

- The middle turbinate is expected to insert into the lateral lamella of the cribriform plate. In many patients, the most anterior aspect of the middle turbinate lies anterior to the cribriform plate and may insert into the floor of the frontal sinus.
- The anterior aspect of the middle turbinate offers a reliable landmark to identify the locations of the frontal sinus and olfactory fossa (Fig. 10.3).

INDICATIONS AND CONTRAINDICATIONS FOR EXTENDED FRONTAL SINUS SURGERY

- Indications for extended frontal sinus surgery include
  - failed prior frontal surgery, often associated with neo-osteogenesis or lateralized middle turbinate remnant (Fig. 10.4)
  - mucocele (Fig. 10.5)
  - frontal sinus unobliteration
  - need for surgical access (treatment of type 3 or type 4 frontal cell, intersinus septal cell)
  - benign or malignant tumor
  - repair of CSF leak or encephalocele
  - select trauma cases
- Relative contraindications for extended frontal sinus surgery include
  - extremely narrow A-P diameter
  - severe bilateral neo-osteogenesis
  - lesions requiring access to the lateral aspect of a well-pneumatized frontal sinus
  - medical comorbidities precluding general anesthesia

PREOPERATIVE CONSIDERATIONS

- The disease process, radiologic findings, and goals of surgery should be reviewed thoroughly before making the decision as to which approach is most favorable.

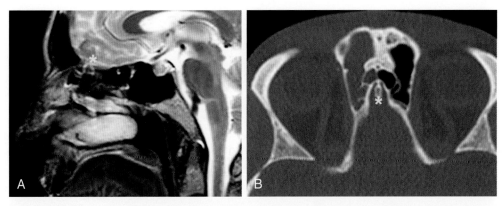

Fig. 10.2. Sagittal magnetic resonance image **(A)** and axial computed tomographic scan **(B)** showing the location of the olfactory fossa *(asterisk)*. The surgeon should recognize the olfactory fossa as the lowest point in the floor of the anterior cranial base **(A)** and be aware of its anterior projection into the frontal sinus **(B)**.

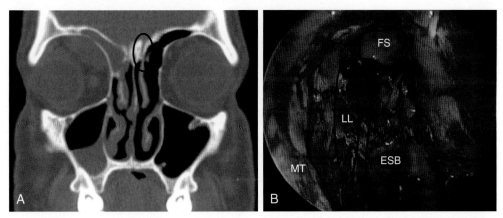

Fig. 10.3. (A) Coronal computed tomographic scan illustrating that the vertical portion of the middle turbinate is the medial boundary of the frontal recess *(black oval)*. **(B)** Endoscopic image showing the middle turbinate *(MT)* attachment at the lateral lamella *(LL)* of the cribriform, which corresponds to the oval area in **(A)**. *ESB,* Ethmoid skull base; *FS,* frontal sinus ostium.

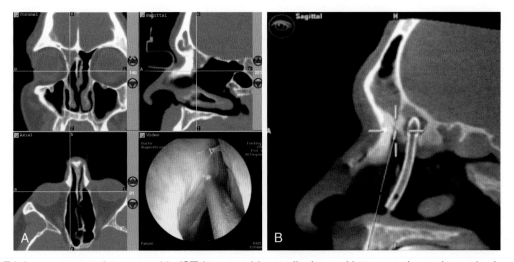

Fig. 10.4. (A) Triplanar computed tomographic (CT) image guidance display and intraoperative endoscopic view for a patient who underwent prior sinus surgery with partial middle turbinate resection. A lateralized middle turbinate remnant with associated osteitis was identified as the cause of his frontal sinus obstruction. **(B)** Sagittal CT scan for a patient who underwent six prior sinus surgeries, most recently with placement of a frontal sinus stent. The stent was located in a supraorbital ethmoid cell with significant surrounding neo-osteogenesis.

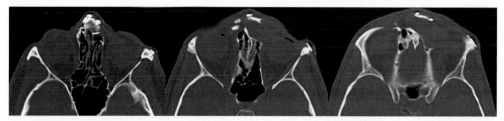

Fig. 10.5. Axial computed tomographic (CT) scans for a patient who underwent extensive repair of traumatic facial fractures over 10 years before developing a frontal sinus mucocele. CT images demonstrate neo-osteogenesis and hardware to be the sources of outflow obstruction.

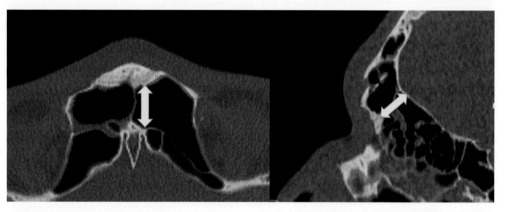

Fig. 10.6. Axial *(left)* and sagittal *(right)* computed tomographic scans for a patient with a frontal sinus fracture in whom hyperpneumatization with a large anterior-posterior diameter *(yellow arrows)* creates a favorable setting for endoscopic access.

- The risks of surgery, including CSF leak, orbital injury, hemorrhage, smell dysfunction, and possible recurrence of disease, should be discussed fully with the patient well in advance of surgery.
- The possible need for adjunctive open approaches should be entertained and discussed.
- Postoperative care expectations should be agreed upon, including follow-up, débridement, and medication regimens.
- Preoperative medical treatment with agents such as antibiotics and systemic corticosteroids may be necessary to optimize intraoperative hemostasis and visualization.

Radiologic Considerations

- Thoroughly review fine-cut computed tomographic (CT) scans in the coronal, axial, and sagittal planes. Actively scrolling through the scans on a computer workstation is helpful to create a three-dimensional understanding of the anatomy.
- Examine the A-P dimension in both axial and sagittal planes. Smaller dimensions indicate a more technically challenging surgery and ultimately a smaller sinusotomy, which may yield a worse long-term prognosis.

- It is often quoted that a minimum A-P dimension of 10 mm is required, but in reality there need only be enough room for the drill to fit comfortably without the back end of the bur violating the cribriform plate or posterior table of the sinus (Fig. 10.6).
- Assess the thickness of the nasofrontal beak because this can be drilled out to increase the A-P dimension.
- Identify the middle turbinate or middle turbinate remnant. This will serve as a surgical landmark. Its anterior insertion is helpful to note preoperatively, as is the presence of lateralization, osteitis, or neo-osteogenesis.
- Establish the location of the anterior ethmoid artery and note its presence within the skull base or hanging in a mesentery. If the anterior ethmoid artery is in a mesentery, bipolar cautery may be used early in the procedure to prevent risk of inadvertent injury.
- Look for the presence of a skull base defect. It is not uncommon for a mucocele or postobstructive tumor secretions to demineralize the anterior and/or posterior table of the frontal sinus. Posterior table dehiscence warrants more careful introduction of instruments (Fig. 10.7).
- In the case of a tumor or CSF leak or encephalocele, determine the presence, location, and size of the potential skull base defect to decide on the

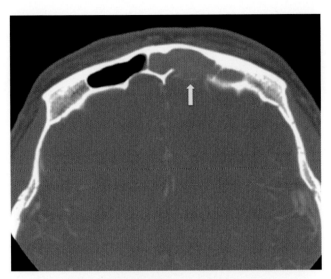

Fig. 10.7. Axial contrast-enhanced computed tomographic scan for a patient with allergic fungal sinusitis and posterior table dehiscence *(yellow arrow)*.

optimal surgical approach. Magnetic resonance imaging (MRI) aids in the diagnosis of mucocele, tumor, and CSF leak or encephalocele. It may also be helpful in postoperative examination of patients who have previously undergone fat obliteration, although findings are highly variable in this population. MRI is helpful to distinguish tumor from inspissated secretions and to identify the location and size of a skull base defect.

- If far lateral dissection is expected, an adjunctive open approach, such as a trephine or osteoplastic flap, may be anticipated.

INSTRUMENTATION

- Overall instrumentation and setup are similar to that described in Chapter 9.
- In extended frontal approaches, certain equipment is particularly important:
  - 45- and 70-degree endoscopes
  - Punches, such as a 45-degree mushroom punch for thinner bone and a Hosemann punch for the thicker bone of the frontal recess
  - Angled irrigating drills: 70-degree diamond drills are the safest and most useful; however, cutting burs may be used for extensive bone removal. Extreme care must be taken with cutting burs, because misplacement or skipping of the bur can have quick untoward effects on both the orbit and dura.
- Image guidance is a surgical tool that is widely accepted by the endoscopic surgeon and used in the majority of frontal sinus surgeries. The use of image guidance can help identify critical structures

and distorted anatomic landmarks, increasing the surgeon's confidence and ability to perform a more complete dissection. Image-guided placement of limited external frontal sinusotomy allows access to and management of frontal sinus pathology that is beyond endoscopic reach while avoiding the need for an osteoplastic flap.

- Mini-trephination set: if difficulty in identification of the frontal sinus ostium is anticipated, fluorescein irrigation through a mini-trephination may be helpful.
- Materials for CSF leak repair according to the surgeon's preferred method: these should be available in case a leak is encountered intraoperatively.

SURGICAL PROCEDURE

Preparation

- The patient's airway is maintained by either an endotracheal tube or laryngeal mask, which is taped to the lower left commissure in an effort to allow unimpeded hand mobility for a right-handed surgeon.
- The patient is prepared topically with 1% ropivacaine and 1:2000 adrenaline-soaked neurosurgical cottonoids placed within the inferior meatus and over the anterior head of the inferior turbinate.
- Endoscopically, the mucosa is injected with 1% ropivacaine and 1:100,000 adrenaline at the middle turbinate, lateral wall anterior to the middle turbinate, and septum near the anterior ethmoid artery or swell body.
- The patient's head is placed in the neutral anatomic position, and the operative bed is placed in 15- to 20-degree reverse Trendelenburg with total intravenous anesthesia.

Surgical Technique

Step 1: Anterior Ethmoid and Frontal Recess Dissection

- If prior sphenoethmoidectomy has not been performed, at least an anterior ethmoidectomy is performed to identify the medial orbital wall. Complete the anterior ethmoid and frontal recess dissection(s) as in the Draf I and IIa procedures.

Step 2: Localization of the Anterior Ethmoid Arteries

- Identify the location of the anterior ethmoid arteries at the skull base. This will be the posterior boundary of the frontal dissection on each side. Attempt to directly visualize and follow the skull base anterior to the artery. This may require opening the supraorbital ethmoid cell(s) and connecting these cells to the frontal ostium if this has not already been done. If this

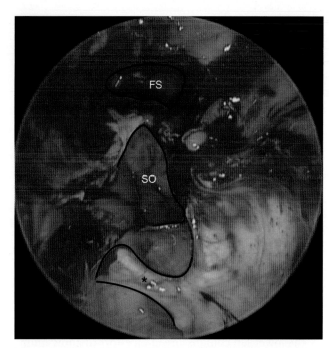

Fig. 10.8. View of the left frontal recess through a 70-degree endoscope. The frontal sinus *(FS)* is anterior to the supraorbital cell *(SO),* and the artery is seen behind a smaller second supraorbital cell *(asterisk).* The artery heads anteriorly as it courses from the orbit into the lateral cribriform.

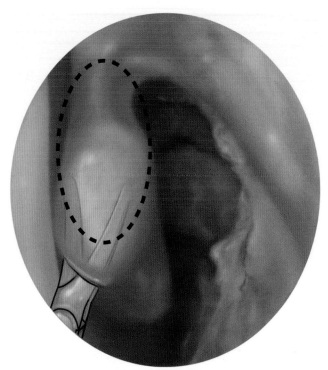

Fig. 10.9. Artist's depiction of resection of the anterior portion of the middle turbinate using curved endoscopic scissors (endoscopic view).

area has been completely replaced by neo-osteogenesis, then stop and attempt to perform this dissection on the contralateral side. Do not hesitate to cauterize the artery if there is a concern it will impede later dissection. It is far better to cauterize early than to injure it later in the dissection (Fig. 10.8).

Step 3: Enlargement of the Frontal Sinus Ostium

- Identify and enlarge the frontal sinus ostium and imagine the horseshoe shape of the floor of the frontal sinus. Mentally trace the path under direct visualization and confirm this with the image guidance probe.
- If the frontal outflow is substantially narrowed, such as in the case of significant neo-osteogenesis, mini-trephination with fluorescein irrigation may be considered to help direct the endoscopic dissection at this point.

Step 4: Partial Resection of the Anterior Middle Turbinate

- Partially resect the anterior middle turbinate. Carry out the resection unilaterally for the Draf IIb approach. The most inferior portion of the middle turbinate can be preserved for potential maintenance of function.
- Use curved endoscopic scissors to make a superior cut just below the anterior attachment at the skull

base toward the level of the anterior ethmoid artery. Make a second cut from the inferior aspect of the turbinate and angle it to meet the first cut. Scissor cuts are generally made conservatively and then refined with through-cutting instruments (Figs. 10.9 and 10.10).

Step 5: Initial Frontal Recess Floor Removal

- Using a 45-degree mushroom punch and more robust punches, such as the Hosemann and/or Bachert variety, punch out the floor of the sinus in an anterior to medial direction. The thickness of the bone will determine the amount of bone removal performed with a punch (Fig. 10.11).

Step 6: Further Bone Removal

- If required for a larger ostium, use a 70-degree diamond drill to gradually expand the ostium in an anterior to medial direction. It is safer to drill anteriorly first to thin out the nasofrontal beak (Fig. 10.12).
- Bone removal in the anterior to medial direction can be performed with improved visualization of the skull base and intersinus septum. As bone is thinned with the drill, reintroduce punches. The serial use of punches aids in both speed and safety.
- When a prominent nasofrontal beak or severe neo-osteogenesis is present, a cutting bur may be

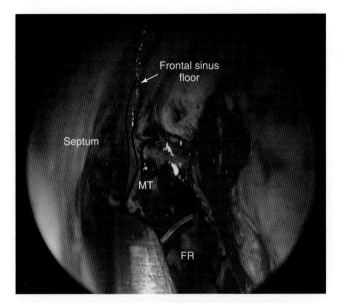

Fig. 10.10. Endoscopic view of the use of through-cutting frontal instruments to remove the anterior portion of the middle turbinate *(MT)* up to the skull base. *FR,* Frontal recess.

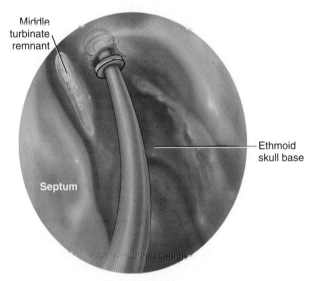

Fig. 10.11. Artist's depiction of the use of a frontal sinus punch to remove the frontal sinus floor after partial middle turbinate resection (endoscopic view).

used carefully to facilitate removal of thick bone. However, the frontal sinus proper and skull base should be definitively visualized before the introduction of the bur.

■ In the Draf IIb procedure, removal of the anterior middle turbinate and ipsilateral frontal sinus floor completes the procedure.

Step 7: Cavity Optimization

■ Optimize the cavity for postoperative success. Clear any purulence, bone chips, or bone dust.

■ Using a bipolar cautery, cauterize the midline soft tissue just anterior to the cribriform; then, cut the edges of the middle turbinates and nasal septum.

■ Medialize the middle turbinate remnants using a transseptal absorbable suture. Consider the need for dressings, such as a temporary silicone elastomer (Silastic) roll.

■ If a stent is used postoperatively, thin, pliable Silastic appears more favorable for wound healing than other more rigid types of stents.

PEARLS AND POTENTIAL PITFALLS

Pearls

■ If maxillary, sphenoid, and ethmoid surgeries are required, these procedures are performed before the frontal dissection.

■ Appropriate visualization is mandatory at all times. 0- and 30-degree endoscopes are used early, when working on the anterior ethmoid and turbinates; 45- or 70-degree endoscopes are used when working within the frontal recess and frontal sinus.

■ Image guidance is frequently used in these cases but is never solely relied upon. When image guidance is used, registration accuracy must be repeatedly checked on fixed landmarks.

■ The working instrument is generally introduced underneath the endoscope. However, when dissecting anteriorly, it may be helpful to work with the endoscope underneath the instrument. Alternatively, the thick bone of the anterior agger nasi region leading to the nasofrontal beak can be removed to facilitate a more direct approach.

Potential Pitfalls

■ Inattention to the location of the posterior surface of the drill can potentially lead to skull base penetration.

■ Excessive removal of mucosa prolongs recovery and increases the potential for stenosis.

■ Irregular postoperative follow-up and/or lack of meticulous medical care and débridement will certainly lead to stenosis. The neo-ostium is still maturing for up to 1 year after surgery and potentially longer if there is ongoing disease.

POSTOPERATIVE CONSIDERATIONS

Complications

■ Possible postoperative complications include
 – bleeding (anterior ethmoid artery, anterior cribriform, cut edge of middle turbinate or septum)

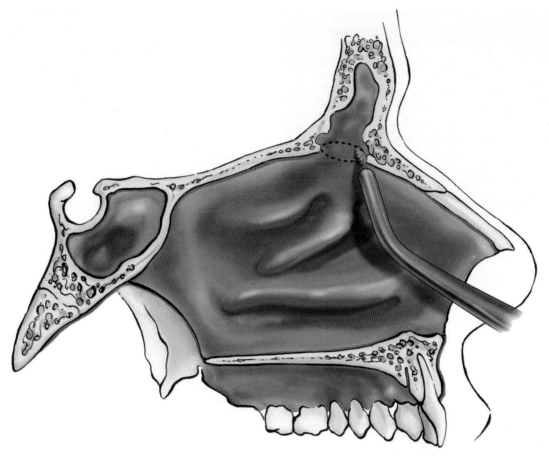

Fig. 10.12. Drawing showing the use of a drill to remove the frontal sinus floor and nasofrontal beak.

- orbital ecchymosis and hematoma, diplopia (direct ocular muscle injury)
- CSF leak, meningitis
- temporary or permanent olfactory dysfunction
- stenosis and disease recurrence

POSTOPERATIVE MANAGEMENT

- Postoperative medical management and appropriate surgical technique are equally important in ensuring long-term patency after extended frontal surgery.
- The following medications are administered postoperatively.
  - Oral steroids are dosed and tapered according to extent of disease at surgery, endoscopic appearance in the postoperative phase, and any patient-specific factors.
  - Oral antibiotics: culture-directed therapy is preferred.
  - Irrigants: gentle saline rinses or sprays are started early.
  - Topical steroids: topical agents are started once oral steroid therapy is completed.

  - For improved frontal sinus penetration, nebulized therapy or steroid drops administered using appropriate head positioning maneuvers should be considered.
- Nasal packing is not necessary. If stents are used, there should be a rationale for their placement and duration of use. Biofilm colonization of stents has been shown at 3 weeks and likely occurs substantially sooner. Common practice is to use Silastic stents for 2 weeks, as described in Chapter 9.
- Patients should be given appropriate instructions upon discharge. Activity restrictions are similar to those for routine sinus surgeries. Patients should be counseled to recognize symptoms and signs of intracranial and orbital complications.
- Patients should receive regular follow-up with débridement as needed. This can require weekly endoscopic examinations in the clinic setting until the cavity is stable. The exact course should be tailored to the degree of disease and the endoscopic appearance of the cavity.
- Débridement may consist of the suctioning of mucus and blood clots, removal of thick fibrinous debris, early takedown of scar bands or circumferential

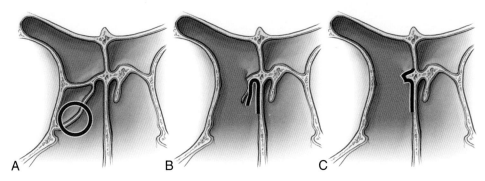

Fig. 10.13. Drawings illustrating the frontal sinus rescue procedure. The procedure begins with identification of the middle turbinate remnant (MTR) **(A)**, elevation of the mucosa and removal of the bony remnant **(B)**, and reapproximation of the mucosal edges **(C)**.

stenosis, irrigation, direct instillation of topical steroids, or treatment of circumferential stenosis with a mushroom punch or balloon in the office.

Frontal Sinus Rescue Procedure

■ The frontal sinus rescue procedure can be used to treat frontal sinus obstruction secondary to prior surgery that resulted in lateralization of a partially resected middle turbinate. In this procedure, a medially based mucosal flap is elevated from the middle turbinate stump and preserved. A Draf IIb procedure is performed, and the mucosal flap is advanced over the denuded bone. Thus, a frontal sinus rescue procedure is a Draf IIb frontal sinusotomy with an advancement flap (Fig. 10.13).

Frontal Sinusotomy—Draf III

E. Ritter Sansoni, Raymond Sacks, and Richard J. Harvey

ENDOSCOPIC COMMON FRONTAL SINUSOTOMY

Introduction

- The common frontal sinusotomy, modified endoscopic Lothrop procedure (MELP), or Draf III procedure, is an adaptation of the technique first described by Dr. Harold Lothrop in 1914.[1] Wolfgang Draf popularized the operation in the 1990s; it has since become an important surgical procedure used in the treatment of a variety of disease processes.
- The fundamental concept of the common frontal sinusotomy is that it converts the complex and limited frontal sinus outflow tracts into a simple common cavity by removing the frontal sinus floor and nasofrontal beak.
- Maximally opening the frontal sinus minimizes the issues of access inherent to the design of the frontal sinus and has been shown to improve the delivery of topical therapies to the frontal sinus when compared to more limited dissections.[2]
- Additionally, the Draf III procedure permits the surgeon to endoscopically access almost the entire frontal sinus, thereby increasing the number of neoplastic lesions involving the frontal sinus or rostral skull base that are amenable to a purely endoscopic resection.[3]
- Traditionally, the MELP has been described as an inside-out approach whereby the surgeon first performs frontal sinus dissections and then commences drilling from the frontal recess. This can be challenging if the frontal recess has significant disease burden, neo-osteogenesis, or scarring from prior surgery. The outside-in approach, which is discussed here, avoids this issue altogether as dissection is not related to frontal recess anatomy. As a result, the outside-in approach offers an efficient, safe, and reliable option to the traditional technique.[4]

ANATOMY

- The frontal sinus is the last sinus to pneumatize and demonstrates a variety of pneumatization patterns. Additionally, the frontal sinuses develop independent of one another and are divided by an intersinus septum that is variable in contour.
- The nasofrontal beak is the midline bony thickening of the nasal process of the frontal bone and is considered to be the anterior boundary of the frontal sinus ostium. The posterior edge of the nasofrontal beak will be anterior to the anterior aspect of the olfactory fossa.[5]
- The olfactory fossa is the lowest portion of the anterior skull base, and the anterior aspect of it projects into the frontal sinus centrally. It is critical for the surgeon to appreciate this to prevent an inadvertent injury. Also, there can be some variability between the two sides, which should be noted on preoperative imaging.
- The outside-in MELP relies on known anatomic landmarks that serve as the boundaries for the common frontal sinusotomy cavity and are identified early in the procedure.[4] The limits of the endoscopic common frontal sinusotomy cavity are as follows:
  - Posteriorly, the first olfactory neuron on each side demarcates the forward projection of the olfactory bulb.
  - Laterally, the orbital plates of the frontal bone and periosteum of the skin covering the frontal process of the maxilla on both sides.
  - Anteriorly, the plane of the anterior table of the frontal sinus.
- A discussion of the complex and varied anatomy of the frontal recess is not necessary here since the outside-in approach does not use frontal recess anatomy to develop the common frontal sinusotomy cavity. However, it is important to have a sound foundation of knowledge of the anatomy of both the frontal recess and osteomeatal complex, specifically their re-

lationship to the medial orbital wall. These relationships have been extensively discussed in prior chapters. At the conclusion of the procedure, the frontal recesses are connected to the common frontal sinusotomy, thus a creating an inverted U shape.

INDICATIONS AND CONTRAINDICATIONS

Indications

- One of the primary benefits of the common frontal sinusotomy is improved access to the frontal sinus and anterior skull base. This offers advantages in numerous clinical situations; consequently, the common frontal sinusotomy is used alone or in conjunction with other surgical procedures to treat a variety of pathologies.
- Inflammatory sinus disease: A mainstay in the management of inflammatory sinus disease is the ability to deliver topical medications—namely, corticosteroids—to the affected sinuses. The common frontal sinusotomy maximally exteriorizes the frontal sinus and allows for a more effective delivery of topical therapies.[2] As our understanding of the pathophysiology of chronic rhinosinusitis (CRS) has evolved, we have become more assertive in our treatment algorithm and use the common frontal sinusotomy as a primary surgical intervention and as a salvage procedure. The common frontal sinusotomy procedure should be considered in the following scenarios:
  - Primary surgery for patients with eosinophilic CRS, the Samter triad, aspirin-exacerbated airway disease, and extensive nasal polyposis, especially in patients with concurrent lower airway inflammatory disease
  - Patients with recalcitrant frontal sinus disease who have failed prior endoscopic sinus surgery or those who have developed iatrogenic frontal sinus disease
  - Salvage for failed osteoplastic flap with sinus obliteration[6]
- Sinonasal and skull base neoplasms: Many frontal sinus neoplasms can be surgically accessed through the Draf III cavity.[3] The lateral orbital roof is an exception, but the common frontal sinusotomy can be expanded with an orbital transposition to access more laterally based lesions.[7] Additionally, the common frontal sinusotomy is an important surgical adjunct during resections of anterior skull base neoplasms because it improves exposure and the angle of surgical access.[8] The common frontal sinusotomy is beneficial for the treatment of neoplastic processes for the following reasons:
  - Enhanced surgical access for tumors involving the frontal sinus, anterior ethmoids, and rostral skull base

- Improved postoperative surveillance
- Simplified posttreatment care after surgery and radiotherapy
- The common frontal sinusotomy can also be used in selected cases for surgical access in the management of cerebrospinal fluid (CSF) leaks, encephaloceles, mucoceles, and postcraniofacial trauma.

Contraindications

- A general contraindication for the common frontal sinusotomy is in the setting of very active inflammatory airway disease that requires systemic steroids. These patients are unlikely to improve with the addition of topical therapy and often heal poorly if there is suboptimal control of their underlying inflammatory condition. As such, wait until the inflammatory airway state has reached a stage at which topical therapies are likely to be the primary modality for disease control before performing a common frontal sinusotomy.
- An extremely narrow anterior-posterior dimension of the frontal recess is often stated as a contraindication, but the outside-in approach negates this issue and the only instances in which anatomy precludes the common frontal sinusotomy is if the posterior table is less than 5 mm to the skin anterior to the nasofrontal beak. This is only rarely seen in instances of prior trauma or craniofacial abnormalities.

PREOPERATIVE CONSIDERATIONS

- As with any procedure, deciding the goals of the operation as well as having a complete discussion of risks and expected postoperative care and maintenance with the patient is imperative.
- Patients need to understand how important postoperative care is to the success of the operation. Strongly reconsider whether to do the operation if a patient is unlikely to follow the recommended postoperative regimen and follow-up schedule.
- Fine-cut computed tomography (CT) and magnetic resonance imaging (MRI), if indicated, should be thoroughly examined in the coronal, axial, and sagittal planes. In addition to the anatomy that is typically reviewed for endoscopic sinus and skull base surgery, the surgeon should assess the following:
  - General size and shape of the frontal sinuses as well as the placement of the intersinus septum
  - Thickness of the nasofrontal beak in the sagittal plane and its relationship to the skull base
  - Projection of the olfactory fossa into the frontal sinus

– Distance between the posterior table and nasofrontal and if there is any dehiscence
– Dehiscence of the lamina papyracea
– Septal deviation or prominent septal body

INSTRUMENTATION

- A standard endoscopic sinus tray with a 2-mm Kerrison rongeur
- Only a 0-degree nasal endoscope is required for the outside-in approach. In Wolfgang Draf's original paper, he performed the procedure with an operating microscope, thus proving that the procedure can be accomplished with a straight line of sight.[9]
- A high-speed, 15-degree, self-irrigating drill with a rough diamond bur. We prefer the Medtronic Straightshot M5 drill (Minneapolis, Minnesota), as it is capable of 30,000 rpm and has an integrated distal suction that allows for improved surgical efficiency. The bur size is 4.5 mm or greater. This ensures that the bur head will work beyond the shaft of the drill and is more ergonomic.
- Image guidance is not necessary but helps to identify where to initiate the mucosal incisions. It is also useful for those who are learning how to do the procedure and for teaching purposes.
- 0.5 mm thick Silastic sheet to create the common frontal sinusotomy dressing
- NasoPore dressing (Polyganics B.V., Netherlands)

SURGICAL PROCEDURE

Step 1: Patient Positioning and Preparation

- The patient is placed in the standard supine position with a shoulder roll to extend the neck. Neck extension allows for better and more comfortable surgical access to the frontal sinus. Secure the endotracheal tube to the lower lip in either corner depending on where the anesthesia team is located. Place cotton pledgets soaked in a 50/50 mixture of 1% ropivacaine and 1:1000 adrenaline into the nasal cavities as soon as possible, and then set up the image guidance system.
- Image guidance is very useful to judge the anterior limit of the septectomy/septal window. It is also useful when first adapting to this technique, as drilling often occurs in solid bone between the established landmarks, which can be unsettling at first.
- Place the surgical bed at 15 to 20 degrees in a reverse Trendelenburg position.
- 1% ropivacaine with 1:100,000 adrenaline is infiltrated into the head and axilla of the middle turbinate, the nasal septum near the swell body, and

insertion of the anterior ethmoid artery, and laterally into the mucosa overlying the frontal process of the maxilla.
- Ideally, the anesthesiologist would use total intravenous anesthesia and maintain the patient bradycardic (55–65 bpm) with mean arterial pressures near 60 throughout the case.

Step 2: Anterior Ethmoid Dissection and Defining the Medial Orbital Wall

- At minimum, an anterior ethmoidectomy is performed to identify the medial orbital wall, which is essential prior to the commencement of any drilling. However, depending on the indications or prior surgery, bilateral sphenoethmoidectomies may be performed or completed thus identifying the skull base and anterior ethmoidal artery.

Step 3: Exposing the Nasofrontal Beak and Defining the Posterior Limit of Dissection (the First Olfactory Neuron)

- The mucosa overlying the nasofrontal beak, frontal sinus floor, frontal process of the maxilla, and area of the septum corresponding to the septal window is raised as a single mucosal flap on both sides.
- Monopolar electrocautery with a needle-tip bent at a 45-degree angle and a setting of 12 on coagulation mode is used to make the mucosal incisions.
- Start at an anterosuperior point below the frontal sinus and in line with the cortex of the anterior table. This is identified using the navigation system or estimated from its position relative to the middle meatus based on sagittal imaging (Fig. 11.1A). Then, make a mucosal incision inferiorly along the frontal process of the maxilla in the same sagittal plane as the medial orbital wall (Fig. 11.1B).
- The anterior septal incision is created by starting at the same anterosuperior point and coursing inferiorly to an anteroinferior point, that is, ~5 mm anterior to the lateral incision and level with the junction of the upper one-third and lower two-thirds of the middle turbinate. This will stagger the incisions to prevent adhesion formation.
- The inferior septal incision is then carried posteriorly to approximately the level of the beginning of the middle meatus. This can vary somewhat, since the septal window should include the entire septal swell body and any high septal deviation.
- The needle-tip cautery is then pushed through the nasal septum at the anteroinferior junction of the septal incisions (Fig. 11.2). This will mark the point on the contralateral side, allowing for creation of mucosal flaps of similar proportions bilaterally, and will make an opening that will serve as the starting point for creating the septal window.

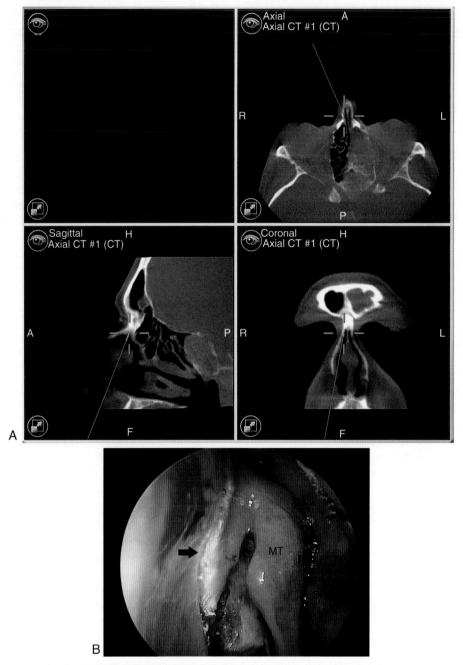

Fig. 11.1. **(A)** Computed tomography images displayed on an image guidance system demonstrating where the anterosuperior mucosal incision should start relative to the anterior table. **(B)** The mucosal incision *(black arrow)* should be carried inferiorly along the same sagittal plane as the medial orbital wall. *MT,* Middle turbinate.

- Use a Cottle elevator to raise the mucosal flaps. This is initiated at the apex, then along the lateral wall and, lastly, the septum. Make sure to divide all bands of tissue prior to elevating the mucosa. The flap is reflected posteriorly until the first olfactory neuron is reached. This is often heralded by a small emissary vein that tends to course laterally. Raising the mucosal flap can be assisted by using a cotton pledget to push the mucosa off the underlying bone if bleeding is troublesome.

- The first olfactory fascicle is tightly adherent to the skull base as there is a sleeve of dura that courses with it through the cribriform plate. This marks the posterior limit of the future frontal sinusotomy (Fig. 11.3).

Step 4: Creation of the Septal Window

- The exposed septum is predominantly bone but does include some of the bony-cartilaginous junction in the area of the swell body.

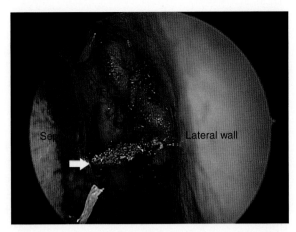

Fig. 11.2. Endoscopic view of the needle-tip electrocautery being pushed through the septum from the contralateral side to mark the anteroinferior corner of the septal window *(white arrow).*

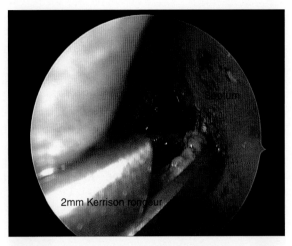

Fig. 11.4. Endoscopic view of a 2-mm Kerrison rongeur being used to help create the septal window.

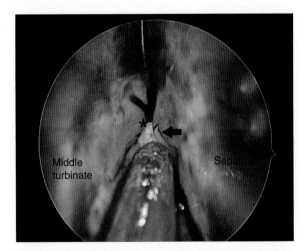

Fig. 11.3. Endoscopic view of the olfactory cleft with the first olfactory neuron exposed *(black arrow).* Note the small emissary vein *(asterisk)* anterior to the neuron, which is often confused with the true olfactory fascicle and tends to course laterally.

- A 2-mm Kerrison rongeur is placed in the previously made opening at the anteroinferior aspect of the exposed septum and carried directly superior along the same line as the mucosal incision (Fig. 11.4).
- Use straight heavy Mayo scissors to make inferior and superior cuts through the septum. Additional intermediate cuts can also be made and the exposed septum is removed, leaving only a small crest of bone septum below the frontal sinus.
- The previously raised mucosal flaps can be removed with a microdébrider. Alternatively, you can harvest them for mucosal grafts, but we find this time consuming and unnecessary. Cauterize the trimmed edges with bipolar electrocautery for improved hemostasis.

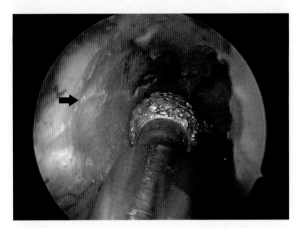

Fig. 11.5. Endoscopic view of the exposed periosteum on the frontal process of the maxilla *(black arrow).* This defines the lateral limits of the future frontal sinusotomy. Note the difference in color compared to the surrounding bone. The residual crest of septum below the frontal sinus has been drilled away *(asterisk).*

Step 5: Drilling to Define the Lateral Limits

- The small crest of septum inferior to the frontal sinus is drilled down first. Then, the bone of the lateral wall is drilled down to the periosteum superiorly. Do this bilaterally. The periosteum is whiter compared to the overlying bone and bleeds more noticeably. This defines the lateral limits of the future frontal sinusotomy (Fig. 11.5).
- The bone inferior to the exposed periosteum is thinned. This move should be done with finesse despite the use of a high-speed drill. Additionally, drill away the bone that is directly anterior to the frontal recess and superior to the axilla of the middle turbinate (Fig. 11.6). This will maximize the width of the dissection and simplify connecting the frontal recesses with the Lothrop cavity later in the case.

Step 6: Drilling Away the Nasofrontal Beak

- This portion of the procedure is often the most disconcerting since it may feel that you are drilling in a block of bone for an extended period. However, it is important to realize that drilling away the nasofrontal beak is done with relative impunity since the limits of the dissection have already been defined and the frontal sinus or frontal recess is between you and the skull base.

- Starting centrally, drill in a sweeping arc through the nasofrontal beak between the defined limits

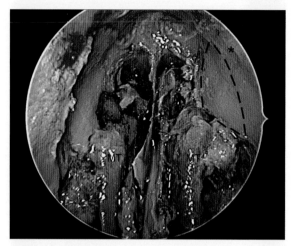

Fig. 11.6. Endoscopic view looking through the septal window at the triangular area of bone (outlined in dashes) that is superior to the axilla of the middle turbinate (MT) and anterior to the frontal recess on the left side. This area bone needs to be removed bilaterally to maximize the width of the neosinus cavity. The exposed periosteum (asterisk) demonstrating the lateral limit of dissection on the left is also seen in this view.

(Fig. 11.7A). Avoid drilling in a small hole toward the frontal sinus by removing the bone along a broad front from both the nasofrontal beak and anterior to the frontal recess. Do not make your vector of drilling too inferior; instead, drill along a more superior and anterior trajectory to avoid entering the sinus near the frontal recess (Fig. 11.7B).

- As the bone over the frontal sinus is thinned and the mucosa becomes visible, avoid the temptation to enter the sinus. The inflamed mucosa will bleed and disturb your visual field. Instead, broadly thin the remainder of the overlying bone, and then enter the sinus.

- Use the equator of the bur to remove the rest of the nasofrontal beak, frontal sinus floor, and bone anterior to the frontal recess.

- Use a 2-mm Kerrison rongeur to connect the frontal recess up to the Draf III cavity and remove any remaining partitions in the frontal recess.

- Drill away any frontal sinus partitions. Also, follow the orbital wall as it turns into the orbital roof. Doing so will "square off" the cavity and maximize the dimensions of the frontal sinusotomy (Fig. 11.8).

- Under direct visualization, carefully drill away the superior aspect of the bony nasal septum back to the origins of the first olfactory neuron. This reveals the T of the upper septum (Fig. 11.9).

- If the heads of the middle turbinates are projecting too far anteriorly, trim them back so that they are posterior to the posterior edge of the septal window. It is important to not have them in the same plane as the nasal septum to prevent formation of synechiae in the olfactory cleft.

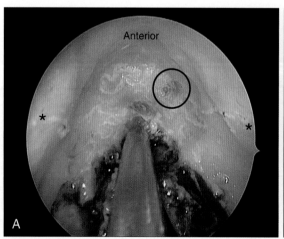
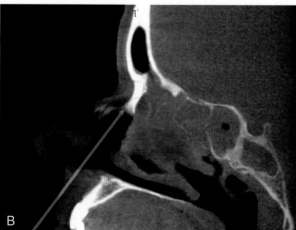

Fig. 11.7. **(A)** Endoscopic view of drilling away the nasofrontal beak along a broad, inverted U-shaped front. The exposed periosteums on either side are the lateral limits of dissection (asterisks). As the bone is thinned, it will be apparent where you are about to enter the frontal sinus because the mucosa will appear darker than the exposed bone (circle). **(B)** Sagittal CT image of the correct vector of drilling through the nasofrontal beak.

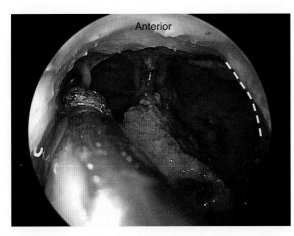

Fig. 11.8. Endoscopic view of drilling laterally over the transition of the medial orbital wall to the orbital roof *(white dashed line)* to "square off" the cavity and maximize the dimensions of the frontal sinusotomy. The intersinus septum *(asterisk)* is drilled away.

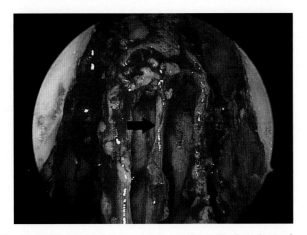

Fig. 11.9. Endoscopic view of the perpendicular plate of the ethmoid *(black arrow),* which forms a T shape with the anterior projection of the olfactory fossa *(asterisk)* once appropriately drilled away. *MT,* Middle turbinate.

Step 7: Closure and Dressing

- Mucosa grafts improve the healing process and minimize crusting.[10] We prefer to use the mucosa from the posterior aspect of the inferior turbinate, as this adds very little morbidity. When harvesting the inferior turbinate graft, do not cut too deep or you will injure the artery that supplies the turbinate and risk a postoperative bleed. "Butterfly" the submucosal surface of the graft, and sharply remove the submucosa. This will give you a large, thin mucosal graft.
- Cut the 0.5-mm Silastic sheet as shown in the template (Fig. 11.10A). Place the Silastic into the cavity with the limbs going into the corresponding cavities (Fig. 11.10B).
- Place the mucosal grafts under the Silastic sheet making sure to cover the exposed bone of the frontal process of the maxilla. This area is more likely to dry out and crust since it is exposed to moving air during respiration.
- Place one-third of a NasoPore dressing under the Silastic stent in the septal window to hold the stent in place and infiltrate it with dexamethasone.

PEARLS AND PITFALLS

- Clearly identify the medial orbital wall prior to any drilling.
- If a septal deviation or the septal swell body impairs visualization of where the mucosal incisions will be, raise the mucosal flap on the more open side and create the septal window to generate more space.
- Use a self-irrigating, high-speed drill with an integrated distal suction. This will obviate the need to have an assistant to suction.

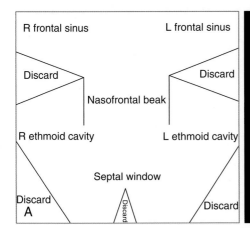

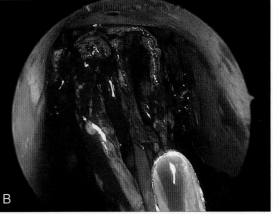

Fig. 11.10. (A) Template of the Silastic sheet with limbs marked with their corresponding locations within the sinonasal cavity. **(B)** Endoscopic view of proper positioning of the Silastic dressing inside the cavity. A piece of NasoPore is placed below the Silastic to provide support. *MT,* Middle turbinate. (B, ©2017 Stryker. Used with the permission of Stryker.)

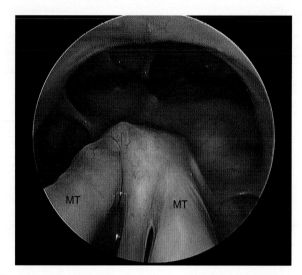

Fig. 11.11. Endoscopic view of a well-healed frontal sinusotomy 12 months after surgery in a patient with eosinophilic chronic rhinosinusitis (CRS) controlled with steroid irrigations. *MT,* Middle turbinate.

- Use a drill bur that is wider than the shaft of the drill and orient the drill so that the bur is angled toward the bone.
- Identify the periosteum on the frontal process of the maxilla as superiorly as possible. This allows for safe removal of any bone inferior and medial to this.
- Use the equator of the drill when possible to maximize efficiency.
- Do not plunge the drill into the frontal sinus. Open the sinus broadly to avoid inadvertently injuring the skull base or olfactory cleft. Also, leave the actual mucosa entry into the frontal sinus as late as possible in the drilling process.
- Maximize the dimensions of the cavity. The larger the frontal sinusotomy, the less likely it will scar down (Fig. 11.11).

POSTOPERATIVE CARE

- Patients go home the same day as surgery, unless there are medical or social reasons that dictate otherwise. Initial follow-up is scheduled for 3 weeks following surgery.
- Patients are placed on high-volume saline irrigations on postoperative day one. Additionally, a 3-week course of oral steroids and 10 days of antibiotics are part of the regimen. Antibiotics should have broad coverage but may be culture directed if needed.
- Leave the Silastic stent in place for a minimum of 3 weeks, but it can be left in for much longer and does not seem to negatively impact the patient's postoperative discomfort.
- It is not uncommon for patients to develop swelling around the nasal dorsum and eyes several days after surgery. This is an inflammatory response related to drilling away the bone in the area and responds well to nonsteroidal antiinflammatory drugs, such as meloxicam.
- Once the Silastic stent is removed, débride the cavity. Remove any granulation tissue or crust and divide any unfavorable synechiae.
- The next review is at 12 weeks. For inflammatory disease, the transition from combination corticosteroid to topical only occurs between weeks 3 and 12. All patients are still doing once-daily corticosteroid irrigations. For patients in which the common frontal sinusotomy was used for access, only simple saline irrigations are used.
- At 12 weeks, if there is thick fibrotic web on the anterior nasofrontal beak, then it is injected with 0.3 to 0.5 mL of triamcinolone 40 mg/mL with a long 25G needle. The area is often not very sensitive and injection is well tolerated.

REFERENCES

Access the reference list online at ExpertConsult.com.

Postoperative Débridement

Arjun Parasher, Robert T. Adelson, Calvin Wei, Noam Cohen, and Nithin D. Adappa

INTRODUCTION

- For many, postoperative débridement is considered a crucial aspect of optimizing endoscopic surgical results.
- The most widely cited study supporting the practice of postoperative débridement is that of Senior et al., which suggested that weekly postoperative débridement was integral to the long-term improvement of symptoms in their series.[1]
- Several advantages to postoperative débridement have been described:
  - Impairment of mucociliary function persists for 3 to 12 weeks after surgery. Stagnant blood and mucus may act as a culture medium for microbes to perpetuate an immune response. Débridement reduces such colonization.
  - The removal of postoperative blood, fibrinous clot, mucus and bone fragments, and residual partitions may diminish the amount of postoperative inflammation and the potential for synechiae formation and middle turbinate lateralization.
  - Débridement improves patients' postoperative symptoms and the endoscopic appearance of a healing sinus cavity.[2]
- The timing of postoperative débridements varies from surgeon to surgeon. In general, the patient returns for the first postoperative visit 5 to 7 days following surgery. A second postoperative visit is scheduled in 1 to 2 weeks, depending on the healing status of the sinonasal cavity. A third postoperative visit is often needed 4 to 5 weeks after surgery when the sinonasal cavity is nearly healed.

ANATOMY

- The nature of the postsurgical cavity depends on the extent of the endoscopic surgery. A thorough understanding of the anatomy and surgical case are necessary before débridement.
- For specific anatomy, refer to Chapters 6 to 9.

PREOPERATIVE CONSIDERATIONS

- Patient discomfort may limit the extent of débridement. The use of topical anesthetics and vasoconstrictive agents is recommended.
  - Topical 4% cocaine solution can act as a potent anesthetic and vasoconstrictive agent.
  - It is often recommended that patients take a narcotic pain reliever before the initial postoperative débridement.
- Minimal débridement should be undertaken if the indication for surgery included repair of cerebrospinal fluid leaks or skull base tumor resections.

INSTRUMENTATION

- 0-degree and various angled endoscopes
- Olive-tip suction
- Frazier-tip suction
- 45-degree Blakesley forceps
- 0- and 45-degree through-cutting forceps

PEARLS AND POTENTIAL PITFALLS

Pearls

- If a frontal sinus dissection has been performed, it is often easier to identify the natural recess in the office if a frontal sinus stent has been placed intraoperatively (Fig. 12.1).
- It is recommended that a full set of functional endoscopic sinus surgery instruments be available in the

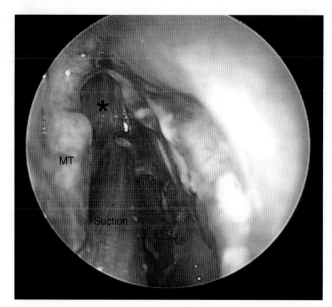

Fig. 12.1. View through a 30-degree endoscope with a malleable, curved suction tube. With this device, the left natural frontal recess can easily be identified by following a stent placed intraoperatively *(asterisk)*. *MT,* Middle turbinate.

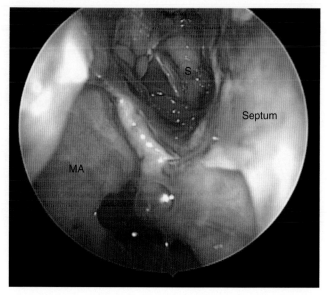

Fig. 12.2. Endoscopic view of a right débridement. After the nasopharynx and nasal cavity are identified, débridement of crust, purulent debris, and tissue should continue until the posterior border of the initial surgery is identified. In this case, it is the sphenoid sinus *(S). MA,* Maxillary antrum.

clinic for resection of retained bone fragments and recurrent polyps.

■ When instrumentation of the sinonasal cavity is performed, the nasal septum should be avoided, because it is often the most sensitive to the healing patient. Moving the instruments along the lateral nasal wall is generally better tolerated than moving them along the septum.

■ Talking to the patient while performing the débridement helps ease patient anxiety and improve patient comfort. A more comfortable patient often translates into a more compliant patient and more effective débridement.

  – For example, when the maxillary sinus is débrided, the patient should be warned that discomfort may be experienced in the teeth.

Potential Pitfalls

■ Crusting at or near the sphenopalatine foramen or a resected middle turbinate should initially be left alone for at least 10 days to avoid a potential sphenopalatine arterial bleed in the office setting.

■ Although removal of denuded bone is recommended, care must be taken in aggressively removing bone from the skull base, especially in cases in which the anterior ethmoid artery is in a mesentery and may potentially be injured.

SURGICAL PROCEDURE

Step 1

■ Remove any nonabsorbable nasal pack or space.

Step 2

■ Aggressively apply a topical decongestant or anesthetic.

■ Allow adequate time for the topical decongestant or anesthetic to take effect.

Step 3

■ Under endoscopic visualization, use a straight Frazier suction tube to suction the nasal cavity and nasopharynx of blood and debris.

■ Using a 30-degree endoscope initially angled inferiorly avoids the need to change to angled endoscopes later in the débridement process.

Step 4

■ Identify the sphenoid sinus (if surgically opened) or the face of the sphenoid and suction debris to identify the posterior limit of débridement (Fig. 12.2).

■ In general, a No. 7 or No. 9 Frazier-tip suction tube is used; initially, a larger-caliber suction tube is often necessary to clear thick inspissated blood and debris.

■ Gently move the middle turbinate laterally with a straight suction device to gain access to the sphenoid sinus.

Step 5

■ Continue to suction debris along the lamina papyracea and skull base, identifying the lateral and superior extent of débridement.

Step 6

■ Change to an angled suction device and continue removal of tissue, secretions, and blood clot from the

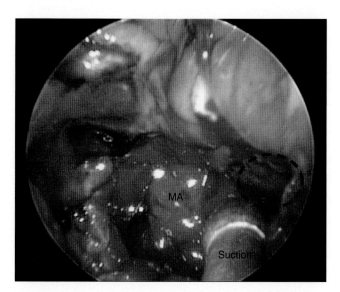

Fig. 12.3. View of a left débridement through a 30-degree endoscope used to visualize the maxillary antrum *(MA)*. A curved suction device is used to clean debris. Special attention should be paid to the natural ostium *(dashed circle)*, because scarring in this area can result in mucus recirculation.

maxillary sinus and then the frontal sinus (if a frontal sinusotomy was performed).

■ A mallcable suction device is often easiest to use because adjustments in curvature can be made depending on patient anatomy.

■ When cleaning out the maxillary sinus, give special care to the anterior aspect at the level of the natural ostium, because this area has a propensity to scar; such scarring can result in a recirculation phenomenon and persistent sinus symptoms (Fig. 12.3).

■ As previously mentioned, a thin silicone elastomer (Silastic) stent can be placed in the frontal recess. This allows straightforward débridement of the frontal recess during the initial postoperative period when visualization is often challenging.

■ Suction debris and blood from the frontal recess. Be careful not to cause new bleeding in the healing frontal recess.

Step 7

■ Remove any recurrent polyps or polypoid tissue.

■ If an area continually develops polyps, it often has retained bone fragments in the area.

Step 8

■ Anticipate potential scarring zones between the middle turbinate and lateral nasal wall, frontal recess, and natural maxillary ostium.

■ Divide any synechiae with through-cutting instruments.

■ The middle turbinate has a propensity to scar to the lateral nasal wall if it has been inadequately medialized during surgery.

– In this situation, place a middle meatal spacer or dissolvable matrix to stent open the region for 1 week while the mucosa heals without adhering.

POSTOPERATIVE CONSIDERATIONS

■ Patients may become light-headed or syncopal; it is important to recognize warning signs, including diaphoresis and skin pallor.

– In such an event, it is advisable to stop the procedure.

– The patient should be placed with the head down and legs elevated. Vital signs should be checked.

– An ice pack can be placed along the patient's forehead, and giving the patient a drink of water may be helpful. The patient should be reassured that the episode will resolve in a few minutes.

– Smelling salts should be available in case the patient has a true syncopal episode.

Postprocedure Epistaxis

■ Initial examination should determine whether the epistaxis is arterial in origin. In the vast majority of cases, the bleeding is mucosal oozing caused by the procedure.

■ If the bleeding is arterial, silver nitrate generally will not be adequate for hemostasis.

■ Arterial bleeding generally requires electrocautery, which may be feasible in the clinic. If not, the sinonasal cavity should be packed and the patient should be taken to the operating room for electrocauterization under anesthesia.

■ Mucosal bleeding will generally slow and then stop after application of additional decongestant.

Postoperative Medical Therapy

■ Nasal saline irrigations are generally well tolerated.

– A high volume (240 mL) of isotonic normal saline is most commonly used.

– Benefits of postoperative nasal saline irrigations include improved early postoperative symptoms and better endoscopic appearance of healing mucosal surfaces.[3]

– Nasal saline irrigations can cause local irritation, nasal burning, headaches, and otalgia; however, these symptoms are most commonly associated with the use of hypertonic solutions.

– It is recommended that patients start normal saline irrigations 24 to 48 hours after surgery.

■ The use of a standard topical nasal steroid spray postoperatively is an option in patients who have severe inflammatory mucosal disease.

- Application of a topical nasal steroid spray has been found to improve symptoms and the endoscopic appearance of the healing sinus cavities, as well as to lengthen the time to polyp recurrence.
- Topical nasal steroid sprays potentially reduce the risk of ostial stenosis and may decrease the need for systemic steroids. Topical nasal steroid sprays are an option in patients with severe mucosal inflammatory disease.[4]
- The use of topical nasal steroid sprays has been found to cause headache, epistaxis, and cough in some patients.
- Potential systemic risks may include adrenal suppression and delayed wound healing, although these risks are poorly defined.
- Alternatively, in patients with severe nasal polyposis, the addition of budesonide to saline irrigations has been used with some success.
- The recommended dosage is one 0.50 mg/2 mL ampule mixed with 240 mL saline used for irrigation one or two times per day.
- Budesonide ampules are not approved by the US Food and Drug administration for nasal lavage; this must be discussed with the patient before initiation of treatment.
- Limited studies have demonstrated no effect on the hypothalamic-pituitary-adrenal axis.[5]

- A short course of postoperative antibiotics is optional after sinus surgery.
  - A study by Albu and Lucaciu showed that postoperative antibiotic therapy improved patient symptoms during the first 5 days, improved endoscopic appearance of the sinus cavities during the first 12 days, and reduced sinonasal crust formation.[6]
  - In cases in which septal splints or other foreign bodies, including spacers or hemostatic agents, are left in the nasal cavities, treatment with an antistaphylococcal antibiotic is recommended to prevent toxic shock syndrome.

- The benefits of reducing early postoperative symptoms and preventing an early postoperative acute bacterial infection, which may trigger inflammation postoperatively, must be weighed against the risk of gastritis, *Clostridium difficile* colitis, anaphylaxis, and the development of bacterial resistance.

- There is limited evidence to support the efficacy of postoperative administration of systemic steroids.
  - In a study by Wright and Agrawal, although systemic steroids administered 5 days before surgery and continued for 9 days after surgery did not improve postoperative symptoms, the group receiving steroids showed significant postoperative improvement in the endoscopic appearance of the sinus cavities compared with the group given a placebo.[7]
  - Although serious adverse effects from the short-term use of systemic steroids are rare, they may include insomnia, mood changes, gastritis, hyperglycemia, increased intraocular pressure, and avascular necrosis of the hip.

SPECIAL CONSIDERATIONS

- Increased crusting is often present when endoscopic medial maxillectomies or Draf III (frontal sinus) drill-out procedures are performed. In these situations, more frequent débridement may be necessary.
- Pediatric patients may not tolerate endoscopic débridement in the office; the procedure may need to be performed under anesthesia. Parents should be counseled beforehand that this may be necessary.

REFERENCES

Access the reference list online at ExpertConsult.com.

Balloon Dilatation of the Maxillary, Frontal, and Sphenoid Sinuses

Aaron N. Pearlman and David B. Conley

INTRODUCTION

- Balloon sinus dilatation is a surgical technique that widens the natural sinus ostium using a balloon catheter.
- Balloon sinus dilatation has been used to address the maxillary, sphenoid, and frontal sinuses. It can be performed as a balloon-only procedure unaccompanied by endoscopic sinus surgery (ESS) in which the sinus ostia are dilated without any removal of bone or redundant mucosa. It can also be combined with ESS, termed a *hybrid procedure,* in which ESS is performed with traditional techniques and balloon dilatation is used as a complementary procedure in various sinuses as needed.
- The basic technique of balloon sinus dilatation involves advancing a balloon catheter over a guidewire through the natural opening of the sinus. The balloons are available in various lengths and widths that have been designed for specific sinus anatomy. A guide catheter is often used that helps direct the guidewire toward the sinus ostium. When positioned, the balloon is inflated with water under pressure. The balloon is then deflated and removed.
- Currently, balloon sinus dilatation is not applied to the ethmoid sinuses. The ethmoid sinuses have multiple septations, with individual ostia that feed into a larger and variable outflow system. There is no one ethmoid sinus ostium that can be dilated with the balloon. Because of this, balloon dilatation is not a treatment modality that directly addresses ethmoid sinus disease.

PREOPERATIVE CONSIDERATIONS

- Determining the applicability of balloon sinus dilatation in the setting of chronic inflammatory disease has been a source of significant contention within the rhinologic community. When balloon sinus dilatation is used in isolation, no bone is removed. Rather, the natural ostium is widened. Surgical objectives of ESS include the restoration of functional mucus flow and air exchange of the sinuses and facilitation of access for topical and irrigated medical treatments. A prevailing principle in ESS is that the bony septations of the sinuses are involved in the chronic inflammatory process and must be removed for the disease process to be adequately impacted. In ESS, the uncinate process is consistently resected, as are the bony septations of the ethmoid sinuses. Balloon sinus dilatation used without traditional ESS techniques does not directly address mucosal and bone inflammation, which is often thought to be a source of continued sinus inflammation.
- For the foregoing reasons, consideration should be given to the severity of the disease present and the extent of surgery necessary to achieve clinical improvement. For balloon sinus dilatation to be performed, the natural ostium must be identified and cannulated. Significant mucosal inflammation may prevent introduction of the guidewire and may be more appropriately treated with a hybrid procedure or ESS without dilatation. Furthermore, bony obstructions and changes caused by osteitis may be present that inhibit the easy placement of the balloon system.
- Patients with nasal polyposis are poor candidates for balloon sinus dilatation without traditional ESS. Nasal polyps may significantly obstruct the natural outflow tracts, and without débridement of the polyps, sinus dilatation is unlikely to adequately address the obstructive aspects of nasal polyps.
- Various anatomic deformities may make balloon dilatation difficult. A deviated nasal septum may make it hard to maneuver the necessary instruments through the nose. Large inferior turbinates or a

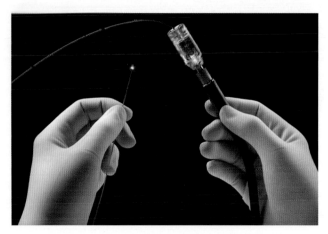

Fig. 13.1. Photograph of an illuminated guidewire. (Courtesy Acclarent Inc., Menlo Park, California. Reproduced with permission.)

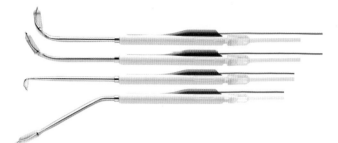

Fig. 13.2. Photograph of image-guided balloons. (©2017 Medtronic. All rights reserved. Used with the permission of Medtronic.)

concha bullosa may also cause difficulty in passing the balloon. Furthermore, a tortuous or complex frontal sinus outflow tract may not allow for easy maneuverability of the guide catheter.

Radiographic Considerations

- Identify the uncinate process and its relation to the orbit and skull base on CT scan. Examine the borders of the frontal outflow tract and, if possible, attempt to determine the location of the frontal recess in three dimensions. Identify significant variations in anatomy that may complicate the ability to pass the balloon, such as a deviated nasal septum, concha bullosa, large ethmoid bulla, agger nasi cell, suprabullar ethmoid cells, complex frontal sinus anatomy, severe inferior turbinate hypertrophy, and nasal polyposis.
- Rule out variants of sinus anatomy that could predispose patients to complications from balloon dilatation. Examples are a dehiscent carotid artery and optic nerve within the sphenoid sinus, herniation of orbital fat into the maxillary sinus or ethmoid complex as a result of prior trauma, the presence of a supraorbital ethmoid cell, or any dehiscence of the skull base.

INSTRUMENTATION

- Guidewire: A flexible guidewire is used to determine the location of the sinus ostia. When the technology was originally introduced, fluoroscopy was necessary to confirm placement of the wire within the desired sinus. Now, both flexible and fixed angle guidewires are available with a fiberoptic core that allows the tip to be illuminated. This permits transillumination of the frontal or maxillary sinus to confirm guidewire placement (Fig. 13.1).

- Guide catheter: The guide catheter is a hollow-bore tube through which the balloon catheter and guidewire are passed. The tip of the catheter is configured at various angles depending on the sinus to be dilated. The purpose of the guide catheter is to make it easy to advance the balloon through the nasal cavity and direct the balloon into the sinus. Newer catheters have been developed that allow for suction to aid in visualization. Another recent innovation is image guidance localized balloons that allow for computed tomographic (CT) image guidance confirmation of sinus anatomy and balloon positioning (Fig. 13.2).
- Balloon: Balloons are available in various diameters and widths. Depending on the sinus to be dilated, a surgeon may choose a wider and longer, or narrower and shorter balloon. Balloons are passed over the flexible guidewire and through a catheter to be introduced into the sinus (Fig. 13.3). Other devices have been designed that combine the balloon and guide catheter into one system (Fig. 13.4).
- Inflation device: An inflation device is attached to the balloon apparatus. The inflation device typically consists of a reservoir filled with water and a pressure gauge (Fig. 13.5). Various configurations of this model exist depending on the manufacturer of the balloon system.
- Irrigation catheters: Catheters have been designed that can be advanced over the guidewire for irrigation of sinuses.
- Image guidance: Stereotactic image guidance systems can be utilized to track certain guide catheters to aid in localization of the sinus outflow tract for balloon placement.

PEARLS AND POTENTIAL PITFALLS

- The frontal anatomy in relation to the ethmoid anatomy should be determined before attempting to dilate the frontal sinus. Frontal recess cells can be mistaken for the true frontal recess.

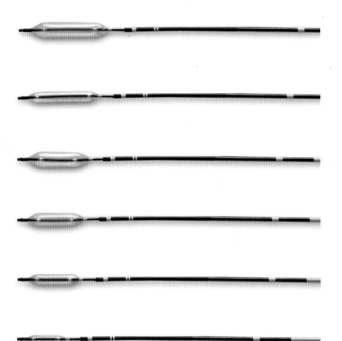

Fig. 13.3. Photograph of balloon dilators. (Courtesy Acclarent Inc., Menlo Park, California. Reproduced with permission.)

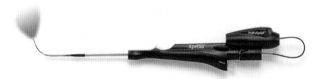

Fig. 13.4. Photograph of balloon and guidewire combined. (Courtesy Entellus Medical Inc., Maple Grove, Minnesota. Used with the permission of Entellus Medical Inc.)

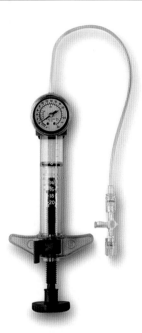

Fig. 13.5. Photograph of an inflation device. (Courtesy Acclarent Inc., Menlo Park, California. Reproduced with permission.)

- Dilating the frontal recess at the beginning of surgery, before traditional ESS dissection, may be easier, because there will be no bleeding to obstruct the field of view. However, at times it can be difficult to introduce the guidewire into the frontal sinus with the uncinate process intact. Thus, dissection of the uncinate process before dilatation of the frontal sinus outflow tract is attempted may, in some cases, provide better access to the recess.
- The risk of submucosal dissection by the guidewire is increased when the wire is placed after surgical dissection. Special care must be taken to appreciate the tactile feel of the wire during advancement to avoid this complication. Advancement with smooth, light pressure is appropriate, and resistance is an indication that the wire may not be in the correct space.
- It is imperative to have a firm understanding of the patient's ethmoid anatomy in relation to the frontal sinus anatomy. If well-pneumatized suprabullar ethmoid cells are present, it is easy to confuse these with the frontal sinus. For this reason, when an attempt is made to dilate the frontal sinus, the suprabullar ethmoid cell may actually be dilated. To prevent this error, it is critical to observe the intensity of the light on the forehead. When the guidewire is properly placed in the frontal sinus, the transillumination from the guidewire light will move as a well-defined spot along the inner surface with wire manipulation. When the wire is placed in the ethmoid or a suprabullar cell, the light will be more generally diffused without a focused, more intense spot that moves with the tip of the catheter.
- A large ethmoid bulla can interfere with the movement of the guide catheter in the anterior to posterior dimension. At times, it may be necessary to dissect the anterior ethmoid cells so that proper positioning of the guide catheter is possible when the frontal sinus is to be dilated.
- When the sphenoid sinus is to be dilated, there should be a firm understanding of the location of the carotid artery, optic nerve, and skull base in relation to the natural ostium. The guidewire is introduced blindly through the sphenoid ostium; if a dehiscent artery or nerve is present, these structures could be at risk. Likewise, the balloon should be subsequently introduced at the appropriate angle and depth. If there is any question as to the location of the guidewire, fluoroscopy can be used to confirm placement.

- If a balloon-only procedure is used to dilate the maxillary sinus, careful attention should be paid to avoid causing mucosal injury to the uncinate process, which could result in adhesion formation and further obstruction.
- When the guidewire is introduced into the maxillary sinus, it is of the utmost importance that the wire pass through the natural maxillary ostium. If the balloon is dilated in a location other than the natural ostium, an accessory ostium can be created or dilated, which may result in a recirculation phenomenon. If this occurs and is recognized at the time of surgery, the natural ostium should be identified and evaluated, and the surgeon should consider connecting the newly formed accessory ostium to the natural ostium.

SURGICAL PROCEDURES

- When planning a balloon sinus dilatation, one must differentiate between a balloon-only procedure and a hybrid procedure in which traditional ESS is combined with balloon dilatation.

Balloon-Only Procedure

- Assemble the inflation device and attach it to the balloon. Pass the guidewire through the balloon and then place the balloon into the guide catheter. Illuminate the guidewire by an external light source.
- Decongest the nose in a typical fashion. The surgery may be performed under local anesthesia, local anesthesia with sedation, or general anesthesia. Local anesthetic, such as 4% tetracaine, is only applied topically. Tetracaine is for topical use only and cannot be injected. If desired, inject 1% lidocaine with 1:100,000 epinephrine in the axilla of the middle turbinate.

Step 1
- Gently medialize the middle turbinate to ensure that the mucosa is not harmed.
- Use an acute-angle maxillary catheter to dilate the maxillary sinus. Place the catheter posterior to the uncinate process and angle it inferolaterally.

Step 2
- Advance the guidewire through the catheter. It is imperative that the guidewire travel through the natural maxillary ostium (Fig. 13.6A). Confirm the correct placement of the guidewire through transillumination. The light will appear focused and move around within the sinus when the guidewire is manipulated or twisted.

Step 3
- Advance the balloon over the guidewire and into the sinus (Fig. 13.6B). A series of markings appear on the balloon catheter that assist in knowing when the desired length of balloon has passed through the ostium. Place the balloon to bridge the natural ostium with enough length on the nasal side that the device does not slip into the maxillary sinus during inflation. Then dilate the balloon to a pressure of 8 to 12 mm H_2O. The diameter of the balloon will determine the size of the antrostomy (see Fig. 13.6).

Step 4
- Deflate the balloon. If irrigation of the sinus is desired, remove the balloon and introduce the irrigation catheter over the guidewire and through the catheter (Fig. 13.6C). Upon completion, remove the entire system. Finally, use a 30-, 45-, or 90-degree telescope to inspect the enlarged antrostomy.

Step 5
- Dilate the frontal recess in a similar fashion. Use a catheter with the angle necessary to approach the frontal recess, usually 70 degrees. Introduce the guidewire and balloon. Multiple attempts may be required to pass the guidewire through the frontal recess into the sinus. Often, both changing the catheter angle and repositioning the guidewire are necessary. Furthermore, slowly spinning the guidewire may help in finding the frontal recess. The tip of the guidewire has a slight bend, and spinning the wire may angle the tip toward the recess without the need to reposition the catheter.

Step 6
- When the wire enters the sinus, confirm placement by identifying focal illumination on the forehead (Fig. 13.7). Once you are satisfied with the placement of the guidewire, advance the balloon. Next, inflate the balloon. If the recess is long or you are not satisfied with the initial placement of the balloon, perform serial dilatations, usually from superior to inferior. Perform direct inspection of the dilatation with a 45- or 70-degree telescope (Fig. 13.8).

Step 7
- To dilate the sphenoid sinus, first identify the natural sphenoid ostium. It usually lies 1 cm to 1.5 cm superior to the choana just medial to the superior turbinate. When it is visualized, pass the guidewire into the ostium.

Step 8
- Introduce, inflate, deflate, and remove the balloon. Perform direct examination of the dilation with a 0-degree endoscope. When sphenoid dilation is performed, it may be difficult to confirm guidewire placement by transillumination. If necessary, confirmation can be achieved with fluoroscopy.

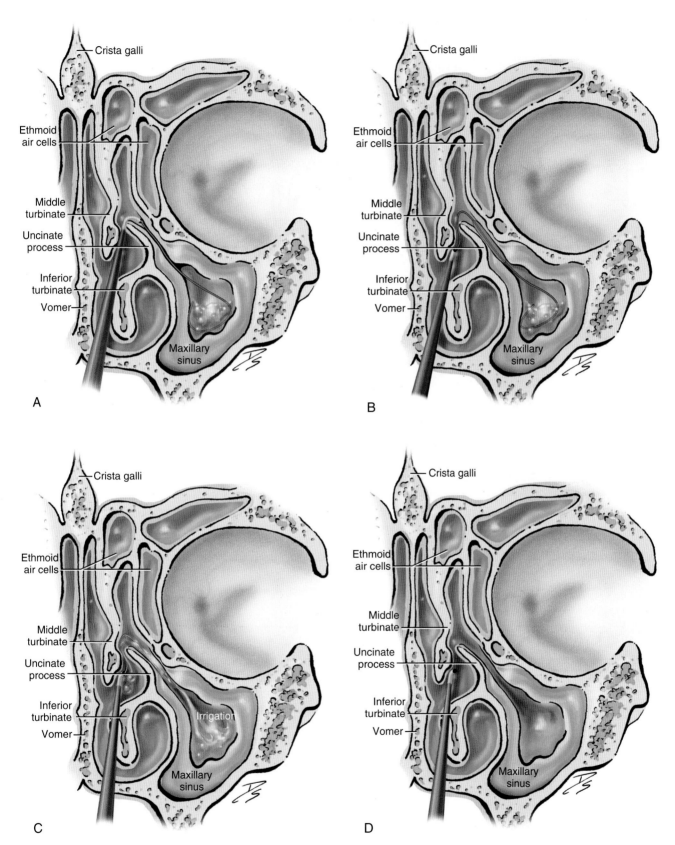

Fig. 13.6. Schematic drawings of maxillary sinus dilatation. **(A)** Introduction of the guidewire into the diseased maxillary sinus. **(B)** Placement of the balloon to dilate the maxillary os. **(C)** Irrigation cannula placed through the maxillary os into the maxillary sinus to wash out infected debris. **(D)** Removal of the catheter and the dilated maxillary os.

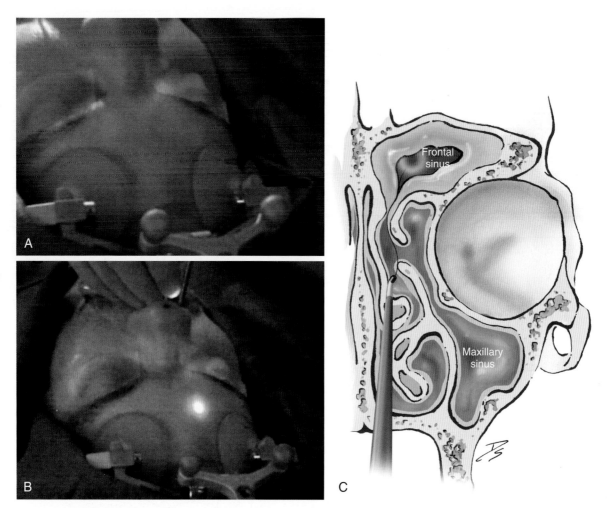

Fig. 13.7. Photographs of transillumination of the frontal sinus with the illuminated guidewire. **(A)** Diffuse illumination of the frontal sinus when the wire is in the anterior ethmoid region. **(B)** Direct point illumination of the frontal sinus when the wire is in the true frontal sinus. **(C)** Schematic drawing of transillumination of the frontal sinus with an illuminated guidewire. See **(A)** and **(B)** to differentiate true frontal sinus illumination from illumination with the guidewire in the anterior ethmoid region.

Balloon Hybrid Procedure

- A hybrid procedure resembles traditional ESS. The dissection of bone and diseased mucosa is performed with blunt, cutting, and mechanized instruments. The balloon dilatation system may be applied at any point during the dissection as a tool to access the maxillary, sphenoid, and/or frontal sinus.

- In hybrid procedures, the most commonly dilated sinus is the frontal sinus (Fig. 13.9). Frontal recess anatomy can be complex, and balloon dilatation tools often aid in identifying the frontal recess quickly and safely. Because most surgeons are more comfortable performing maxillary sinus surgery with traditional techniques, the balloon is less often used to access the maxillary sinus.

- Typically, after dilatation, there are bony overhangs and mucosal irregularities that have been created. In a hybrid procedure, these overhangs are removed either bluntly or with mechanized débridement. Careful attention should be given to sparing the mucosa and avoiding circumferential trauma because injury may cause postoperative stenosis.

- The most important difference between the balloon-only and hybrid procedures is in their ability to address the ethmoid sinuses. A balloon-only procedure cannot treat ethmoid disease directly, whereas a hybrid procedure can access the ethmoid complex and dissection can be performed as needed.

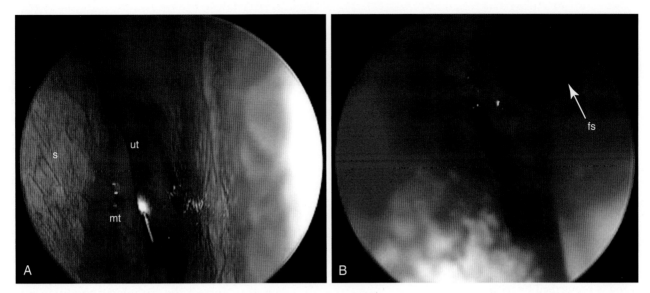

Fig. 13.8. Endoscopic photographs of balloon dilatation of the frontal sinus. **(A)** Illuminated guidewire and catheter placement behind the uncinate *(ut)*. **(B)** Seventy-degree angled endoscope visualization of dilated frontal sinus *(fs)*. *mt,* Middle turbinate; *s,* septum.

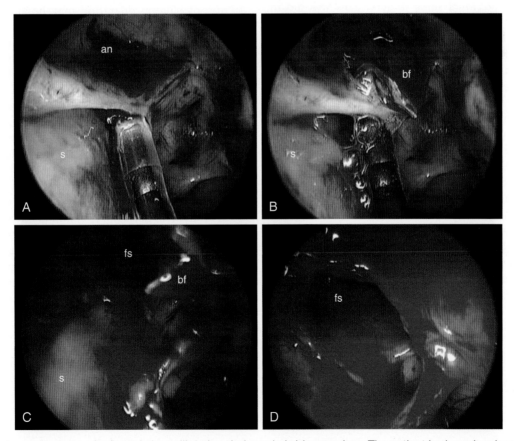

Fig. 13.9. Endoscopic views of a frontal sinus dilatation during a hybrid procedure. The patient had previously undergone ethmoidectomy. **(A)** Balloon in the frontal recess just posterior to the residual agger nasi *(an)* cell. **(B)** Inflated balloon displacing ethmoid bone fragments *(bf)*. **(C)** Angled endoscopic view after balloon removal. **(D)** View of the frontal sinus *(fs)* after removal of free bone fragments. *s,* Septum.

POSTOPERATIVE CONSIDERATIONS

- Postoperative considerations are similar for the balloon-only and hybrid procedures. Immediately after surgery, pain and bleeding are the most important considerations. Adequate pain control should be ensured with acetaminophen with or without an opiate. Aspirin and other nonsteroidal antiinflammatory drugs should be avoided because of the increased risk of bleeding. Bleeding usually resolves quickly after minimal oozing for 24 to 48 hours postoperatively. Packing is rarely necessary to control bleeding and should be reserved for patients with significant intraoperative bleeding.

- Antibiotics are often administered for 5 to 10 days after surgery. Although no consensus has been reached as to their necessity, such therapy is the convention and is prescribed by most surgeons.

- Oral steroids are often administered to patients after surgery. A prolonged course of oral steroids may be used if severe edema or polypoid burden was present intraoperatively.

- Saline irrigations can be used to lavage the nasal cavity as in traditional sinus surgery. This will aid in return to function of the nasal mucosa as well as the clearing of postoperative debris and blood clot.

- Patients should be followed with postprocedural examinations, as in traditional ESS. Endoscopy with débridement of blood crusts and static secretions will help improve healing. The patient should be monitored for stenosis of the ostia, infection, and the recurrence of symptoms.

- As with traditional ESS, complications can occur when balloon sinus dilatation is performed. Although there are few reports of complications directly attributed to balloon sinus instrumentation, one should always keep the differential diagnosis broad when approaching the postoperative patient. Severe bleeding that is uncontrolled by standard techniques may be the result of arterial injury. The anterior and posterior ethmoid arteries and sphenopalatine artery should be considered. If an orbital complication is present, the surgeon should be diligent in preserving vision in the affected eye, performing a lateral canthotomy and cantholysis if a significant orbital hematoma occurs.

- Cerebrospinal fluid leak is always a consideration in a patient with unilateral clear nasal discharge following surgery. Furthermore, conditions that narrow the frontal outflow tract, such as the presence of anterior osteitis or an osteoma, could possibly result in transmission of increased pressure to the posterior table when balloon inflation is performed. This may be a possible source of a cerebrospinal fluid leak if a fracture occurs.

SPECIAL CONSIDERATIONS

- The extent of sinus disease and the extent of surgery required to correct the pathologic condition is the most important consideration in selecting balloon sinus dilatation for a patient. Balloon-only procedures may be well suited for patients with focal disease that compromises the mucus outflow of a sinus. In carefully selected patients, the in-office application of balloon dilatation may be appropriate and can help avoid the morbidity of general anesthesia and recovery from more invasive procedures. However, it is more common in chronic inflammatory sinus disease that extensive mucosal pathology is present.

- The ethmoid sinuses likely play a key role in the perpetuation of the inflammatory process. For this reason, if ethmoid disease is present, it is important to understand that a balloon-only procedure will not directly address this problem. Traditional ESS opens the ethmoids and other sinuses widely to allow for delivery of topical and irrigated medications.

- In a hybrid procedure, balloon catheters can be used as a tool to dilate the maxillary, sphenoid, and frontal sinuses when used in conjunction with traditional ESS and give the sinus surgeon greater flexibility in properly addressing this complex anatomic system.

Revision Endoscopic Sinus Surgery for Inflammatory Disease

Revision Functional Endoscopic Sinus Surgery: Completion Sphenoethmoidectomy

Randy Leung and Rakesh Chandra

INTRODUCTION

- *Completion sphenoethmoidectomy* refers to a revision sinus procedure in a patient in whom a maxillary antrostomy and partial ethmoidectomy have been previously performed.
- Patients with nasal polyposis and moderate to severe inflammatory disease commonly have persistent symptoms despite a partial ethmoidectomy and limited sinus surgery. Completion sphenoethmoidectomy is often combined with a frontal recess dissection in hopes that it will be the last surgery ever needed by the patient.
- Often in these cases, there are remnant osteitic ethmoid bony partitions along the medial orbital wall and skull base that can be a source of persistent overlying mucosal inflammation (Fig. 14.1).
- Persistent inflammation in the bone and sinuses can often result in a bloody visual field. Surgeons must be careful and meticulous in their technique to achieve a safe and effective surgery.

ANATOMY

- See Chapters 7 and 8 for the anatomy of the ethmoid and sphenoid sinuses.

PREOPERATIVE CONSIDERATIONS

- Medical optimization should be accomplished.
  - Preoperative administration of an oral corticosteroid may lessen surgical difficulty both subjectively[1] and in terms of blood loss.[2]

- Decongesting agents may be applied to minimize bleeding and facilitate surgical access. Options include the following:
  - Topical α-agonists, including pseudoephedrine, oxymetazoline, xylometazoline
  - Topical cocaine, 4%
  - Topical adrenaline, 1:1000

Radiographic Considerations

- Computed tomography (CT) scans of the sinuses with coronal reformats should be available for review intraoperatively. Resolution should be at least 2 to 3 mm per slice.
- Preoperative review of images is critical to identify danger areas, as detailed later.
- Review preoperative CT scans.
  - Evaluate for the presence of bony dehiscences in the orbit and skull base.
  - Identify the depth of the lateral lamella to avoid inadvertent intracranial entry and cerebrospinal fluid (CSF) leak during dissection along the skull base.
  - Identify remnant ethmoid partitions along the medial orbital wall and skull base.
  - Identify the presence of a lateralized middle turbinate remnant.
  - Diagnose polypoid disease within the maxillary and/or sphenoid sinuses.
- Evaluate the path of the anterior ethmoid artery as it courses between the orbit and the skull base. If it has a long course through the sinonasal cavity, it may be at risk of injury during ethmoid dissection along the ethmoid skull base. Retraction of the artery into the orbit may risk retro-orbital hematoma.

- Identify the presence of Onodi cells, which are posteriorly pneumatized posterior ethmoid cells. Recognition of such cells is important, because the optic nerve may be dehiscent into these sinuses and vulnerable to injury. Equally important is evaluation of the skull base. Identification of a low-lying skull base or asymmetry is critical to avoid inadvertent injury.
- Look for a short posterior ethmoid height, particularly in the context of a well pneumatized maxillary sinus. If the ratio of the maxillary sinus height to the height of the posterior ethmoid exceeds 2:1, the surgeon may be led erroneously on a trajectory to the skull base instead of the sphenoid sinus, which puts the patient at risk of CSF leak.[3]
- Identify bony dehiscences of the optic nerve and internal carotid artery in the sphenoid sinus.
  - Carotid dehiscences in the sphenoid sinuses have been found in 5% to 25% of cases in radiographic and cadaveric examinations.[4,5]
  - Note the sphenoid intersinus septum. When the sphenoid sinuses are asymmetric, the intersinus septum typically attaches to the carotid canal on one side.

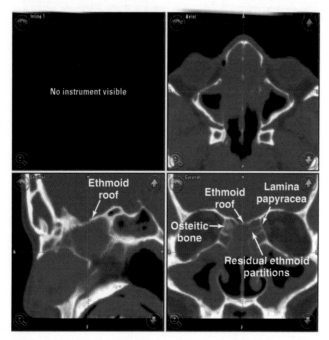

Fig. 14.1. Triplanar computed tomography images for a patient scheduled to undergo a revision completion sphenoethmoidectomy. Note the presence of numerous osteitic ethmoid partitions along the medial orbital wall and skull base.

INSTRUMENTATION

- 0- and 30-degree rigid endoscopes
- Manual instruments
  - Straight and 90-degree J-curettes
  - Straight and 45-degree Blakesley forceps
  - Straight and 45-degree through-cutting forceps
  - Kerrison rongeur
- Powered instruments
  - Straight and 40-degree microdébriders

SURGICAL PROCEDURE

Step 1: Debulk Polyps in the Nasal Cavity With a Microdébrider

- Make sure to débride just the polyps; leave the bony dissection to hand instruments, which have a greater tactile feel (Fig. 14.2).

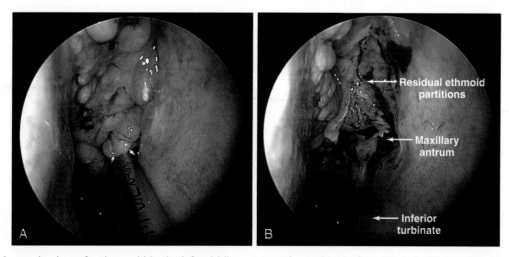

Fig. 14.2. Endoscopic view of polyps within the left middle meatus of a patient before (A) and after (B) débridement of polyps with a straight microdébrider.

Step 2: Revise the Maxillary Antrostomy

- Nasal polyps from the ethmoid cavity can often block the maxillary sinus, which results in the presence of polyps and allergic mucin within the sinus itself (Fig. 14.3).
- Revising the maxillary antrostomy often requires removing the remnant uncinate process with a backbiter, which maximizes the antrostomy size (Fig. 14.4).

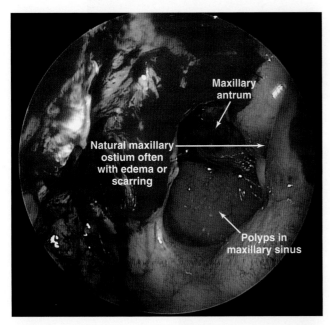

Fig. 14.3. Thirty-degree endoscopic view of the left maxillary sinus with polyps and allergic mucin.

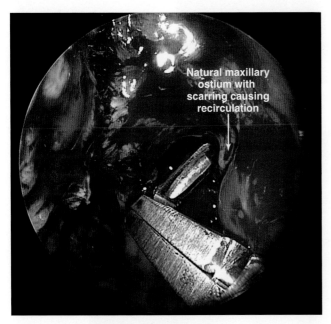

Fig. 14.4. Endoscopic view of the use of a backbiter to remove the remnant left uncinate process back to its attachment to the lacrimal bone.

- Débride polyps and mucin within the maxillary sinus. It is important to flush out any remaining mucin in the sinus. This can be accomplished using a 60-mL syringe of saline attached to a curved olive-tip suction.

Step 3: Remove the Posterior Maxillary Air Scoop

- The posterior maxillary sinus often becomes osteitic and polypoid; the posterior fontanelle can often act as an air scoop and serve as a persistent nidus for inflammation.
- Use straight through-cut forceps to remove the posterior fontanelle back to the posterior wall of the maxillary sinus (Fig. 14.5).

Step 4: Skeletonize the Medial Orbital Wall

- Osteitic bony partitions along the medial orbital wall are another persistent nidus of inflammation.
- Failure to remove the osteitic bone will often result in persistent mucosal edema and nasal polyposis.
- The curvature of the orbital floor is contiguous with the medial orbital wall. Follow this curvature to help in anticipating the medial orbital contour.
- 2- and 4-mm Kerrison punches and 45-degree through-cutting forceps are useful to remove these hard partitions (Fig. 14.6).

Step 5: Dissect the Remaining Posterior Ethmoid Air Cells Down to the Sphenoid Face

- The last posterior ethmoid cell typically has the appearance of a pyramid, formed by the junction of the basal lamella of the superior turbinate with the skull base.
- The posterior maxillary wall will curve posteriorly and approximate the location of the face of the sphenoid, which provides another clue to the location of the sphenoid sinus.

Step 6: Enlarge the Sphenoidotomy

- In many patients with nasal polyposis, allergic mucin resides in the bottom of the sphenoid sinus, causing persistent mucosal edema. Maximally enlarging the sphenoid can make it easier to remove the mucin postoperatively and allow the patient to irrigate the sphenoid more efficiently.
- Posterior ethmoid bony partitions and the lateral sphenoid face are often left behind. Removal is best performed with a Kerrison punch or straight mushroom punch. Dissect from medial to lateral starting with the natural os of the sphenoid sinus (Fig. 14.7).
- Enlarging the sphenoidotomy often requires removing the inferior face of the sphenoid with a Kerrison punch.
- Use a suction elevator to retract the mucosa inferiorly, in turn protecting the septal branch of the

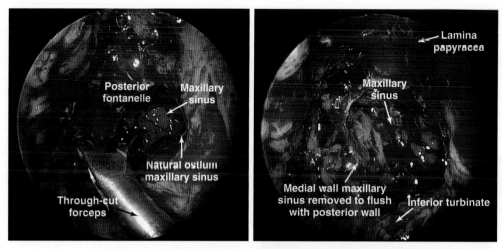

Fig. 14.5. Endoscopic view of the removal of the left posterior maxillary bone and polypoid tissue with through-cut forceps.

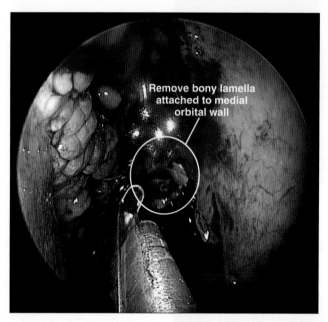

Fig. 14.6. Endoscopic view of skeletonization of the left medial orbital wall using a Kerrison rongeur.

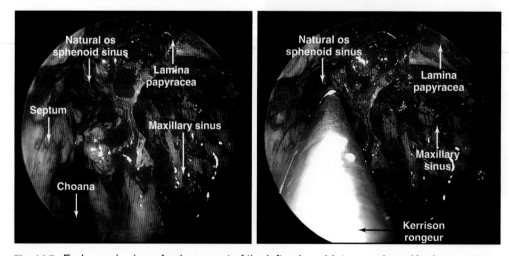

Fig. 14.7. Endoscopic view of enlargement of the left sphenoidotomy using a Kerrison rongeur.

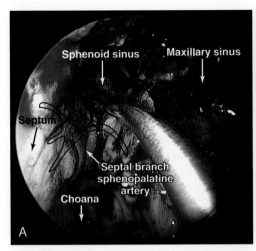 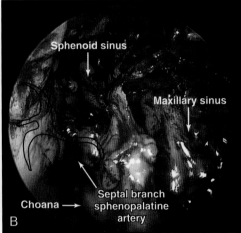

Fig. 14.8. Endoscopic view of the technique for enlarging the left sphenoidotomy while avoiding the posterior septal branch of the left sphenopalatine artery. (A) A Freer elevator is gently used to inferiorly retract the mucosa of the inferior sphenoid face bone. A Kerrison rongeur can then be employed to remove the bone only. (B) Endoscopic view after resection of the inferior sphenoid face. Black outline is location of the septal branch of the sphenopalatine artery running through the mucosa of the anterior-inferior face of the sphenoid sinus.

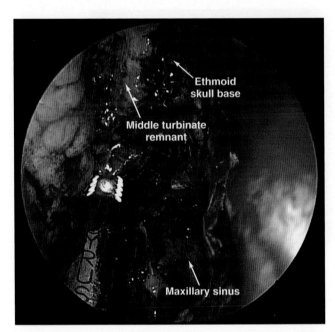

Fig. 14.9. Endoscopic view of the use of a curved 40-degree microdébrider to gently débride polyps off of the ethmoid bony partitions along the left ethmoid skull base.

sphenopalatine artery. Use a Kerrison rongeur to remove the underlying bone (Fig. 14.8).

Step 7: Skeletonize the Skull Base of Superior Ethmoid Partitions

- Identify the skull base within the sphenoid sinus.
- The bone of the skull base is typically thicker and more ivory colored than the ethmoid septations, although this is not always true, particularly in cases of chronic infection or revision surgery.

- Recall that the posterior ethmoid skull base is shaped like a cone or pyramid, which tapers to a point at the skull base and posterior-superior orbit.
- Dissect in a posterior-to-anterior direction along the skull base to minimize the risk of CSF leak. Because the skull base slopes inferiorly in the medial portion of the ethmoid cavity, dissection should also err laterally against the lamina, which is skeletonized and preserved throughout.
- Dissection is best done using a microdébrider to remove nasal polyps while leaving bone behind (Fig. 14.9), and then using 45-degree through-cut forceps to remove the bone. If you can feel behind and see in front of the bone, the partition is safe to remove (Fig. 14.10).

Step 8: Remove the Superior Uncinate Process

- Working anteriorly, make sure to remove the superior uncinate process as it lies against the anterior-medial orbital wall (Fig. 14.11).

POSTOPERATIVE CONSIDERATIONS

- The patient should avoid nose blowing for the following reasons:
  - To minimize the risk of postoperative bleeding
  - To minimize orbital or subcutaneous emphysema in case an inadvertent breach of the orbit has occurred
- Intranasal dressing, packing, and spacers can be considered.
  - Depending on the structural integrity of the middle turbinates and their ability to stay medialized, the

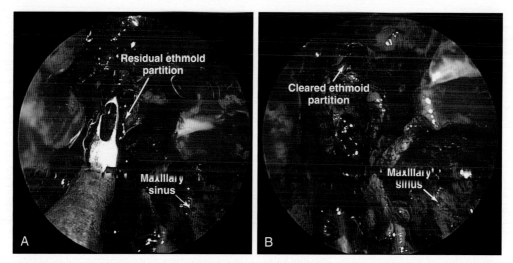

Fig. 14.10. (A) Endoscopic view of the use of a 45-degree through-cut forceps to feel behind, see in front, and remove the ethmoid bony partitions along the left ethmoid skull base. (B) Endoscopic view after removal of the partition.

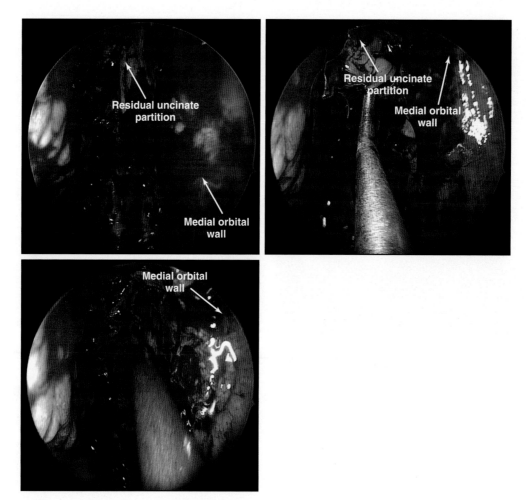

Fig. 14.11. Endoscopic views of removal of the remnant left superior uncinate process along the superior medial orbital wall.

surgeon may elect to place middle meatal spacers or gels to help reduce the risk of synechiae formation.

- If there is concern about hemostasis, a variety of absorbable and nonabsorbable packing materials and hemostatic agents may be considered at the surgeon's discretion.

- Routine use of packing is likely unnecessary. Orlandi and Lanza reported that 87% of 165 patients did not require use of any hemostatic agents or packing.[6] A review of the use of nasal spacers after surgery demonstrated little effect on postoperative bleeding. However, there was a significant reduction in postoperative synechiae formation.[7]

- Overall, selection of a postoperative intranasal dressing should consider the benefits and risks of bleeding, synechiae formation, ease of removal and débridement, and patient discomfort.

REFERENCES

Access the reference list online at ExpertConsult.com.

Modified Medial Maxillectomy for Recalcitrant Maxillary Sinusitis

Bradford A. Woodworth and Jessica Grayson

INTRODUCTION

- The modified medial maxillectomy entails removing a large portion of the medial maxillary wall to gain wide access to the maxillary sinus. It is primarily used for the removal of benign tumors, such as inverted papillomas and juvenile nasopharyngeal angiofibromas.[1–12]
- The modified medial maxillectomy can also be used to treat chronic maxillary sinusitis refractory to maximum medical management and standard maxillary antrostomy. Modified medial maxillectomy creates a wide opening into the maxillary sinus that may allow improved mucus clearance and better penetration of topical medication and lavages.[13–15] This procedure can be used in the management of those sinuses in which infected secretions and mucin are persistently found in the floor or along the anterior wall and lateral wall of the sinus. Markedly enlarging the sinus will allow for improved distribution of nasal irrigation and easier access for in-office débridements and suctioning.
- This procedure is commonly used for chronic maxillary sinusitis associated with cystic fibrosis, biofilms, extensive allergic mucin, or polyps of the anterior wall and floor of the sinus.
- The procedure is also useful for treatment of chronic maxillary sinusitis caused by prolapsed orbital fat from previous medial orbital decompression surgery or inflammation from previous mucosal stripping from other sinus procedures (e.g., Caldwell-Luc).[13,16]
- Modified medial maxillectomy differs from a traditional endoscopic medial maxillectomy by preserving the nasolacrimal duct and a portion of the inferior turbinate.

ANATOMY

- The lateral nasal wall includes the inferior turbinate, infundibulum (with maxillary ostium), uncinate process, and nasolacrimal duct.

- The boundaries for a modified medial maxillectomy are the nasolacrimal duct anteriorly, the posterior maxillary wall posteriorly, the nasal floor and inferior turbinate medially, the lateral maxillary wall laterally, the agger nasi cell and lamina papyracea superiorly, and the maxillary sinus floor inferiorly (Figs. 15.1 and 15.2).
- The nasolacrimal duct runs anteriorly in the bony lateral nasal wall and empties into the inferior meatus (Hasner valve) just inferior to the attachment of the inferior turbinate.
- The inferior turbinate spans the length of the nasal cavity. The majority of the maxillary sinus cavity lies inferior to the superior attachment of the inferior turbinate to the lateral nasal wall. Removal of the midportion of the inferior turbinate significantly improves exposure of the maxillary sinus.[3]

PREOPERATIVE CONSIDERATIONS

- If pathology or inflammatory disease exists in other sinuses, these areas can be addressed before or after performing a modified medial maxillectomy depending on the indication or exposure.[3,14]

Radiographic Considerations

- Study both the axial and coronal computed tomography (CT) scans.
- Identify the course of the nasolacrimal duct and its position in the lateral nasal wall.
- Identify the extent and origin of the tumor preoperatively so that appropriate instrumentation can be made available for adequate removal, including angled endoscopes, microdébriders, and drills.

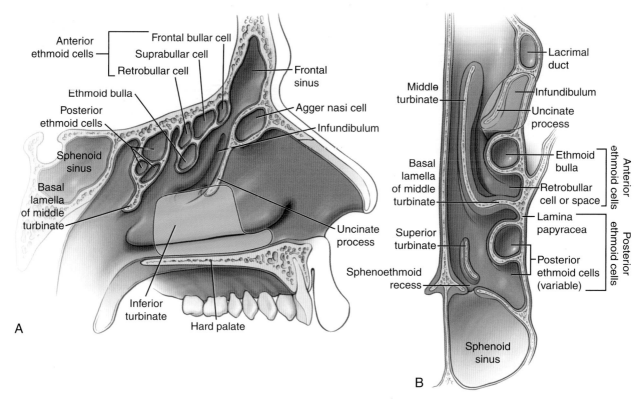

Fig. 15.1. Schematic drawings in sagittal (A) and axial (B) views showing the region removed *(shaded area)* when a modified medial maxillectomy is performed.

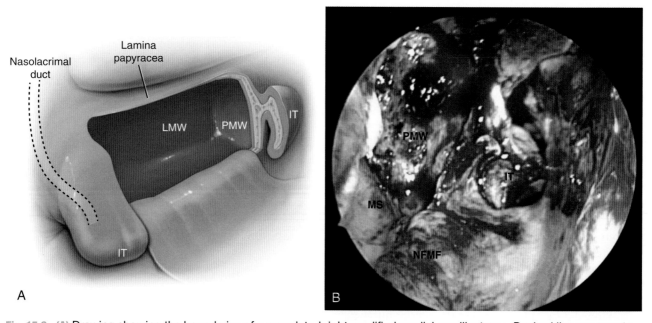

Fig. 15.2. (A) Drawing showing the boundaries of a completed right modified medial maxillectomy. *Dashed line* represents the course of the nasolacrimal duct within the medial maxillary wall. The posterior boundary is the posterior maxillary wall *(PMW)*. The superior boundary is the lamina papyracea. The inferior boundary is the maxillary sinus floor. The medial boundary is the inferior turbinate *(IT)* and nasal floor. The lateral boundary is the lateral wall of the maxillary sinus *(LMW)*. (B) Endoscopic image showing a completed modified medial maxillectomy. *MS,* Maxillary sinus wall; *NFMF,* nasal floor mucosal flap.

INSTRUMENTATION

- 0-degree and 30-degree endoscopes
  - 45-degree or 70-degree endoscope to remove allergic mucin or polyps along the anterior or lateral maxillary wall
- Curved and straight Beaver blades
- J-curette
- Suction Freer elevator
- Turbinate scissors
- Through-cut instruments (Blakesley, backbiting, side-biting)
- 15-degree drill
- Small hemostat
- Suction Bovie electrocautery

PEARLS AND POTENTIAL PITFALLS

Pearls

- Raising a medially based mucosal flap off the floor of the nasal cavity allows complete coverage of the exposed bone of the inferior maxillary ridge and helps prevent postoperative crusting and contracture.

Potential Pitfalls

- Be sure that the remnant end of the inferior turbinate is cauterized adequately to prevent postoperative epistaxis from the posterolateral nasal branch of the sphenopalatine artery.
- Aggressive postoperative débridement of the posterior inferior turbinate remnant should be avoided for 2 weeks following surgery. There is an increased risk of postoperative epistaxis that can result from clot dissolution or débridement within this time period.
- If the nasolacrimal duct is resected, be sure that the duct is cut obliquely or opened with anterior and posterior flaps to prevent stenosis of the duct and postoperative epiphora.[1,2,10]
- Avoid stripping maxillary sinus mucosa. Damage to the sinus mucosa can lead to extensive inflammation, poor mucociliary clearance postoperatively, and contracture of the maxillary cavity.[16]
- If the operation is being performed to treat chronic maxillary sinusitis secondary to orbital fat herniation or prior medial orbital decompression, create the inferior and anterior maxillary wall bone incisions first to provide an endoscopic view of where the mucosalized fat fills the infundibulum. The medial maxillary wall can then be reflected away from the orbital fat in a lateral to medial direction, which helps avoid inadvertent orbital entry.

SURGICAL PROCEDURE

- Inject 1% lidocaine with 1:100,000 epinephrine into the superior attachment of the middle turbinate, inferior turbinate, and medial maxillary wall. A sphenopalatine block may also be performed by injecting lidocaine with epinephrine transorally into the greater palatine foramen.

Step 1: Perform a Maxillary Antrostomy With Complete Removal of the Uncinate Process

- See Chapter 8.

Step 2: Resect the Posterior Two-Thirds of the Inferior Turbinate (Fig. 15.3)

- Begin by using a Freer elevator to medialize the inferior turbinate along its length.
- Use a hemostat to clamp just posterior to the anterior ⅓ portion of the inferior turbinate in preparation for cutting the turbinate. Keep it clamped for at least 30 seconds to decrease blood supply to the turbinate.
- Use turbinate scissors to cut the anterior portion of the inferior turbinate, angling the cut posterior to the distal end of the nasolacrimal duct (Hasner valve).

Step 3: Resect the Inferior Turbinate and Cauterize the Inferior Turbinate Remnant

- Use turbinate scissors to cut the posterior portion of the inferior turbinate flush with the posterior maxillary wall (Fig. 15.4).
- The posterior inferior turbinate remnant tends to bleed from the posterolateral nasal artery. Use the suction Bovie device to cauterize the residual posterior portion.

Step 4: Create a Nasal Floor Mucosal Flap

- Use a curved Beaver blade to make the anterior incision by incising the mucosa just inferior to the attachment of the inferior turbinate and slightly posterior to the Hasner valve. Carry the cut medially onto the nasal floor, ending at the base of the septum (Fig. 15.5).
- Begin the posterior incision at the level of the posterior maxillary wall, again just inferior to the attachment of the inferior turbinate and extending onto the nasal floor, ending at the base of the septum (Fig. 15.6).
- Use a straight Beaver blade to connect the anterior and posterior incisions by incising the mucosa just inferior to the attachment of the inferior turbinate along its whole length. Making the incision as close as possible to the attachment of the inferior turbinate will create greater flap length.

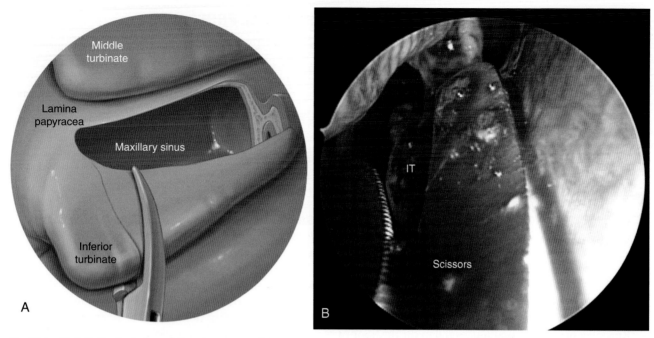

Fig. 15.3. (A) Artist's depiction of the placement of the anterior cut on the inferior turbinate (IT) after the turbinate has been clamped with a hemostat (endoscopic view). (B) Endoscopic view of resection of the inferior turbinate with turbinate scissors.

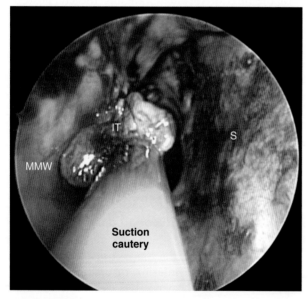

Fig. 15.4. Endoscopic view of cauterization of the posterior remnant of the inferior turbinate after resection. IT, Inferior turbinate; MMW, medial maxillary wall; S, septum.

- Use a suction Freer elevator to elevate the mucosal flap off of the nasal floor and roll it medially toward the septum (Fig. 15.7).

Step 5: Identify the Location of the Anterior Cut of the Medial Maxillary Wall

- Identify the inferior meatus (Hasner valve) just inferior to the attachment of the inferior turbinate at its anterior end.

- Using a J-curette, punch through the medial maxillary wall into the maxillary sinus just posterior and inferior to the inferior meatus (Hasner valve) to identify the site of the anterior cut (Fig. 15.8).

Step 6: Create an Inferior Osteotomy

- Extend the antrostomy in the lateral nasal wall posteriorly through the posterior fontanelle with through-cut forceps (or scissors).
- Use backbiting forceps to enlarge the cut anteriorly (inferior to the Hasner valve) to a level flush with the anterior maxillary wall (Fig. 15.9).

Step 7: Make the Anterior Osteotomy in the Medial Maxillary Wall

- Use angled through-cut forceps, scissors, or side-biting forceps to incise just posterior to the nasolacrimal duct and connect with the maxillary antrostomy (Fig. 15.10).
- Be sure to angle the cut posterior to the Hasner valve and the nasolacrimal duct to avoid transecting the duct.

Step 8: Reflect the Wall Medially

- The medial maxillectomy is now attached only posteriorly.
- Use a Freer elevator to push the wall medially and provide an improved view of any polyps or mucin.

Step 9: Make the Posterior Cut of the Medial Maxillary Wall

- Use angled through-cut forceps or turbinate scissors angled from an inferior to superior direction to incise

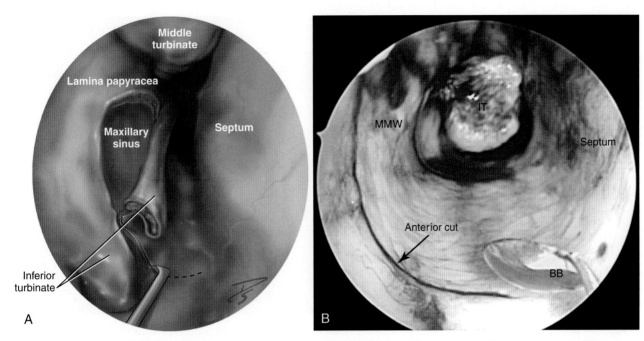

Fig. 15.5. (A) Artist's depiction of the placement of the anterior cut of the nasal floor mucosal flap using a curved Beaver blade (*BB;* endoscopic view). Note that, in the drawing, the inferior turbinate has not been resected. (B) Endoscopic image showing the anterior cut of the nasal floor mucosal flap. *IT,* Inferior turbinate; *MMW,* medial maxillary wall.

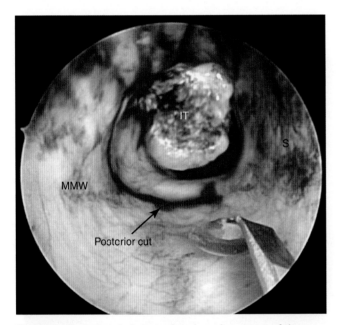

Fig. 15.6. Endoscopic image showing placement of the posterior cut of the nasal floor mucosal flap. *IT,* Inferior turbinate; *MMW,* medial maxillary wall; *S,* septum.

flush with the posterior maxillary wall through the inferior turbinate (Fig. 15.11).

Step 10: Remove the Medial Maxillary Wall (With or Without the Inferior Turbinate; Fig. 15.12)

- After completing this step, proceed to the next step.

Step 11: Drill the Remainder of the Inferior Maxillary Ridge Flush With the Nasal Floor If Necessary

- An inferior ridge of the medial maxillary wall will still be present after the osteotomies. Use the 15-degree diamond bur to drill this flush with the nasal floor (Fig. 15.13).
- The nasal floor will be flush with the maxillary sinus floor only in the presence of a hypoplastic or contracted sinus (e.g., in patients who have cystic fibrosis or have undergone prior mucosal stripping).[17–19]

Step 12: Replace the Nasal Floor Mucosal Flap

- Using a Freer elevator, lay the nasal floor mucosal flap back in place. The flap should lie partially on the floor of the maxillary sinus completely covering the area of exposed bone left behind after removal of the medial maxillary wall (Fig. 15.14).

POSTOPERATIVE CONSIDERATIONS

- Inspect the nasolacrimal duct upon completion to ensure that the apparatus was not accidently transected or damaged during the procedure. If so, a dacryocystorhinostomy may be required (see Chapter 18).
- Ensure that hemostasis is achieved at the cut ends of the inferior turbinate.
- Two quarter-inch polyvinyl acetal sponges (cut to size) in a pinky finger of a nonlatex glove may be

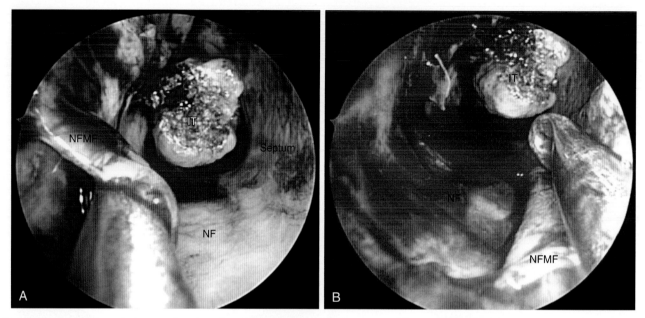

Fig. 15.7. (A) Endoscopic image showing elevation of the nasal floor mucosal flap between the anterior and posterior cuts using a suction Freer elevator. *IT,* Inferior turbinate; *NF,* nasal floor; *NFMF,* nasal floor mucosal flap. (B) Endoscopic view of the nasal floor mucosal flap *(NFMF)* being elevated and rolled toward the septum. *IT,* Inferior turbinate; *NF,* nasal floor.

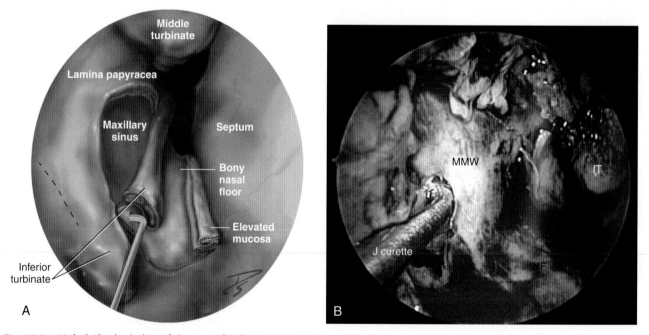

Fig. 15.8. (A) Artist's depiction of the use of a J-curette to make an inferior osteotomy in the medial maxillary wall (endoscopic view). *Dashed line* shows the course of the nasolacrimal duct in the medial maxillary wall. Note that, in the drawing, the inferior turbinate has not been resected. (B) Endoscopic view of the use of a J-curette to make an inferior osteotomy in the medial maxillary wall *(MMW)*. *IT,* Inferior turbinate; *NF,* nasal floor.

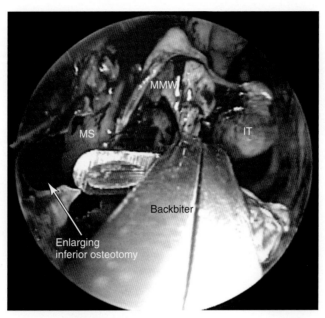

Fig. 15.9. Endoscopic view of the use of a backbiter to enlarge the inferior osteotomy of the medial maxillary wall *(MMW). IT,* Inferior turbinate; *MS,* maxillary sinus.

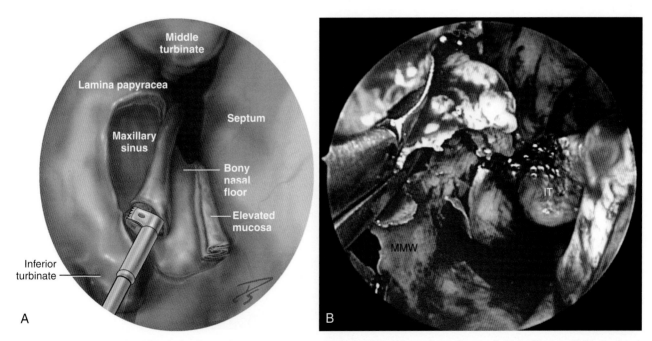

Fig. 15.10. (A) Artist's depiction of a through-cut instrument making an anterior cut on the medial maxillary wall (endoscopic view). Note that, in the drawing, the inferior turbinate has not been resected. **(B)** Endoscopic view of an endoscopic scissor making the anterior cut of the medial maxillectomy. *IT,* Inferior turbinate; *MMW,* medial maxillary wall.

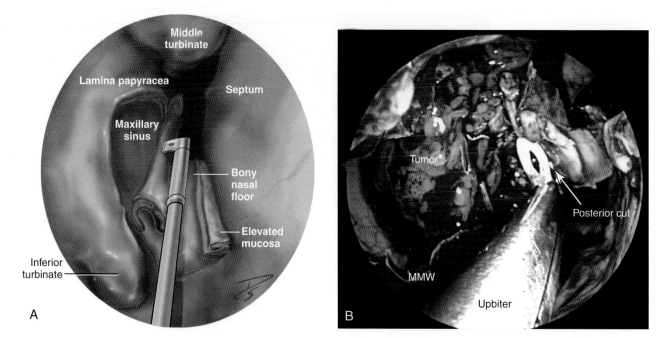

Fig. 15.11. **(A)** Artist's depiction of the posterior cut of the medial maxillectomy using a through-cut instrument (endoscopic view). **(B)** Endoscopic view of the posterior cut of a medial maxillectomy using a Tru-Cut instrument. *MMW,* Medial maxillary wall.

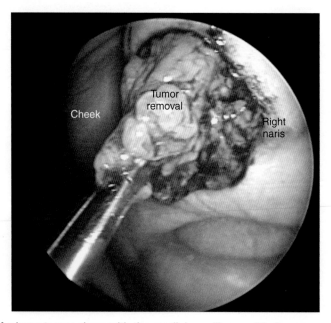

Fig. 15.12. Endoscopic view of a large tumor along with the medial maxillary wall being removed from the right naris using the medial maxillectomy approach.

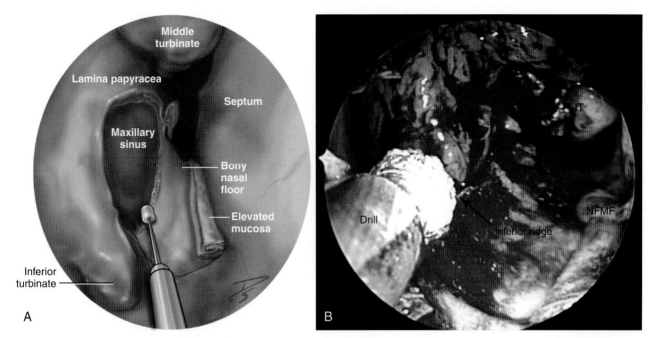

Fig. 15.13. **(A)** Artist's depiction of the use of a 15-degree drill to drill down the inferior ridge of the medial maxillary wall flush with the nasal floor (endoscopic view). **(B)** Endoscopic view of the drilling down of the inferior ridge of the medial maxillary wall. *IT,* Inferior turbinate; *NFMF,* nasal floor mucosal flap.

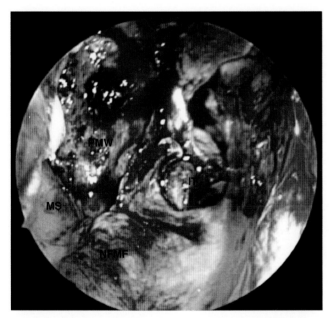

Fig. 15.14. Endoscopic view of a completed modified medial maxillectomy with the nasal floor mucosal flap *(NFMF)* in place. *IT,* Inferior turbinate; *MS,* maxillary sinus wall; *PMW,* posterior maxillary wall.

placed loosely within the cavity to put mild pressure on the nasal mucosal flap and decrease crusting before the first postoperative visit. Alternatively, dissolvable spacers may be used and placed against the posterior inferior turbinate remnant. Leaving this to dissolve on its own will minimize postoperative débridement along the posterior inferior turbinate remnant.

SPECIAL CONSIDERATIONS

- Multiple variations of the modified medial maxillectomy can be performed to increase access to difficult areas of the maxillary sinus, such as the lateral maxillary wall and anterior maxillary wall.
- For more anterior access, the medial buttress of the medial maxillary wall may be completely removed, including resection of the nasolacrimal duct. If the nasolacrimal duct is resected, measures should be taken to prevent stenosis and postoperative epiphora.
- The entire inferior turbinate may be removed for more exposure. However, leaving the anterior head of the inferior turbinate helps to preserve the nasal airway and normal airway turbulence.
- A canine fossa puncture can be used as an auxiliary site for instruments (endoscopes or débrider) to provide increased visibility and access.[2,14]

REFERENCES

Access the reference list online at ExpertConsult.com.

Extended Sphenoid Sinus Antrostomy and Radical Sphenoidectomy

John M. Lee and Jonathan Yip

INTRODUCTION

- Endoscopic sphenoidotomy has become the most common surgical approach for management of inflammatory and neoplastic diseases of the sphenoid sinus largely due to its excellent outcomes and low morbidity.
- Long-term outcomes of endoscopic sphenoidotomy in the context of isolated sphenoid sinus disease (ISSD) have demonstrated patency rates of greater than 90% at a follow-up of up to 4 years.[1,2]
- However, chronic rhinosinusitis with sphenoid involvement is more challenging to treat. Although it is typically the least common sinus involved, additional surgery is necessary in 34% to 65% of revision cases due to persistent/recurrent disease and stenosis.[3,4]
- Given this, it is important to consider potential causes for sphenoidotomy failure. The most commonly cited reasons include
  - circumferentially denuded bone
  - inadequate size
  - bony osteitis
- While circumferentially denuded bone and inadequate size can often be managed with more mucosal-sparing techniques and wider sphenoid antrostomies, the issue of underlying bony osteitis may require modifications to the traditional endoscopic sphenoid sinus procedure.
- Hierarchy of surgical management of chronic sphenoid sinusitis[5]:
  - Standard sphenoidotomy
  - Sphenoid "drill-out" (wide removal of bilateral sphenoid faces and intersinus septum)[5]
  - Radical sphenoidectomy or sphenoid marsupialization[6]

- Sphenoid drill-out is associated with low nasal morbidity. One study demonstrated a 100% patency rate in nine patients at a mean-follow-up of 17.1 months.[5]
- This chapter aims to highlight the techniques of extended sphenoid sinus antrostomy and radical sphenoidectomy as alternatives for the management of severe chronic sphenoiditis with associated bony inflammation.
- The use of a modified short/mini-pedicled nasal septal flap will also be highlighted as an adjunctive procedure to cover areas of denuded bone. This technique has previously been described through a case series of nine patients and resulted in 100% patency at a mean postoperative follow-up at 8.4 months. The most common indication for its use was fungal rhinosinusitis.[7]
- The steps of an extended sphenoid sinus antrostomy may also serve as the foundation for endoscopic transsphenoidal approaches for management of sphenoid sinus and skull base tumors.

ANATOMY

- Most of the relevant anatomy of the sphenoid sinus is reviewed in Chapter 8.
- For the procedures described in this chapter, it is important to understand the location of the septal branch of the nasoseptal artery.
- The nasoseptal artery is the main blood supply for the pedicled nasoseptal flap described by Hadad et al.[8]
- Arising as a terminal branch of the sphenopalatine artery, it commonly takes a horizontal course along the sphenoid face, midway between the natural

sphenoid ostium and the arch of the choana before branching and supplying the septal mucosa.

■ The location of this artery must be considered because inferior widening of the sphenoid antrostomy may inadvertently compromise and sacrifice the main blood supply for the nasoseptal flap.

PREOPERATIVE CONSIDERATIONS

■ Extended sphenoid sinus antrostomy or radical sphenoidectomy may be performed in isolation or as part of a complete functional endoscopic sinus surgery procedure.

■ The presence of bony osteitis can be appreciated when preoperative computed tomography (CT) scans are reviewed.

■ As with other elements of endoscopic sinus surgery, it is imperative to allow adequate time for mucosal decongestion.

■ This decongestion can be accomplished with pledgets soaked in either topical oxymetazoline or topical epinephrine at a concentration of 1:1000.

■ Topical pledgets should be placed medial to the superior turbinate and in the sphenoethmoidal recess to enhance identification of the sphenoid ostium.

Preoperative Radiographic Considerations

■ As in a standard endoscopic sphenoidotomy procedure, preoperative CT imaging is useful for recognizing the presence of Onodi (sphenoethmoidal) cells and a dehiscent carotid artery or optic nerve.

■ There are two variations of the extended sphenoid sinus antrostomy procedure.
  − The first is a modification to the traditional unilateral endoscopic sphenoidotomy.
  − This procedure is often indicated for bony osteitis secondary to an isolated sphenoid mycetoma.
  − In Fig. 16.1, note the extensive bony thickening in the right sphenoid sinus compared to the left side.

■ The second variation of the extended sphenoid sinus antrostomy procedure involves the creation of a single combined sphenoid sinus by joining the left and right sides together (sphenoid "drill-out").
  − This procedure is most often indicated for bilateral chronic sphenoiditis with extensive bony thickening that has failed previous endoscopic attempts (i.e., the sinus is deemed to be nonfunctional).
  − In Fig. 16.2, note the extensive bony osteitis in both sphenoid sinuses.

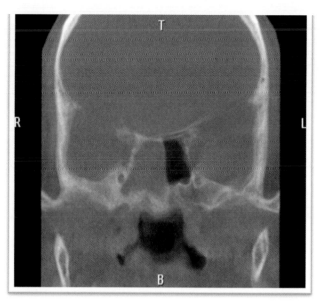

Fig. 16.1. Coronal CT image demonstrating extensive bony osteitis of the right sphenoid sinus compared to the left.

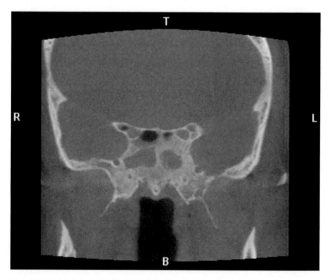

Fig. 16.2. Coronal CT image demonstrating bilateral chronic sphenoiditis with associated bony thickening.

  − For this procedure, the sphenoid intersinus septum needs to be removed; thus, it is important to note its location relative to the carotid artery.
  − This is best appreciated on an axial CT image.
  − Note the intersinus septum curving toward the right carotid artery in Fig. 16.3.

■ Radical sphenoidectomy ensures total marsupialization of the sphenoid cavity.
  − It eliminates the reliance of ciliary action of the mucosa to carry mucus up and out of the sinus cavity and reduces the impact of postoperative cicatrization.[6]
  − It can perform unilateral or bilateral sphenoid marsupialization.

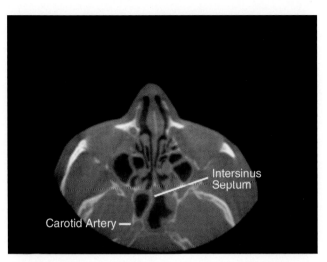

Fig. 16.3. Axial CT image demonstrating the sphenoid intersinus septum curving toward the right carotid canal.

INSTRUMENTATION

- 0-degree and 30-degree endoscopes
- J-curette
- Straight through-cutter
- Upbiting through-cutter
- Rotating sphenoid Hajak punch or 2-mm and 4-mm Kerrison rongeurs
- Straight-microdébrider
- Straight suction irrigation drill
- Freer elevator
- 15-blade and round knife on extended handles

PEARLS

- The sphenoid sinus ostium is often at the same vertical level as the roof of the maxillary sinus (a good landmark for the relative height of entry into the sphenoid sinus).
- If present, the superior turbinate is the best landmark for the sphenoid ostium and is often just posterior-medial to the superior turbinate.
- If the sphenoid ostium cannot be easily identified because of previous surgery or inflammatory disease, the use of image guidance may help identify the floor and roof of the sphenoid sinus before surgical entry.
- The sphenoid rostrum will need to be removed if both sides of the sphenoid sinus will be joined together; the rostrum resembles the keel of a ship.
- If required, the sphenoid intersinus septum should be removed precisely either with straight through-cutting instruments or with an irrigating diamond drill bur.
- The majority of the endoscopic dissection can be accomplished with a 0-degree endoscope.

- The 30-degree endoscope is useful for inspecting the floor, roof, and lateral recesses of the sphenoid sinus to make sure that all disease has been evacuated.
- Repeated saline irrigations of the sinus are imperative to ensure that all disease has been removed.

POTENTIAL PITFALLS

- When landmarks such as the superior turbinate are missing from previous surgery, it is imperative to not venture too high superiorly, because the skull base slopes from anterior to posterior toward the sphenoid sinus.
- If you open the sphenoid sinus inferiorly before a pedicled nasoseptal flap is raised, the blood supply to the flap may be inadvertently divided.
- The sphenoid intersinus septum often curves toward the carotid canal in the sphenoid sinus. Blunt manipulation of the septum may lead to unpredictable bony breaks near the carotid artery.
- If a microdébrider is used to remove polyps near the sphenoid ostium, it is important *not* to engage the microdébrider within the sphenoid sinus itself.

SURGICAL STEPS, VARIATION 1: UNILATERAL EXTENDED SPHENOID ANTROSTOMY

Step 1: Identify the Natural Sphenoid Ostium
- A standard sphenoidotomy can be performed as long as it is not widened inferiorly.

Step 2: Harvest a Short Pedicled Nasoseptal Flap (Figs. 16.4 and 16.5)
- The pedicle of the nasoseptal flap is usually found midway between the sphenoid os and the arch of the choana.
- Using a No. 15 blade on an extended handle, make two parallel horizontal incisions across the sphenoid face (one at the level of the ostium and one at the level of the arch of the choana).
- Using a round knife on an extended handle, flare the incisions onto the posterior septum like a fan to make a wider flap.
- The length of the flap does not need to be greater than 5 to 10 mm along the posterior septum.
- Use a round knife to connect the two horizontal incisions vertically along the posterior septum.
- Use a Freer elevator to elevate the short pedicled nasoseptal flap across the sphenoid face.
- Leave the flap in the nasopharynx to be used at the end of the procedure.

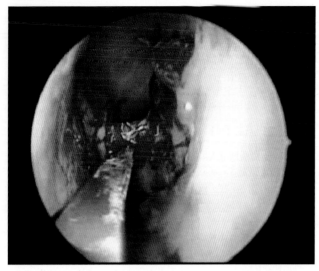

Fig. 16.4. Using a No. 15 blade to make the superior horizontal incision for the nasoseptal flap at the level of the sphenoid ostium.

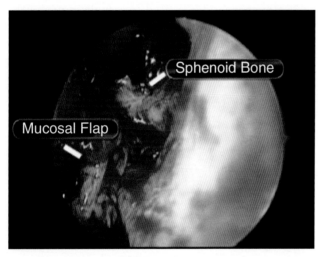

Fig. 16.5. Harvest of a right-sided short nasoseptal flap while exposing osteitic sphenoid bone inferiorly.

Step 3: Widely Open the Sphenoid

- Upbiting through-cutters can be used to enlarge the sphenoid opening to the skull base superiorly.
- Use a rotating sphenoid punch to open the sphenoid laterally to the medial orbital wall.
- Rotate the sphenoid punch inferiorly to widen the sphenoid face inferiorly down to the floor of the sphenoid sinus. Depending on the degree of osteoneogenesis and fibrosis, this portion of the procedure can be performed using a combination of the microdébrider, Kerrison punches, straight mushroom punch, and straight suction irrigation drill. This step is especially important if the patient has a large inferior sphenoid recess with evidence of fungal debris.

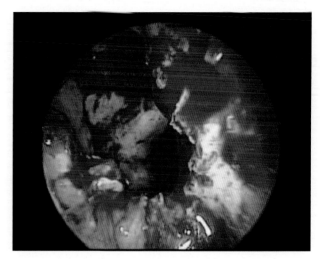

Fig. 16.6. Placement of the nasoseptal flap across the inferior bony edge of the sphenoid opening.

Step 4: Irrigate the Sphenoid Sinus

- Irrigate the sphenoid sinus with a malleable-tip suction attached to a syringe filled with saline.
- Aim the tip toward the sphenoid floor to help evacuate any trapped debris.
- Inspect the sinus with a 30-degree endoscope to ensure that all disease has been removed.

Step 5: Place the Nasoseptal Flap Across the Inferior Bony Opening of the Sphenoid Sinus (Figs. 16.6 and 16.7)

- Once all disease has been removed, carefully place the nasoseptal flap across the inferior bony sphenoid opening.
- This mucosal coverage will prevent a circumferential bony opening, which may be prone to stenosis because of the significant underlying osteitis.

SURGICAL STEPS, VARIATION 2: BILATERAL EXTENDED SPHENOID ANTROSTOMY (SPHENOID "DRILL-OUT")

Step 1: Raise a Single Pedicled Nasoseptal Flap

- The side in which the flap is raised depends on which sphenoid sinus is larger and will have more areas of exposed bone inferiorly.
- Follow the same steps for harvest of the pedicled nasoseptal flap as previously described.
- The length of the flap may need to be extended 1 to 2 cm along the posterior septum depending on how much inferior bone coverage is needed (the flap can always be trimmed after it is harvested).
- Place the flap into the nasopharynx for use at the end of the procedure.

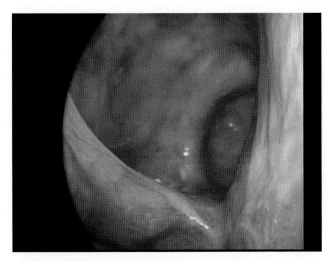

Fig. 16.7. One month postoperative view of the unilateral extended sphenoid antrostomy.

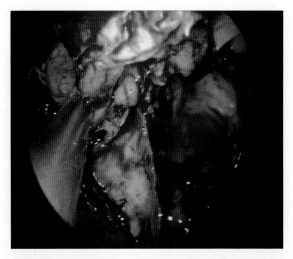

Fig. 16.8. Endoscopic view of the sphenoid rostrum that resembles the keel of a ship.

Step 2: Perform Bilateral Wide Sphenoid Antrostomies as Previously Described

■ After completing this step, proceed to the next step.

Step 3: With Both Sphenoid Sinuses Opened, a Posterior Septectomy Can Be Performed

■ One side of the posterior septum will already have been denuded of mucosa because of the harvest of the nasoseptal flap.

■ Use a microdébrider to remove the same area of mucosa from the contralateral posterior septum.

■ Use a J-curette to break across the posterior bony septum (at a level no higher than the sphenoid ostium).

■ Perform a posterior septectomy using either straight through-cutting instruments or a suction irrigation drill (cutting drill bur).

■ The size of the posterior septectomy needs to be approximately 2 cm in anterior-posterior length so that one can visualize both sphenoid sinuses with an endoscope through one nostril.

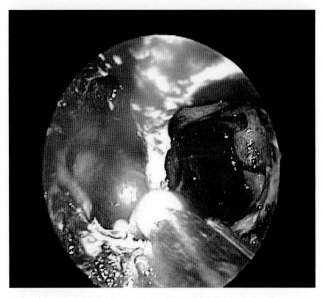

Fig. 16.9. Using a suction irrigation drill to remove the sphenoid intersinus septum and rostrum.

Step 4: Remove the Sphenoid Rostrum and Connect the Right and Left Sphenoid Openings

■ The sphenoid rostrum resembles the keel of a ship when viewed directly with a 0-degree endoscope (Fig. 16.8).

■ The right and left sphenoid openings previously created should be on each side of the rostrum.

■ Using a suction irrigation bur (cutting drill bit), remove the sphenoid rostrum and connect the left and right sphenoid openings.

■ Note that the sphenoid rostrum can be very thick, especially in the presence of significant osteitis.

■ Lower the entire face of the sphenoid sinus down to the floor of the sphenoid sinus.

Step 5: Remove the Sphenoid Intersinus Septum (Fig. 16.9)

■ Removal of the sphenoid intersinus septum is best accomplished using either a through-cutting instrument or a suction irrigation bur (diamond drill bit).

■ Remove the intersinus septum almost flush with the posterior sphenoid wall (i.e., flush with the planum sphenoidale, face of the sella, and the clival recess) and floor. This creates a single combined-sphenoid sinus.

■ Do not bluntly twist the intersinus septum, especially if it is angled toward the carotid canal.

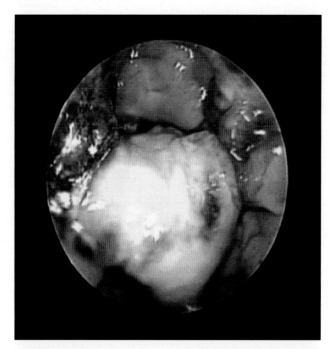

Fig. 16.10. Two-week postoperative view of a newly created unisphenoid sinus with a short nasoseptal flap inferiorly to prevent stenosis.

Step 6: Remove All Disease From the Sphenoid Sinus

- Once again, irrigate the sphenoid sinus with copious amounts of saline so that any retained secretions or debris is removed.
- Use a 30-degree endoscope to inspect all sides of the sphenoid sinus.

Step 7: Place the Pedicled Nasoseptal Flap Across the Inferiorly Exposed Bone of the Newly Created Unisphenoid Sinus (Fig. 16.10)

- Consider adding absorbable nasal packing and tissue glue to assist in setting the flap in the sphenoid cavity.

RADICAL SPHENOIDECTOMY OR SPHENOID MARSUPIALIZATION

Step 1: Apply Local Anesthesia and Perform an Ethmoidectomy on the Diseased Side

- Inject 1% lidocaine with 1:100,000 epinephrine into the mucosa of the sphenoid rostrum.
- Remove residual disease in the ethmoid sinuses using standard techniques.

Step 2: Identify and Ligate the Nasoseptal Artery

- Remove bony partitions over the anterior sphenoid face but be diligent not to strip overlying mucosa.
- Cauterize and transect the nasoseptal artery as it crosses the sphenoid face.

Step 3: Create a Nasopharyngeal Mucoperiosteal Flap (Figs. 16.11 and 16.12)

- Identify the sphenoid os and use stereotactic guidance if necessary.
- Using a No. 15 blade on an extended handle, make two vertical incisions in the lateral recesses of the nasopharyngeal roof extending from the edge of the sphenoid ostium to a point in the nasopharyngeal roof that marks the posterior termination of the sphenoid sinus.
- Lift the inferiorly based mucoperiosteal flap using a Freer or Cottle elevator.
- Leave the flap in the nasopharynx to be used at the end of the procedure.

Step 4: Remove Bone of the Sphenoid Sinus Floor (Fig. 16.13)

- Strip the remaining mucosa off the sphenoid face.
- Remove the exposed sphenoid bone with a high-speed suction irrigation bur (cutting drill bit) until the bone of the sphenoid floor is flush with the posterior wall of the sphenoid sinus.
- Concurrently, suction and irrigate the sphenoid sinus to evacuate any residual disease.

Step 5: Set the Nasopharyngeal Mucoperiosteal Flap (Fig. 16.14)

- Inset the mucoperiosteal flap from the inferior sphenoid rostrum into the marsupialized cavity.
- Instill absorbable sphenoid packs ± tissue glue to tack down the flap.
- Apply separate nasal packs to gently push against flap and remove them at 3 to 5 days postoperatively.

Step 6: Repeat Aforementioned Steps on Contralateral Side If Necessary

- The posterior 1 to 2 cm of the nasal septum can be removed to facilitate bone removal and allow removal of the intersphenoid septum in order to create a wide common aperture.

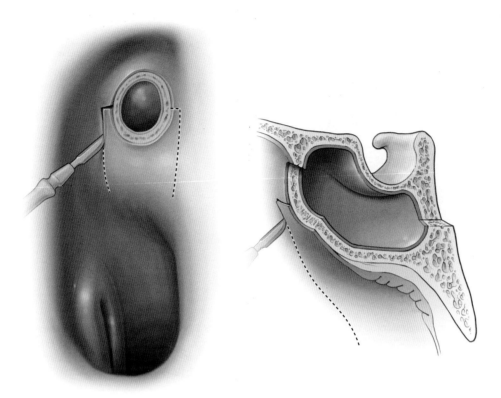

Fig. 16.11. Incisions on anterior sphenoid face extending to the nasopharynx in order to create the inferiorly based mucoperiosteal flap. (From Donald PJ. Sphenoid marsupialization for chronic sphenoidal sinusitis. *The Laryngoscope.* 2000;110:1349–1352.)

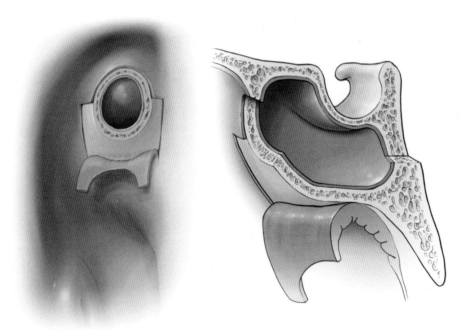

Fig. 16.12. Elevation of the nasopharyngeal mucoperiosteal flap. (From Donald PJ. Sphenoid marsupialization for chronic sphenoidal sinusitis. *The Laryngoscope.* 2000;110:1349–1352.)

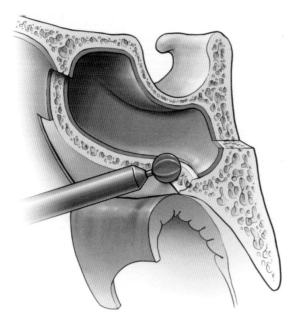

Fig. 16.13. Bone of the sphenoid floor is removed with high-speed suction irrigation bur (cutting drill bit). (From Donald PJ. Sphenoid marsupialization for chronic sphenoidal sinusitis. *The Laryngoscope.* 2000;110:1349–1352.)

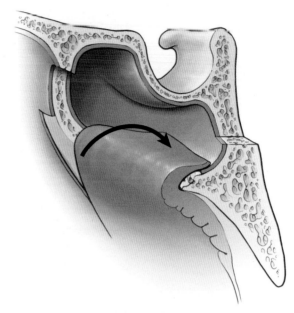

Fig. 16.14. Nasopharyngeal mucoperiosteal flap is inset into marsupialized cavity. (From Donald PJ. Sphenoid marsupialization for chronic sphenoidal sinusitis. *The Laryngoscope.* 2000;110:1349–1352.)

POSTOPERATIVE CONSIDERATIONS

▪ As with other types of endoscopic sinus surgery, postoperative care and débridement are paramount to the success of the endoscopic extended sphenoid antrostomy.

▪ Old blood and debris should be suctioned from the sphenoid sinus approximately 1 week after surgery.

▪ Care must be taken not to disturb the nasoseptal flap on the inferior portion of the sphenoid opening.

REFERENCES

Access the reference list online at ExpertConsult.com.

Orbital Surgery

Endoscopic Dacryocystorhinostomy

Raymond Sacks and Yuresh Naidoo

INTRODUCTION

- Endoscopic dacryocystorhinostomy (DCR) is a well-established treatment for epiphora caused by anatomic or functional obstruction of the nasolacrimal apparatus.
- A thorough understanding of the endonasal anatomy, wide marsupialization of the lacrimal sac, and meticulous care of the mucosa are critical for success.

ANATOMY

- The lacrimal sac extends approximately 10 mm above the axilla of the middle turbinate.
- The common canaliculus opens high up on the lateral wall of the sac. This area must be exposed during a DCR for best results.
- The lacrimal bone extends from the frontal process of the maxilla anteriorly to the attachment of the uncinate process posteriorly.
- This retrolacrimal region of the lamina papyracea is extremely thin; inadvertent disturbance of the uncinate at this point can lead to orbital penetration.
- It is important to recognize that the lacrimal bone and sac lie anterior to the orbit; therefore, the orbit is not at risk unless the surgeon is inadvertently posterior to these landmarks (Fig. 17.1).

PREOPERATIVE CONSIDERATIONS

- Surgery is performed under general anesthesia.
- The nose is prepared with local injections and vasoconstrictive neurosurgical cottonoids.
- With a dental syringe, 2 mL of 1% lidocaine with 1:100,000 epinephrine is infiltrated into the axilla of the middle turbinate and frontal process of the maxilla (Fig. 17.2).

- Three neurosurgical cottonoids soaked in 1:3000 epinephrine are then placed in the middle meatus, along the frontal process of the maxilla and adjacent to the septum.
- A septoplasty is performed if a septal deflection is preventing access to the middle meatus and lateral nasal wall. The septal incision is ideally placed on the side contralateral to the DCR, because this prevents inadvertent trauma to the septal flap when the endoscope is inserted into the nasal cavity. It also minimizes clouding of the endoscope with blood from the septal incision as well as the potential for the development of postoperative synechiae between the septum and lateral nasal wall.

Radiographic Considerations

- A dacryocystogram and lacrimal scintigraphy can be of some use preoperatively. They often provide some idea as to the level of obstruction and whether a tight common canaliculus is contributing to epiphora.
- For patients with concomitant sinus disease, the relevant computed tomographic scans should be reviewed in the usual fashion. The sinuses can be addressed at the same time as the DCR in most cases.

INSTRUMENTATION

- 0-degree and 30-degree endoscopes
- Scalpel with a No. 11 blade or Beaver blade
- Hajek-Koffler punch or 2-mm upbiting Kerrison rongeur
- DCR spear knife
- Bellucci micro ear scissors (from micro ear tray)
- Round knife (from micro ear tray)
- Punctum dilators
- Bowman lacrimal probes (sizes 00 and 000)
- DCR sickle knife
- Lusk pediatric through-biting forceps

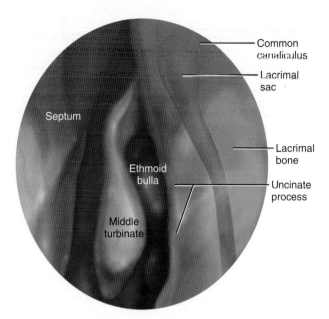

Fig. 17.1. Artist's depiction of an endoscopic view of the left middle turbinate, frontal process of the maxilla, lacrimal bone, and insertion of the uncinate. The lacrimal sac extends above the axilla of the middle turbinate and the opening of the common canaliculus is high up on the lateral wall of the sac.

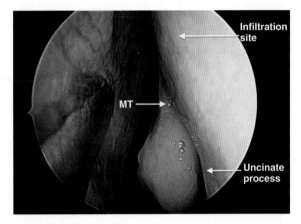

Fig. 17.2. Endoscopic view showing site of infiltration with a local anesthetic and vasoconstrictor. *MT,* Middle turbinate.

- DCR bur
- Crawford silicone elastomer (Silastic) tubes

PEARLS AND POTENTIAL PITFALLS

- Have a low threshold for performing a septoplasty. Limited access restricts the surgeon in making the precise surgical cuts required for the mucosal flaps.
- Use a 30-degree endoscope to perform the DCR. This will provide a better view of the lateral nasal wall than a 0-degree endoscope.

- The Hajek-Koffler punch and/or Kerrison rongeurs are faster at removing bone than the DCR bur. Perform as much of the removal of the hard bone of the frontal process of the maxilla with the hand instruments and move to the DCR bur only when the punch is unable to grip the bone adequately.
- When using the Hajek-Koffler punch, release the jaws after each bite. If a small amount of lacrimal sac has been caught inadvertently between the jaws of the punch, it can be released and only the bone removed. This will prevent inadvertent trauma to the sac.
- Use the DCR bur on the bone–sac interface to expose the sac in its entirety but never between the sac and the bone, because this can potentially traumatize the sac.
- Remove all of the lacrimal bone up to the insertion of the uncinate, but do not disturb the uncinate itself. This retrolacrimal region where the uncinate inserts into the lamina papyracea is extremely thin, and inadvertent orbital injury might result.
- When probing the lacrimal system, do so delicately so that a false passage is not created. The upper and lower canaliculi have an angulated course that must be carefully navigated to avoid creating a false passage. Working on a team with an oculoplastic surgeon will enable the ear, nose, and throat surgeon to obtain the requisite skills in probing and examining the lacrimal system.
- Make an incision into the sac only when the lacrimal probe can be clearly seen through the sac wall.

SURGICAL PROCEDURE

Step 1: Create a Posteriorly Based Mucosal Flap to Expose the Lacrimal Bone and Frontal Process of the Maxilla

- Make a superior incision that runs horizontally 10 mm above the axilla of the middle turbinate. Extend the incision from 2 to 3 mm posterior to the axilla and run it forward for approximately 10 mm onto the frontal process of the maxilla.
- Now, turn the blade vertically and make a cut on the frontal process of the maxilla from the superior incision to just above the insertion of the inferior turbinate.
- Next, turn the blade horizontally and make the inferior mucosal incision from the insertion of the uncinate to join the vertical incision (Fig. 17.3).

Step 2: Raise the Mucosal Flap

- Use a suction Freer elevator to elevate the flap (Fig. 17.4). Stay directly on bone to avoid losing the surgical plane in the transition from the hard bone of the frontal process of the maxilla to the soft lacrimal bone.

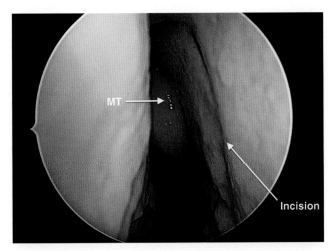

Fig. 17.3. Endoscopic view showing incision to create a posteriorly based mucosal flap to expose the lacrimal bone and frontal process of the maxilla. *MT,* Middle turbinate.

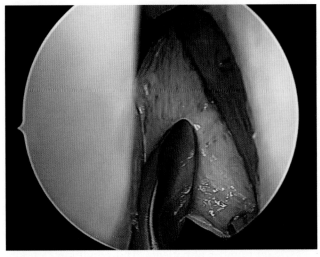

Fig. 17.4. Endoscopic view of the raising of the mucosal flap.

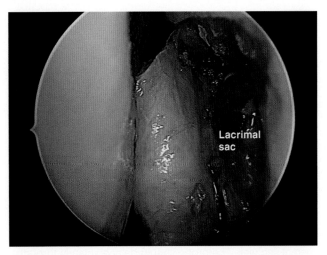

Fig. 17.5. Endoscopic view of the completely exposed sac. The lacrimal sac is seen bulging into the nasal cavity.

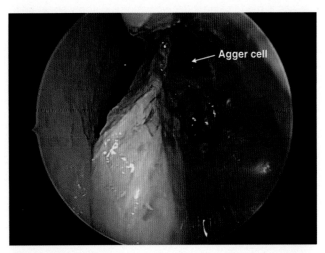

Fig. 17.6. Endoscopic view of exposure of the agger nasi cell.

Step 3: Remove Overlying Bone

- Use a round knife from the ear tray to flake off the lacrimal bone overlying the anterior-inferior portion of the lacrimal sac.

Step 4: Use a Hajek-Koffler Punch to Remove the Hard Bone of the Frontal Process of the Maxilla Overlying the Anterior-Inferior Aspect of the Lacrimal Sac

- When the punch can no longer grip the frontal process, change over to the DCR bur. Fully expose the sac by further removing bone up to the mucosal incisions. The sac should form a prominent bulge into the nasal cavity (Fig. 17.5).

Step 5: Expose the Agger Nasi Cell

- Expose the agger nasi cell (Fig. 17.6). This will allow the mucosa of the lacrimal sac to lie against the mucosa of the agger nasi cell, which allows healing by primary intention.

Step 6: Marsupialize the Lacrimal Sac

- Use a lacrimal probe to tent the lacrimal sac. Make sure that the probe is clearly visible through the mucosa of the sac before incising the sac to prevent inadvertent trauma to the common canaliculus. Use a DCR spear knife to incise the sac as far posteriorly as possible to create the largest possible anterior flap (Fig. 17.7).
- Use Bellucci micro ear scissors to create upper and lower releasing incisions in the posterior flap and use a DCR sickle knife to create the corresponding incisions in the anterior flap.
- The sac should now be completely marsupialized and lying flat on the lateral nasal wall (Figs. 17.8 and 17.9).

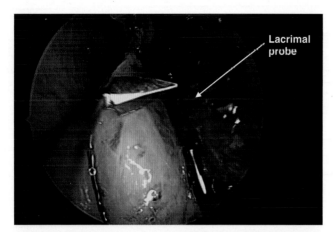

Fig. 17.7. Endoscopic view of lacrimal probe tenting of the medial sac wall. The probe should be seen clearly through the mucosa of the sac before incision to avoid inadvertent injury to the common canaliculus. A vertical incision into the sac is made using a dacryocystorhinostomy spear knife and a gentle rotating movement.

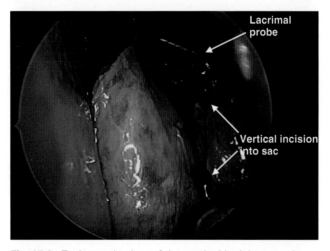

Fig. 17.8. Endoscopic view of the vertical incisions made superiorly and inferiorly into the lacrimal sac to fully marsupialize the sac.

Step 7: Trim the Mucosal Flap to Appose the Lacrimal Sac Mucosa

- Trim the mucosal flap so that only a superior and inferior limb remain, which can be positioned to approximate the corresponding superior and inferior borders of the marsupialized sac (Fig. 17.10).
- Confirm that the agger nasi cell is open and that its mucosa is opposing the posterior-superior aspect of the sac.

Step 8: Pass Crawford Silastic Tubes

- Pass Silastic lacrimal tubes into the nasal cavity via the superior and inferior puncta (Fig. 17.11). Slide a small piece of absorbable gelatin sponge (Gelfoam)

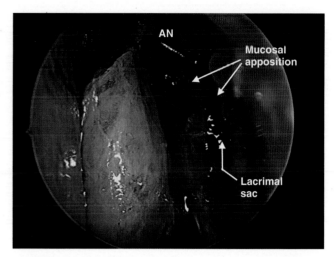

Fig. 17.9. Endoscopic view of the lacrimal sac fully marsupialized and lying flat against the lateral nasal wall. *AN,* Agger nasi.

up the Crawford tubes to hold the flaps in place (Fig. 17.12). Secure the tubes either by placing a ligating clip or by simply tying the tube ends together.

POSTOPERATIVE CONSIDERATIONS

- Before the procedure is completed, all flaps are checked to ensure that they are sitting **perfectly** to allow healing to occur by primary intention.
- Some surgeons use Crawford tubes routinely in their surgery for three reasons:
  1. They dilate the common canaliculus, the narrowing of which contributes to epiphora in a significant number of patients. This condition can only be diagnosed intraoperatively, but a negative result on dacryocystography with penetration of the sac on scintigraphy is highly suggestive of this problem.
  2. It facilitates the positioning of the flaps by allowing a piece of Gelfoam to be slid up along the Crawford tubes onto the mucosal edges.
  3. The tubes promote tear drainage through the canalicular system by capillary action along the tubes.
- The patient is discharged with instructions to use a saline spray, complete a 5-day course of oral antibiotics, and apply antibiotic eye drops for 2 weeks. The patient is examined at 2 weeks, and crusting is removed.
- The Crawford tubes are removed after 4 weeks, and the patency of the lacrimal system is checked using the fluorescein dye disappearance test and the Valsalva bubble test.

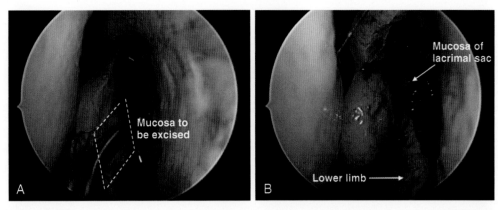

Fig. 17.10. (A) Before: area of mucosal flap to be trimmed to allow for precise apposition to mucosa of lacrima sac. **(B)** After trimming of mucosal flap.

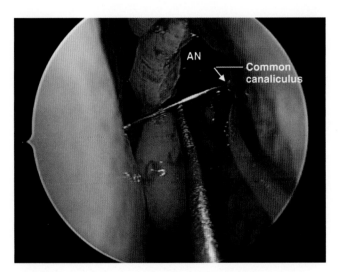

Fig. 17.11. Endoscopic view of Crawford tubes passing through the common canaliculus. *AN,* Agger nasi.

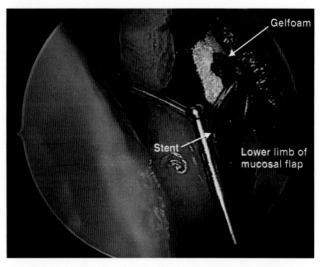

Fig. 17.12. Endoscopic view of the Gelfoam slid up the Silastic stents. The mucosal flaps are carefully positioned to ensure mucosa-to-mucosa apposition.

SPECIAL CONSIDERATIONS

Revision Surgery

■ Make mucosal cuts onto the remaining bone. DCR surgery usually fails because of inadequate exposure of the common canaliculus and lacrimal sac. Palpate the bone above the axilla of the middle turbinate and frontal process of the maxilla to assess the size of the previous osteotomy and make the new mucosal cuts directly onto the bone.

■ Sharply dissect a mucosal flap from the underlying prelacrimal sac.

■ A free mucosal graft harvested from the agger nasi cell can be used to prevent secondary fibrosis and formation of granulation tissue.

■ Application of mitomycin C has been shown to be of some benefit in revision endoscopic DCR.[1-3]

■ Crawford stents should remain in situ for 4 to 6 weeks postoperatively.

■ The patient should use topical steroid drops for 1 week postoperatively.

REFERENCES

Access the reference list online at ExpertConsult.com.

Endoscopic Orbital Decompression

Brian C. Lobo and Raj Sindwani

INTRODUCTION

- For more than 100 years, surgical decompression of the orbit has been used to treat severe proptosis and optic neuropathy associated with Graves disease, also known as Thyroid Eye Disease (TED).
- Although decompression techniques involving removal of each of the four walls of the orbit had been described,[1–4] the transantral approach reported by Walsh and Ogura in the 1950s had been favored by most otolaryngologists.[5]
- Soon after the introduction of transnasal endoscopic sinus surgery in the mid-1980s, surgeons began to experiment with endoscopic orbital surgery.
- Endoscopic orbital decompression was first described by Kennedy et al. and Michel et al. in the early 1990s.[6,7]
- The enhanced visualization of key anatomic landmarks permits safe and thorough decompression of the entire medial orbital wall and the medial portion of the orbital floor.
- This improved visualization is most notable in the region of the orbital apex, a critical area of decompression in patients with optic neuropathy and a region poorly visualized with conventional external approaches.
- These marked advantages have allowed the endoscopic approach to replace previously described techniques as the technique of choice for orbital decompression.

ANATOMY

- Anatomy is best addressed in relation to the individual sinuses and is important to identify on preoperative imaging (Fig. 18.1).[8] The orange shading in Fig. 18.1 indicates the structures removed as part of an endoscopic orbital decompression.

Maxillary Sinus Landmarks

- The maxillary line corresponds to the junction of the uncinate process and the maxilla.[9]

- The *maxillary sinus roof* (orbital floor) is an important landmark because it is a boundary of decompression.
- The *infraorbital nerve* courses through the maxillary roof and innervates the lower lid, the upper lip, and a portion of the vestibule (V2 distribution).

Ethmoid Sinus Landmarks

- The *skull base* is known to have a variable vertical height with an anterior to posterior downward slope.
- The posterior skull base meets the anterior face of the sphenoid sinus where it is relatively thick.
- The angle created at the junction of the sphenoid face and posterior skull base creates the sphenoethmoid angle, which represents the posterior limit of orbital decompression.[10]
- The *lamina papyracea* is the thin orbital plate of the ethmoid bone, which forms the medial wall of the orbit that is removed during decompression surgery.
- In patients with TED, the lamina papyracea often has a bowed or convex appearance secondary to increased intraorbital pressures.

Sphenoid Sinus Landmarks

- Important sphenoid sinus landmarks include the following:
  - The sphenoid face
  - The superior turbinate, because the ostium is medial and inferior to this landmark
  - The sphenoid ostium

PREOPERATIVE CONSIDERATIONS

- Endoscopic orbital decompression is indicated for patients with moderate to severe symptoms of Graves orbitopathy, commonly known as Thyroid Eye Disease (TED). These indications include exophthalmos (including for cosmesis), exposure keratopathy, diplopia, and optic neuropathy.

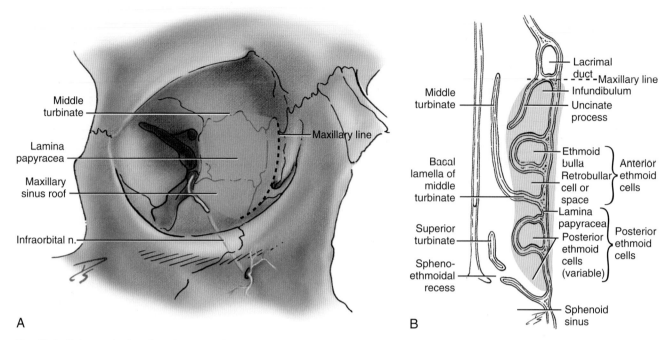

Fig. 18.1. Schematic drawings in coronal **(A)** and axial **(B)** view showing the boundaries of endoscopic orbital decompression. Boundaries are for a standard endoscopic medial and inferior floor decompression; the area to be resected is shaded in yellow. *n.,* Nerve.

- Endoscopic orbital decompression is also used to gain access to the orbit for the removal of benign orbital tumors,[11,12] decompression of orbital abscesses and hematomas, biopsy of indeterminate lesions, palliative therapy for malignant tumors causing visual symptoms, transnasal endoscopic intraorbital ligation of the anterior ethmoid artery,[13] and as the approach for optic nerve decompression.[14]
- The endoscopic technique allows unmatched visualization of critical anatomic landmarks, including the skull base and orbital apex, while avoiding external or sublabial incisions.
- The procedure is usually performed under general anesthesia; however, local anesthesia with sedation can be used in patients with significant medical comorbidities or for surgery on a patient's only seeing eye (depending on surgeon preference).
- Endoscopic orbital decompression may be performed unilaterally, bilaterally, or in a staged fashion and can be combined with lateral decompression.
- The risks, benefits, and alternatives should be discussed with the patient and ophthalmology team, but performance of bilateral decompressions as a single-setting procedure is generally recommended.
- Common practice is to perform endoscopic orbital decompression in a patient's only seeing eye under general anesthesia.
- For severe disease, the recommended procedure is a balanced three-wall decompression, which combines

an endoscopic medial wall and medial orbital floor decompression with an external-approach lateral wall decompression via lateral cathotomy.[14]
- It is imperative to discuss the nuances of endoscopic orbital decompression with the anesthesia team preoperatively. This will limit potential aggressive postextubation bag-mask ventilation, which can result in subcutaneous and/or orbital emphysema.

Radiographic Considerations: Computed Tomography Checklist

- Evaluate the skull base orientation.
- Examine the middle turbinate attachment.
- Identify the location and course of the anterior ethmoid artery.
- Evaluate for the presence of an *Onodi cell,* or sphenoethmoid air cell—a posterior ethmoid cell that is positioned superolateral to the sphenoid sinus.
  - The existence of an Onodi cell is important because the optic nerve can often course through the lateral aspect of this cell instead of through the sphenoid sinus proper.
  - Suspect an Onodi cell when a four-quadrant sphenoid sinus is observed on coronal computed tomographic (CT) views, although this is best evaluated on sagittal CT imaging.

- Identify the location of the *anterior ethmoid artery* to prevent inadvertent injury intraoperatively.
  - On coronal CT, the most posterior view of the globe demonstrates the anterior ethmoid artery within its canal as a nippling at the confluence of the medial rectus and superior oblique muscles.
  - The artery is particularly at risk when a prominent supraorbital cell is present and the artery is located below the level of the skull base, within the ethmoid sinus.
- Evaluate the middle turbinate for the presence of a concha bullosa and note the attachment to the skull base.

INSTRUMENTATION (FIG. 18.2)

- Standard endoscopic sinus surgery set used to perform standard maxillary antrostomy, sphenoethmoidectomy, and middle turbinectomy
- 0-degree and 30-degree rigid nasal endoscopes
- Image guidance system—recommended but not required
- Key instrumentation for the decompression portion of the procedure:
  - Sickle or arachnoid knife
  - Cottle elevator
  - Straight through-cutting forceps
  - 90-degree curette

PEARLS AND POTENTIAL PITFALLS

Pearls

- Middle turbinate resection allows optimal exposure of the medial orbital wall, permits maximal decompression of orbital contents, and facilitates postoperative débridement.
- A 30-degree endoscope should be used during resection of the orbital floor.
- A double-ball probe will elevate the periorbita off the medial orbital floor and provide a pocket for the curette to enter during orbital floor downfracture.
- A small strip of the lamina papyracea should be left intact near the skull base (especially anteriorly). This avoids intraoperative skull base injury, potential cerebrospinal fluid (CSF) leak, and postoperative frontal recess obstruction.
- The sphenoethmoidectomy, lamina resection, and hemostasis should be performed before incising the periorbita.
- The initial periorbital incision should start posteriorly, because fat and orbital contents will herniate into the cavities and obstruct posterior views.
- An arachnoid knife or the very tip of a sickle knife should be used when opening the periorbita to avoid

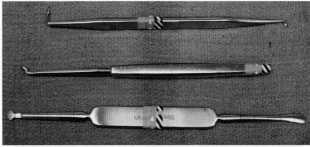
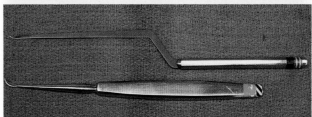

Fig. 18.2. Photographs of instruments used for endoscopic orbital decompression. *Top,* Ninety-degree curette, straight curette, and Cottle elevator. *Bottom,* Arachnoid knife and sickle knife.

injury to deeper structures, including the extraocular muscles and optic nerve.
  - Recent use of carpal tunnel release blades may provide a new tool for periorbital incision.[15]

Potential Pitfalls

- Bleeding may occur from the anterior ethmoid artery or the sphenopalatine artery if they are not avoided.
- Optic nerve injury may occur during incision of the periorbita.
- Nasolacrimal duct injury can result if dissection proceeds too far anteriorly.
- Skull base injury and CSF leak may arise during superior lamina papyracea resection.
- Extraocular muscle injury to the medial or inferior rectus muscle can occur during resection of the periorbita or downfracture of the orbital floor.
- Postoperative maxillary sinus obstruction and sinusitis may be present when there is an inadequate maxillary antrostomy or sphenoidotomy.
- Postoperative frontal sinusitis may occur when there is decompression of the orbital contents into the frontal recess.
- An imbalanced decompression may result in enophthalmos or an asymmetry of the eyes.

SURGICAL PROCEDURE

- The technique for endoscopic orbital decompression, as described in the literature,[14] is as follows with modification by the authors.

- The patient is positioned in the standard supine fashion. The eyes are maintained in the sterile field with lateral taping.
- Topical vasoconstriction is accomplished with oxymetazoline (0.05%) or cocaine (4%) pledgets.
- Local anesthetic (lidocaine 1% with epinephrine 1:100,000) is injected along the lateral nasal wall, at the maxillary line, and into the middle turbinate.

Step 1: Resection of the Middle Turbinate, Maxillary Antrostomy, Complete Ethmoidectomy, and Sphenoidotomy

- Removal of the middle turbinate during decompression is recommended.
- Medialize and remove the uncinate process.
- Perform a maximally wide maxillary antrostomy in the posterior direction to achieve access to the orbital floor, prevent blockage of the ostium by orbital fat, and preserve the nasolacrimal duct.
- Using a 30-degree endoscope, examine the infraorbital nerve, which should be observed coursing along the floor of the orbit.
- Perform a standard total ethmoidectomy and wide sphenoidotomy to avoid future obstructive disease from prolapsed orbital fat (Fig. 18.3A,B).
- An image guidance system may be used to confirm removal of all ethmoid cells along the medial orbital wall and to ensure complete dissection of the sphenoid face and skull base.

Step 2: Penetration of the Medial Orbital Wall

- Carefully penetrate the medial orbital wall in a controlled fashion using a spoon curette (Fig. 18.3C,D).
- The periorbital fascia should not be violated with this maneuver, and orbital fat should not be observed at this point.
- Elevate the thin bone of the lamina papyracea while preserving the underlying periorbita (Fig. 18.3E,F).

Step 3: Removal of Medial Orbital Wall Fragments

- Remove bone fragments using Blakesley forceps.
- Proceed with bone removal superiorly toward the ethmoid roof, inferiorly to the orbital floor, anteriorly to the maxillary line, and posteriorly to sphenoid face.

Step 4: Downfracture of the Orbital Floor

- Elevate the periorbita off the medial orbital floor.
- Use a spoon curette to engage the orbital floor at its medial extent and forcefully downfracture it (Fig. 18.4).
- The bone of the orbital floor is thicker than that of the medial orbital wall, and significant force may be required for this maneuver.
  - It is often necessary to resect the orbitoethmoid strut to achieve this maneuver.
- The bone may fracture in one large piece along the cleavage plane at the infraorbital nerve canal.
- Use of a 30-degree endoscope and angled forceps may facilitate bone removal.

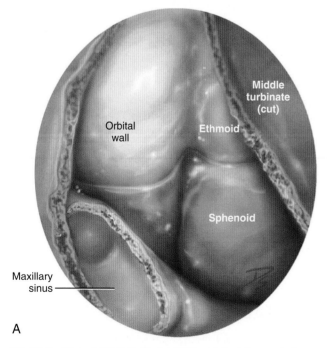

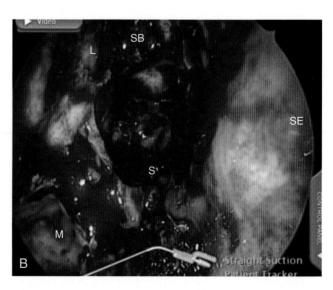

Fig. 18.3. (A) and **(B)** Artist's depiction and endoscopic image, respectively, of a maxillary antrostomy with middle turbinate removed and sphenoethmoidectomy.

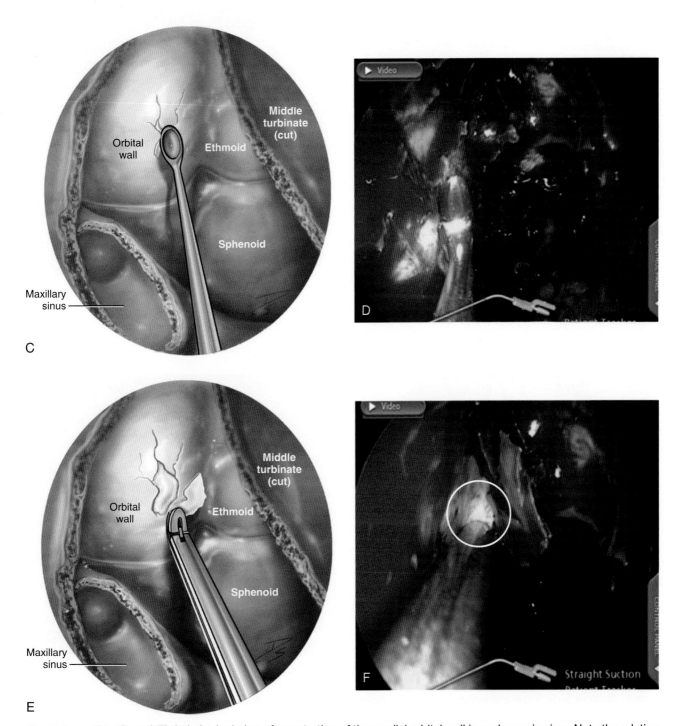

Fig. 18.3. cont'd. **(C)** and **(E)** Artist's depiction of penetration of the medial orbital wall in endoscopic view. Note the relationship with the skull base and maxillary sinus. **(D)** and **(F)** Endoscopic views of the removal of medial orbital wall fragments. Note the underlying periorbita [*circle* in **(F)**]. *L,* Lamina papyracea; *M,* maxillary sinus; *S,* sphenoid ostium; *SB,* skull base; *SE,* septum.

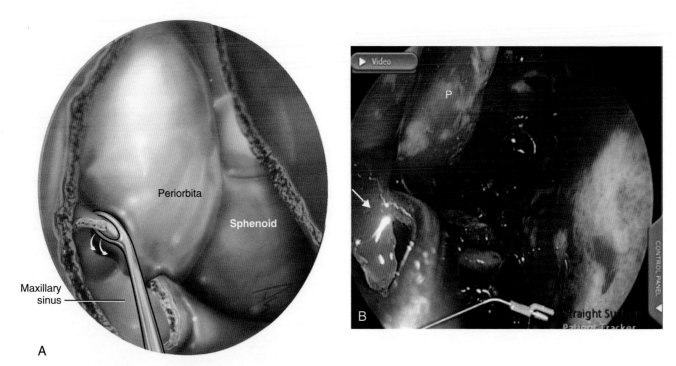

Fig. 18.4. Artist's depiction **(A)** and endoscopic image **(B)** of downfracture of the medial orbital floor (*arrow* in B). *P,* Periorbita.

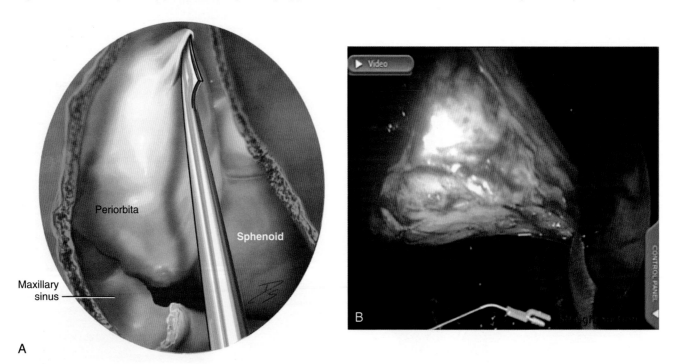

Fig. 18.5. (A) Artist's depiction of incision of the periorbita in endoscopic view. **(B)** Endoscopic view of incision of periorbital fibrous bands.

Step 5: Incision of the Periorbita (Fig. 18.5)

- Once the lamina papyracea and medial orbital floor have been removed and the periorbita is fully exposed, use a sickle knife to open this fascial layer.
- Begin the periorbita incision at the posterior limit of the decompression and bring it anteriorly to

prevent prolapsing fat and contents from obscuring visualization.
- Use a ball-tip probe and sickle knife to identify and incise remaining fibrous bands that course superficially between lobules of fat.

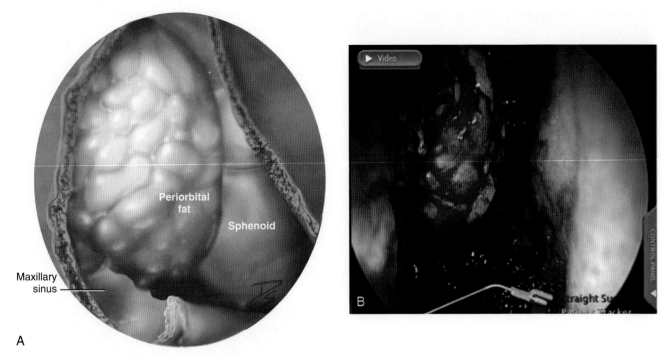

Fig. 18.6. Artist's depiction **(A)** and endoscopic image **(B)** of prolapse of orbital fat.

Step 6: Orbital Fat Prolapse Into the Ethmoid and Maxillary Cavities

■ Upon completion of the procedure, a generous prolapse of fat into the opened ethmoid and maxillary cavities will be observed (Fig. 18.6A,B).
  – Ideally, the maxillary and sphenoid ostium, as well as the frontal outflow tract, should still be visible.
■ Blot the globe to confirm an increase in retropulsion and encourage maximal fat herniation.

Hemostasis

■ Bleeding encountered during endoscopic orbital decompression is best managed with bipolar cautery. Monopolar cautery should be avoided because of possible injury to intraorbital structures.
■ At the conclusion of the procedure, packing should be avoided to ensure maximal decompression and prevent compression of exposed orbital contents.

POSTOPERATIVE CONSIDERATIONS

Postoperative Care

■ The patient is discharged the first postoperative day with a prescription for oral antistaphylococcal antibiotics.
■ Discharge instructions include the following:
  – No nose blowing
  – Mouth open for sneezing
  – No heavy lifting or straining for 5 to 7 days

  – Hold continuous positive airway pressure (CPAP) and bilevel positive airway pressure (BIPAP) use for 1 week postprocedure.
  – Twice-daily nasal saline irrigations
■ At the first postoperative visit 1 week after surgery, crusts and debris are removed from the surgical site under endoscopic guidance. The débridement is repeated 1 week later if necessary.

Outcomes

■ Representative results of endoscopic orbital decompression are shown in Fig. 18.7.
■ Ocular recession as a result of endoscopic decompression averages 3.5 mm (range, 2–12 mm). The addition of concurrent lateral decompression to the endoscopic procedure provides an additional 2 mm of globe recession.[16]
■ Diplopia is not uncommon following orbital decompression and is believed to be a result of the vector change in the pull of the extraocular muscles. Diplopia can be expected in up to $\frac{1}{3}$ of patients. It is temporary in most patients and resolves spontaneously over weeks to months.
  – New evidence suggests that preservation of the inferomedial orbital strut can reduce rates of diplopia.[17,18]
  – All patients should be informed of the possibility of postoperative diplopia and the potential need for surgical intervention if this persists.

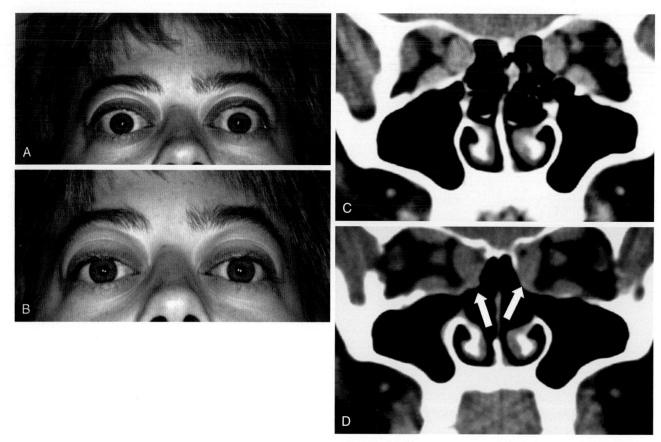

Fig. 18.7. Preoperative **(A)** and postoperative **(B)** photographs and preoperative **(C)** and postoperative **(D)** computed tomographic scans of a patient undergoing endoscopic orbital decompression. Note the removal of the medial orbital wall and fat herniation (*arrows* in D).

- Extraocular muscle, or strabismus, surgery may be considered for correction of persistent diplopia 8 to 10 months after decompression.

SPECIAL CONSIDERATIONS

- Epiphora may develop if the maxillary antrostomy is extended too far anteriorly with transection of the nasolacrimal duct. This complication is treated with an endoscopic dacryocystorhinostomy.
- Counseling regarding diplopia, postobstructive sinusitis should be performed by the surgeon.
- Leakage of CSF and blindness are very rare complications. Risk of intraoperative skull base injury can be minimized by leaving a small margin of lamina papyracea superiorly.

CONCLUSIONS

- The endoscopic transnasal approach is well suited for decompression of both the orbit and the optic canal.
- High-resolution endoscopes provide excellent visualization for bone removal along the orbital apex and skull base.
- Endoscopic orbital decompression has proven to be safe and effective for the treatment of TED.
- Recent evidence demonstrates that endoscopic decompression is no more expensive than open decompression, which may reduce opposition to use of this technique in geographic areas with low penetration.[19]

REFERENCES

Access the reference list online at ExpertConsult.com.

Optic Nerve Decompression

Henry P. Barham, Vijay R. Ramakrishnan, and Todd T. Kingdom

INTRODUCTION

- Endoscopic transnasal surgery has become an effective approach to the surgical management of diseases of the sinuses, orbit, and anterior skull base. Technologic advances have been critical in advancing endoscopic surgical procedures, with the introduction of improved optics and lighting, advanced instrumentation, and image-guided surgical navigation.
- Multiple approaches to the optic nerve have been described, ranging from endonasal endoscopic to open craniotomy. The endonasal endoscopic approach offers many advantages, which makes this the preferred method for optic nerve decompression. Advantages include avoidance of external incisions, preservation of olfaction, superior visualization, and access to the medial optic nerve.
- A close working relationship with an ophthalmologist or neuro-ophthalmologist is recommended. The surgical approach presented is familiar to the otolaryngologist, but experience is recommended before this procedure is attempted.
- Indications for this procedure are limited. The decision to proceed with medical rather than surgical treatment is controversial in many cases.

ANATOMY

Orbit and Orbital Apex

- The extraconal space consists mostly of orbital fat encased within the periorbita.
- The intraconal space is located within the fascia of the extraocular muscles. It contains the muscles, retrobulbar fat, optic nerve, and ophthalmic artery (Fig. 19.1).
- The annulus of Zinn is the fibrous thickening formed by the fusion of the pia and arachnoid. This is the most constricting portion of the fibrous tissue around the nerve. It is also a site of attachment of the extraocular muscles.

- The superior orbital fissure is located superolateral to the optic foramen, and the inferior orbital fissure is located inferolateral to the foramen.

Optic Nerve

- There are four segments of the optic nerve: intracranial, intracanalicular, intraorbital, and intraocular (Fig. 19.2).
- The optic canal is formed by two struts of the lesser wing of the sphenoid. Within it are the optic nerve and ophthalmic artery. The intracanalicular segment is the target of optic nerve decompression surgery.
- The optic nerve is a direct extension of the brain, with its three meningeal layers and cerebrospinal fluid (CSF)–containing subarachnoid space. The dura splits to form an outer layer, which contributes to the periorbita, and an inner layer, which fuses to the arachnoid (Fig. 19.3). The ophthalmic artery travels inferolateral to the nerve in 85% of cases and is located inferomedial to it in 15% (Fig. 19.4).

Sinus

- The transethmoid route to the sphenoid sinus provides the pathway to the optic nerve. The middle and superior turbinates, skull base, and lamina papyracea form the boundaries of this pathway.
- The sphenoid sinus may be variably pneumatized. In the lateral aspect of the sphenoid sinus, the optic nerve (superior) and carotid artery (inferior) impressions are usually visible, as is the opticocarotid recess (Fig. 19.5).
- An Onodi cell is a posterior ethmoid cell that pneumatizes superolaterally into the sphenoid. This cell will contain a portion of the optic nerve.

INDICATIONS AND CONTRAINDICATIONS FOR OPTIC NERVE DECOMPRESSION

- Indications for optic nerve decompression include traumatic optic neuropathy, thyroid eye disease associated

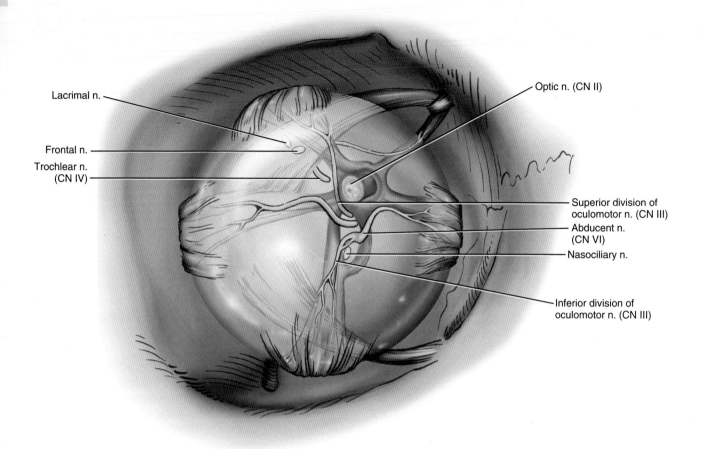

Lacrimal n.

Frontal n.

Trochlear n.
(CN IV)

Optic n. (CN II)

Superior division of
oculomotor n. (CN III)

Abducent n.
(CN VI)

Nasociliary n.

Inferior division of
oculomotor n. (CN III)

Fig. 19.1. Drawing of the posterior orbit in coronal view. *CN,* Cranial nerve; *n.,* nerve.

with optic neuropathy, vision loss secondary to idiopathic intracranial hypertension, fibro-osseous lesions, and other neoplasms (sinonasal tumor, meningioma, orbital apex tumor).

- Contraindications for optic nerve decompression include complete disruption of the nerve or chiasm, complete atrophy of the nerve, carotid-cavernous fistula, and other medical comorbidities precluding the use of general anesthesia.
- If appropriate, a trial of medical therapy should precede consideration of decompression. Decompression for traumatic optic neuropathy is considered controversial. Patients with severe vision loss not improved with high-dose steroid therapy may benefit from surgery.
- Timing of decompression is also controversial for traumatic optic neuropathy. In general, earlier decompression is associated with a higher chance of recovery of vision.

PREOPERATIVE CONSIDERATIONS

- A complete ophthalmologic physical examination should be performed, including pupil examination,

assessment of proptosis, measurement of intraocular pressure, visual field testing (confrontation, formal testing), visual acuity testing, color vision testing, funduscopic examination (to look for nerve atrophy and papilledema and to rule out other causes of vision loss), measurement of visual evoked potentials if the patient is unconscious, and ultrasonography if a hematoma is suspected.

- Optional medical therapies include
  - trial of steroids for traumatic optic neuropathy: methylprednisolone 30 mg/kg loading dose, then 5.4 mg/kg/hr × 48 hours
  - radiation therapy for thyroid eye disease
  - diuretics for idiopathic intracranial hypertension.
- The natural history of the disease process should be considered. The expected results of nonsurgical management should be balanced against those of surgical decompression.

Radiographic Considerations

- Use a fine-cut computed tomographic (CT) scan of the sinus and orbits for the following: evaluation of optic canal compression, fracture or bone displacement,

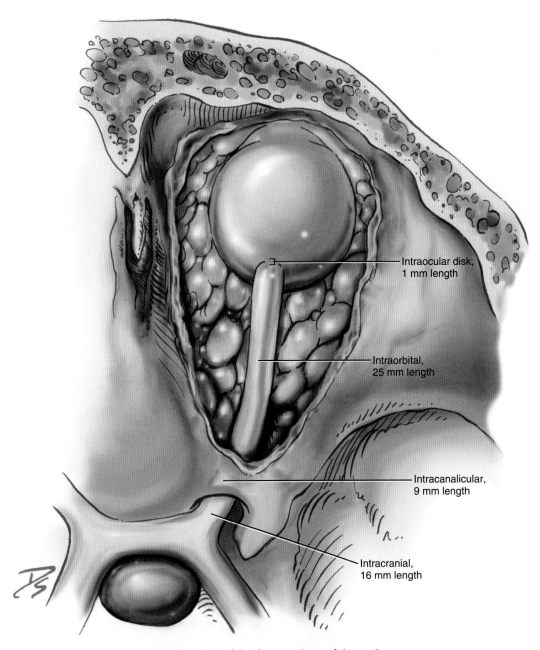

Intraocular disk,
1 mm length

Intraorbital,
25 mm length

Intracanalicular,
9 mm length

Intracranial,
16 mm length

Fig. 19.2. Drawing of the four portions of the optic nerve.

evaluation of sinus anatomy for surgery, and for use with image guidance.

- Review coronal and axial images (Fig. 19.6), and obtain a magnetic resonance image of the orbits when compression of the optic nerve is suspected based on history, physical examination findings, and CT scan (Fig. 19.7).

INSTRUMENTATION (FIG. 19.8)

- 0-degree and 30-degree endoscopes
- Kerrison rongeur or sphenoid punch

- J-curette, elevator, ball-tip probe
- 15-degree irrigating diamond drill
- sharp sickle knife
- fibrin glue
- Bone removal may also be achieved by ultrasonic bone aspirator, according to surgeon preference.

Image guidance is a surgical tool that is widely accepted by the endoscopic surgeon and used in the majority of extended endonasal approaches. The use of image guidance can help identify critical structures and distorted anatomic landmarks, increasing the surgeon's confidence and ability to perform a more complete dissection.

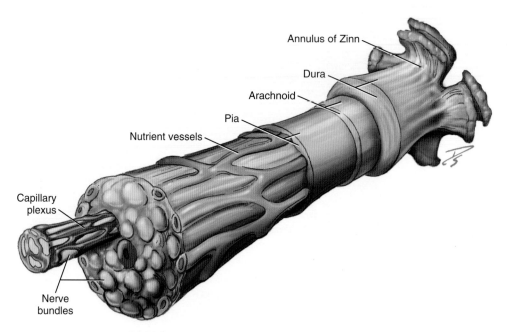

Fig. 19.3. Drawing of the layers of the optic nerve.

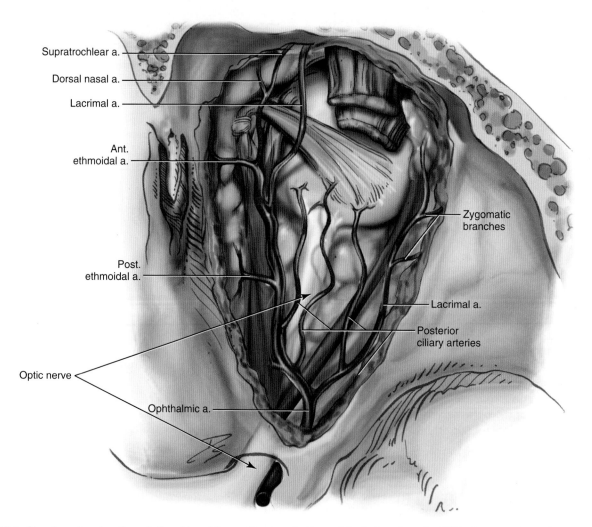

Fig. 19.4. Drawing showing the relationship of the optic nerve to the ophthalmic artery. In 85% of cases, the ophthalmic artery runs inferolateral to the optic nerve. In 15% of cases, it runs inferomedial to the nerve. *A.,* Artery; *Ant.,* anterior; *Post.,* posterior.

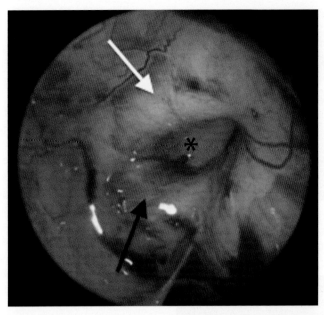

Fig. 19.5. Endoscopic view of a left sphenoid sinus with optic nerve *(white arrow)* and carotid artery *(black arrow)* impressions on the lateral wall. The asterisk indicates the opticocarotid recess.

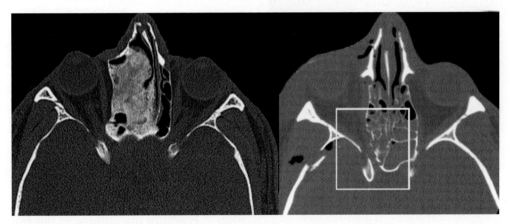

Fig. 19.6. *Left,* Axial computed tomographic (CT) scan for a patient with fibrous dysplasia causing papilledema. *Right,* Axial CT scan for a patient with traumatic optic neuropathy and fractures along the canalicular segment of the nerve *(white box).*

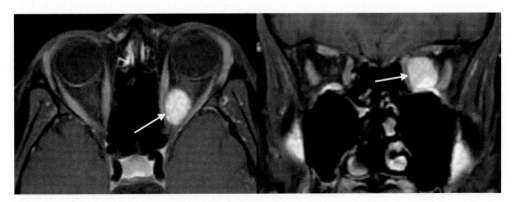

Fig. 19.7. Axial *(left)* and coronal *(right)* T1-weighted contrast-enhanced magnetic resonance images for a patient with progressive vision loss and a large cavernous hemangioma of the left orbital apex *(white arrows).*

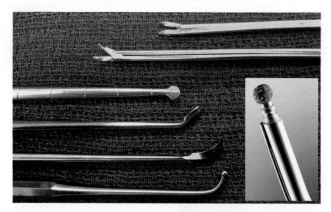

Fig. 19.8. Photograph of instruments commonly used in optic nerve decompression. (Inset photograph courtesy Medtronic, Jacksonville, Florida, with permission.)

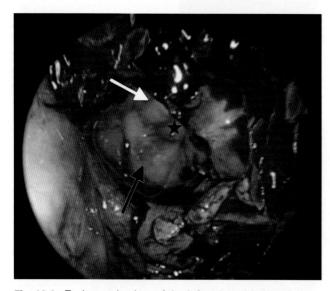

Fig. 19.9. Endoscopic view of the left sphenoid sinus from the ethmoid cavity. The optic nerve *(white arrow)* and carotid artery *(black arrow)* impressions are seen, as is the opticocarotid recess *(asterisk).*

PEARLS AND POTENTIAL PITFALLS

Pearls

- The lamina papyracea should be identified early and a complete ethmoidectomy performed.
- A maximally wide sphenoidotomy will facilitate insertion of the drill and optimize visualization.
- A drill with simultaneous suction and irrigation is favored, given the accumulation of irrigant within the sphenoid. The necessary equipment and personnel should be available in case a complication is encountered.
- A bi-nostril, two-surgeon approach utilizing a posterior septectomy can be useful in challenging cases.

Potential Pitfalls

- Visualization is critical. If necessary, a middle turbinectomy or middle turbinate swing procedure may be performed to aid in visualization and instrument placement.
- Accidental violation of the periorbita in the posterior ethmoid will hamper visualization due to fat prolapse and bleeding.
- Bone removal should be done gently. A diamond drill bit can "eggshell" the bone before removal. Conduction of heat along the nerve can occur when drilling if irrigation is not continuously administered.
- If incising the optic sheath, be sure to make the incision on the medial or superomedial aspect to avoid injury to the ophthalmic artery. CSF may egress after incision of the sheath and can be treated with topical fibrin glue sealant or loose placement of a free mucosal graft.

SURGICAL PROCEDURE

Step 1: Perform a Complete Ethmoidectomy

- After completing this step, proceed to the next step.

Step 2: Perform a Wide Sphenoidotomy

- Use a mushroom punch or Kerrison rongeur to maximally widen the sphenoid opening.
- The posterior nasal branch of the sphenopalatine artery may be crossed at the inferior aspect; be prepared to cauterize if bleeding occurs.

Step 3: Identify the Optic Nerve, Carotid Prominence, and Opticocarotid Recess (Fig. 19.9)

- After completing this step, proceed to the next step.

Step 4: Fracture the Lamina in the Posterior Ethmoid

- Use a J-curette, elevator, or ball-tip probe to fracture the lamina in the posterior ethmoid roughly 1 cm anterior to the sphenoid face (Fig. 19.10).
- Flake away this portion of the lamina with the ball-tip probe or Freer elevator until the optic strut is reached.
- The bone of the lamina papyracea will get progressively thicker as you move from anterior to posterior along the lamina. Once the bone is too thick for hand instruments, a drill or ultrasonic aspirator is needed for bony removal.
- Attempt to keep the periorbita intact.

Step 5: Remove Bone Overlying the Intracanalicular Segment of the Nerve

- Use a diamond drill with copious irrigation for bone removal.

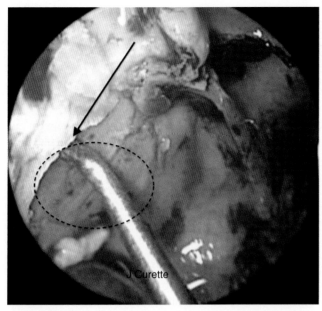

Fig. 19.10. Endoscopic view of right medial orbital wall. Note the fractured lamina papyracea *(arrow)* and the underlying periorbital *(dashed oval).*

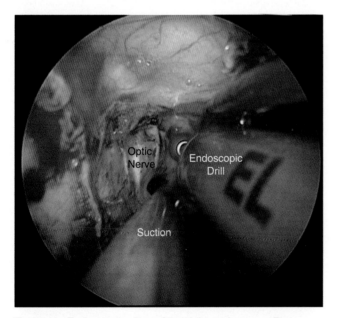

Fig. 19.11. Endoscopic view of the right optic nerve. Bone overlying the optic sheath is drilled along the axis of the nerve. (Courtesy Vijay R. Ramakrishnan, MD, University of Colorado, Denver, Colorado; and Henry P. Barham, MD, Sinus and Nasal Specialists of Louisiana, Baton Rouge, Louisiana.)

- Drill along the axis of the nerve, not across it.
- Flake away bone in the medial direction as it is thinned (Figs. 19.11 and 19.12).
- Attempt to achieve 180 degrees of decompression (Fig. 19.13). Observe for the presence of an intra-neural hematoma.

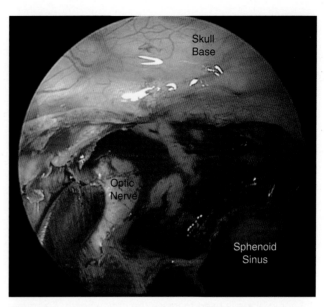

Fig. 19.12. Endoscopic view after bone thinning. The freer elevator is used to gently fracture the bone medially. (Courtesy Vijay R. Ramakrishnan, MD, University of Colorado, Denver, Colorado; and Henry P. Barham, MD, Sinus and Nasal Specialists of Louisiana, Baton Rouge, Louisiana.)

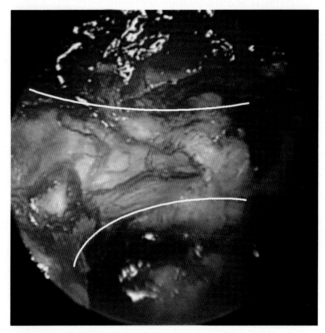

Fig. 19.13. Endoscopic view after the right optic nerve has been decompressed nearly 180 degrees. The sheath was not incised in this case. *White lines* indicate the decompressed optic nerve.

Step 6: Consider the Need to Incise the Optic Sheath

- Incision of the optic sheath is rarely required. If it is to be done, place the incision in the superomedial quadrant to avoid potential injury to the ophthalmic

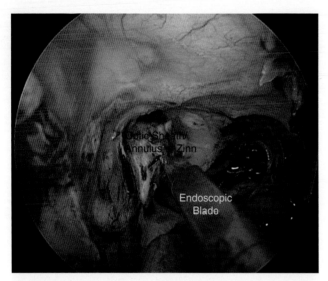

Fig. 19.14. Endoscopic view of the right optic nerve. An endoscopic blade is used to incise the optic sheath. (Courtesy Vijay R. Ramakrishnan, MD, University of Colorado, Denver, Colorado; and Henry P. Barham, MD, Sinus and Nasal Specialists of Louisiana, Baton Rouge.)

artery. It should include the annulus of Zinn (Fig. 19.14).

- Observe for the presence of a CSF leak. If a leak is present, place a small piece of free mucosa or fibrin glue over the nerve with minimal dissolvable packing (e.g., Gelfoam) to stop the leak.

Step 7: Dressings
- Nasal packing is not needed in most cases.

- Suture medialization or reattachment (if middle turbinate swing procedure is performed) of the middle turbinate may be performed.

COMPLICATIONS

- Complications that can occur in association with endoscopic optic nerve decompression include bleeding from the sphenopalatine artery, carotid injury, ecchymosis and hematoma, diplopia caused by medial rectus injury or incision through annulus of Zinn, vision loss or lack of improvement of vision, CSF leak, and meningitis.

Postoperative Considerations
- The following medications are generally prescribed: high-dose oral steroids, tapered carefully; oral antibiotics; gentle saline rinses or sprays, started early.
- Nasal packing should be avoided.
- Serial eye examinations should be performed to help guide the steroid taper.
- Patient instructions should include to limit activity and avoid nose blowing and straining. The patient should also be instructed to recognize and report symptoms and signs of intracranial and orbital complications.
- Postoperative débridement should be limited.
- The patient should receive continued follow-up care from an ophthalmologist.

Endoscopic Approach and Removal of Orbital Tumors

Marcel Menon Miyake and Benjamin S. Bleier

INTRODUCTION

- The endoscopic transnasal approach to the orbit is indicated for tumors located medially and/or inferiorly to the optic nerve.[1]
- This anatomic site is deep, poorly illuminated, and obscured by orbital fat when approached through a standard external approach.
- Globe and optic nerve manipulation required for external access are also avoided using the endoscopic approach.[2]

ANATOMY

- The extraconal space consists primarily of orbital fat between the periorbita and the medial rectus muscle. The ethmoidal neurovasculature may cross from lateral to medial over the superior border of the medial rectus muscle.
- The intraconal space is surrounded by the six extraocular muscles and is divided into medial/lateral and superior/inferior by the optic nerve (Fig. 20.1).
- The medial intraconal space is divided into three conceptual compartments of increasing technical difficulty with regard to surgical approach[3] (Fig. 20.2):
  - Zone A: Anterior to the inferomedial muscular trunk of the ophthalmic artery and inferior to an imaginary line dividing the upper and lower half of the medial rectus muscle belly. It is the most favorable zone to approach due to its relative ease of access and the paucity of neurovascular structures. A branch of the inferior division of the oculomotor nerve inserts along the posterior third of the lateral aspect of the medial rectus muscle.
  - Zone B: Anterior to the inferomedial muscular trunk of the ophthalmic artery and superior to an imaginary line dividing the upper and lower half of the medial rectus muscle belly. Dissecting tumors

within zone B is more challenging due to their proximity to the ethmoid vasculature and the occasional necessity to work above the medial rectus.
  - Zone C: Posterior to the inferomedial muscular trunk of the ophthalmic artery. This region is the most technically challenging to address due to its small volume and proximity to the optic nerve and ophthalmic artery.
- The inferior intraconal space contains branches of the oculomotor nerve to the inferior rectus and inferior oblique muscles.

INDICATIONS AND CONTRAINDICATIONS

- The endoscopic approach may be considered for primary orbital tumors that lie medial to the optic nerve.
- Tumors extending lateral to the optic nerve may be addressed via an endoscopic approach provided it lies beneath the "plane of resectability." This plane may be drawn from the contralateral nare through the long axis of the optic nerve. Structures inferior to this plane may be safely dissected without requiring nerve retraction.
- Tumors that lie lateral to the optic nerve or superior to the plane of resectability are currently not candidates for an exclusive endoscopic approach.

PREOPERATIVE CONSIDERATIONS

- All patients should be evaluated by a multidisciplinary team, including an otolaryngologist and ophthalmologist. A neurosurgeon should also be involved if an adjunctive craniotomy approach or dural transgression is required.
- A complete ophthalmologic physical examination should be performed, including formal visual field testing.

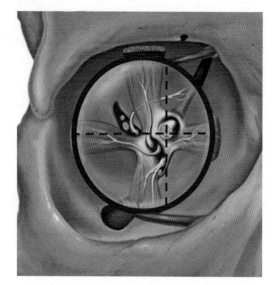

Fig. 20.1. Illustration of the limits of the intraconal space *(continuous blue line)*. The horizontal and vertical dashed lines that cross the optic nerve divide the intraconal space in superior/inferior and lateral/medial, respectively. (Courtesy of Yale Medical School.)

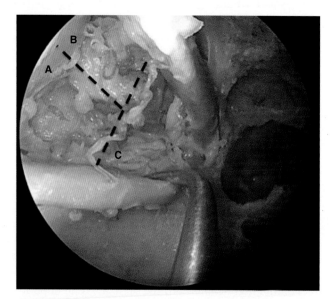

Fig. 20.2. Endoscopic view of the medial intraconal space divided into three conceptual zones A, B, and C by the inferomedial muscular trunk of the ophthalmic artery.

- The natural history of the tumor should be considered.
- The multidisciplinary team and the patient should discuss the goals of surgery, the approach, and the anticipated outcomes.

Radiographic Considerations

- Computed tomography (CT) scan and magnetic resonance imaging (MRI) may be used for the following (Figs. 20.3A and 20.3B):

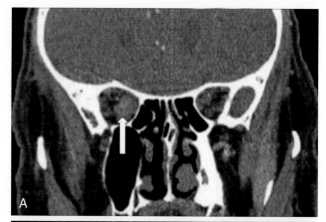

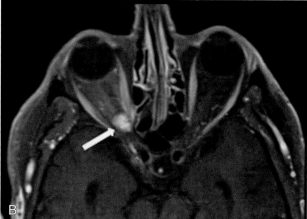

Fig. 20.3. **(A)** Coronal computed tomography (CT) scan and **(B)** axial magnetic resonance imaging (MRI) of a right orbital apex cavernous hemangioma *(white arrow)* and its relationship with the surrounding bony and neurovascular structures.

- Evaluation of the relationship between the lesion and the surrounding bony and neurovascular structures
- Evaluation of the course of the ophthalmic artery relative to the optic nerve (may be determined by the MRI)
- Image guidance
- A three-dimensional (3D) reconstruction based on the CT and MRI provides the following (Fig. 20.4):
  - Delineation of the relationship between the tumor and the course of the optic nerve
  - Accurate estimation of the tumor volume and morphology
  - Determination of the "plane of resectability," which predicts the tumor volume lateral to the optic nerve that may still be resectable via an endoscopic approach
- Angiography is not routinely required but may be useful if a vascular lesion or ophthalmic artery aneurysm is suspected.

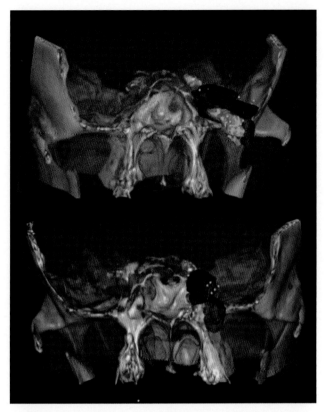

Fig. 20.4. Two views of a three-dimensional (3D) reconstruction showing the optic nerve *(blue),* medial *(green)* and lateral *(purple)* aspects of the tumor based on the optic nerve and inside the plane of resectability *(dashed lines),* and the aspect of the tumor that is outside the plane of resectability *(red).*

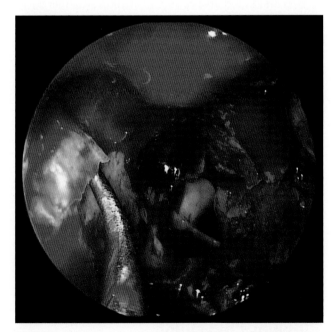

Fig. 20.5. Endoscopic view of the right orbit demonstrating the removal of the lamina papyracea with a double-ball probe.

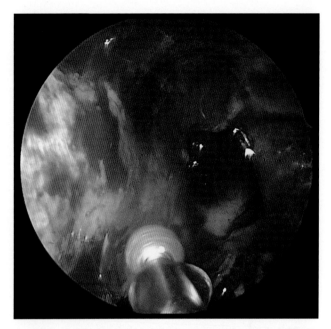

Fig. 20.6. Endoscopic view of the right orbit with the orbital process of the palatine bone being drilled.

INSTRUMENTATION

- The medial intraconal space is located lateral to a plane parallel to the lateral nasal wall. As such, the choice of instrumentation must include angled instruments and endoscopes to visualize and work within this space.
- The initial approach to the medial intraconal space requires a complete functional endoscopic sinus surgery and thus requires all the instrumentation commensurate with this technique, which has been shown in previous chapters.
- The bony resection of the lamina papyracea requires fine dissecting instruments, such as a cottle elevator and double-ball probe (Fig. 20.5).
- Removal of the thicker bone of the palatine and sphenoid bone requires an angled high-speed, 4-mm diamond bur (Fig. 20.6).
- Following bone removal, the periorbita may be incised with a disposable sickle knife (Fig. 20.7).
- Dissection and retraction of the extraocular muscles may be achieved using a combination of the double-ball probe, Freer elevator, and angled Penfield dissector (Fig. 20.8).
- A ½- by 3-inch neuropatty may be used for retraction of orbital fat and diversion of blood (Fig. 20.9).
- Once exposed and dissected out, the tumor may be grasped and removed with a small cupped forcep.

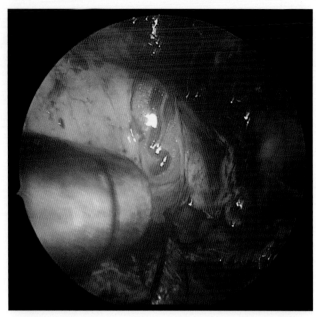

Fig. 20.7. Endoscopic view of the right orbit showing the reverse "hockey stick"–shaped incision of the periorbita with a sickle knife.

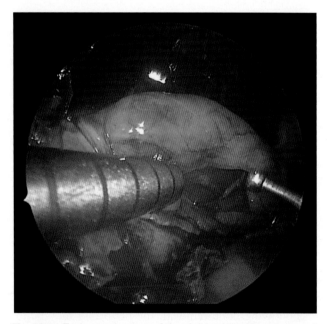

Fig. 20.8. Endoscopic view of the right orbit with extraconal fat dissection.

PEARLS AND POTENTIAL PITFALLS

Pearls

- A binarial, 4-handed approach is recommended for all endoscopic orbital tumor resections, particularly for intraconal lesions.[4] The advantages are:
    - Provides bimanual dissection
    - Greater access for more instruments
    - Wider working angle for improving the dissection of the lateral aspect of the lesion

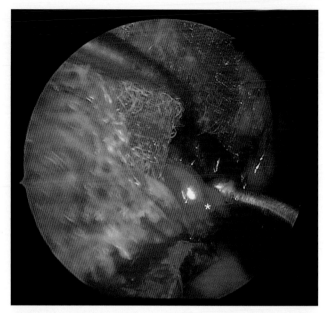

Fig. 20.9. Endoscopic view of the right orbit showing the medial rectus *(asterisk)* muscle retraction with a double-ball probe and the tumor exposure using a neuropatty.

- Enables a more rapid response in case of bleeding
- Retracting the medial rectus muscle with a blunt probe provides dynamic, targeted, and intermittent medial displacement, thereby maximally protecting the neurovascular contributions to the muscle.
- A saline soaked patty is helpful for both fat retraction and blood absorption, providing a cleaner surgical field.
- Warm water irrigation is also useful for hemostasis.

Potential Pitfalls

- The periorbita incision should be performed just anterior to the tumor in order to preserve the anterior periorbita and prevent fat prolapse, which will impair visualization.[5]
- Thermal damage to the optic nerve can occur when drilling the optic canal if irrigation is not continuously administered.
- Bipolar cautery may be judiciously used only in the extraconal space. Monopolar cautery should not be used in order to avoid electrical and thermal spread with attendant injury.

SURGICAL PROCEDURE

Step 1: Perform a Complete Ethmoidectomy, Maxillary Antrostomy, and Sphenoidectomy

- Please see Chapters 6, 7, and 8.

Step 2: Fracture and Remove the Lamina Papyracea (See Fig. 20.5)

- The underlying periorbita should be kept intact.
- Drilling the orbital process of the palatine bone and pterygoid wedge may be required to approach the orbital apex and the optic canal, respectively (see Fig. 20.6).

Step 3: Incise the Periorbita With a Sickle Knife (See Fig. 20.7)

- A reverse "hockey stick"–shaped incision preserves the periorbita, which can assist in the healing process.

Step 4: Dissect the Extraconal Fat (See Fig. 20.8)

- Every attempt should be made to reflect and preserve the extraconal fat. However, in the setting of significant prolapse or bleeding, bipolar electrocautery may be used to reduce extraconal fat.
- Extraconal tumors should be identified and resected at this step.

Step 5: Identify the Inferior Border of the Medial Rectus Muscle and Retract It With a Double-Ball Probe (See Fig. 20.9)

- A septal window should be performed through which the probe will be inserted.
- Superomedial medial rectus muscle retraction allows for exposure of the intraconal space.

Step 6: Identify the Oculomotor Nerve, the Inferomedial Trunk of the Ophthalmic Artery, and the Tumor

- Unlike the extraconal fat, intraconal fat should not be cauterized or resected.

Step 7: Bluntly Dissect the Tumor Using a Binarial, 4-Handed Approach

- One surgeon holds the endoscope and retracts the medial rectus muscle while the other surgeon dissects and suctions the pooled blood.
- The tumor should be separated from its medial, superior, and inferior surrounding attachments.
- Manipulation of the optic nerve should be avoided.

Step 8: Gently Retract the Lesion Anteriorly in a Plane Parallel to the Optic Nerve (Fig. 20.10)

- The final lateral attachments will be detached.
- If any resistance is perceived, the tumor should continue to be further dissected.

Step 9: Reconstruct the Orbit With a Nasoseptal Flap, If Required

- The flap may be harvested from the contralateral nare at the same time as the creation of the septal window.

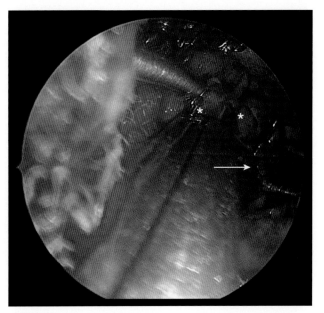

Fig. 20.10. Endoscopic view of the right orbit demonstrating the lesion *(asterisk)* being retracted anteriorly in a plane parallel to the optic nerve *(arrow)*.

- Strong consideration of reconstruction should be given following extensive dissection of lesions of the mid and anterior orbit. Dissection adjacent to the annulus of Zinn and optic canal may not mandate reconstruction. The goals of reconstruction are to prevent postoperative loss of orbital volume with resultant enophthalmos and/or diplopia.

Step 10: Nasal Packing May Be Cautiously Used

- While packing can help keep the nasoseptal flap in place, it can also increase the intraocular pressure in the setting of progressive postoperative bleeding and edema. If packing is used, the direct pressure applied to the orbitotomy should be minimized.

COMPLICATIONS

- Bleeding
- Diplopia
- Enophthalmos
- Incomplete resection
- Visual impairment
- Ophthalmic artery or internal carotid injury
- Cerebrospinal fluid (CSF) leak

POSTOPERATIVE CONSIDERATIONS

- In the immediate postoperative period, the greatest concern is for bleeding or swelling, resulting in optic nerve impingement. Serial eye exams should be performed, and the surgeon should have a low threshold for exploration if nerve compression is suspected.

■ In the setting of evidence of significant intraoperative edema, postoperative corticosteroids may be utilized, although this has not been directly examined in any study to date.

■ The patient may begin gentle saline sprays in the immediate postoperative period; however, high-volume irrigations should be deferred for at least 2 weeks to allow the orbitotomy to heal.

■ The initial débridement between postoperative days 5 to 8 should focus on establishment of an inferior nasal airway. Débridement of clot and fibrinous debris adjacent to the orbitotomy should be deferred until postoperative weeks 3 to 4.

REFERENCES

Access the reference list online at ExpertConsult.com.

Sinonasal Tumors

Endoscopic Medial Maxillectomy

Elisabeth H. Ference and Kevin C. Welch

INTRODUCTION

- Medial maxillectomy is a procedure historically used for the removal of benign and low-grade malignant tumors of the medial aspect of the maxilla, lateral nasal wall, ethmoid sinuses along the lamina papyracea, and the lacrimal sac.[1,2]
- The endoscopic approach allows superior illumination and magnification as well as the ability to treat diseases that extend beyond the limits of the traditional external medial maxillectomy.[3,4]
- The endoscopic medial maxillectomy (EMM) procedure extends maxillary antrostomy (i.e., mega-antrostomy) that is typically performed in endoscopic sinus surgery for chronic rhinosinusitis.
- Indications for EMM are comparable to those indicated for a conventional medial maxillectomy: sinonasal neoplasms, inverted papilloma, and intractable inflammatory maxillary disease.

ANATOMY[5]

- The maxillary sinus usually consists of a single pyramidal chamber with an adult volume of approximately 15 mm.
- The medial maxillary wall contains the natural ostium of the maxillary sinus and includes the uncinate process (mucosa and bone), posterior fontanelle (mucosa only), the inferior turbinate, the perpendicular plate of the palatine bone, and the lacrimal bone. The natural ostium of the maxillary sinus is located along the inferior ⅓ of the medial maxillary line (Fig. 21.1).
- The uncinate process is a thin, sagittally oriented sickle-shaped bone that forms the medial boundary of the infundibulum, which is a functional space into which the maxillary sinus and anterior ethmoid sinuses drain.
- The lateral apex of the sinus extends into the zygomatic process of the maxillary bone. The roof of the

maxillary sinus is formed by the bony orbital floor, and the floor is formed by the alveolar and palatine processes of the maxilla.
- The inferior turbinate arises from the medial maxillary bone as the maxilloturbinal.
- The distal opening of the lacrimal apparatus is the Hasner valve, located in the inferior meatus, 30 to 35 mm posterior to the limen nasi.

PREOPERATIVE CONSIDERATIONS

- An endoscopic medial maxillectomy is performed with hypotensive anesthesia, as it has been shown to improve the intraoperative field. The use of total intravenous anesthesia (TIVA) has been shown to reduce intraoperative blood loss in a number of studies.[6]
- Preoperatively, the nose is decongested topically with 0.05% oxymetazoline or 4% topical cocaine or 1:1000 epinephrine prior to endoscopy. The mucosa of the inferior turbinate and lateral nasal wall is infiltrated with 1% lidocaine with 1:100,000 epinephrine, which can reduce the amount of bleeding during resection.
- A transoral pterygopalatine injection can be performed by inserting a 25-gauge needle bent at 2.5 cm into the greater palatine foramen, opposite the second molar to provide additional vascular control. Alternatively, sphenopalatine injection can be performed by inserting a 25-gauge spinal needle bent at 1 cm inferior to the junction of the middle turbinate and lateral wall in the mucosa overlying the crista ethmoidalis. Care must be taken to avoid an intravascular injection of this local anesthetic.
- A septoplasty may be performed if a septal deflection is preventing access to the middle meatus. However, consideration must be given to the potential need for a septal window, which can be used to access the lateral and anterior portions of the maxillary sinus.[7]

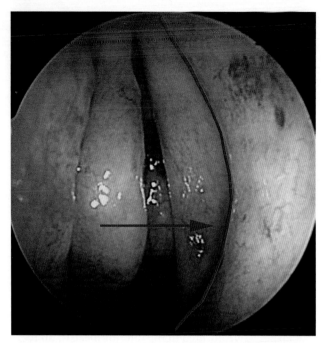

Fig. 21.1. Endoscopic view of the left middle meatus with a 0-degree telescope. The maxillary line *(curved red line)* marks the attachment of the uncinate process. The arrow points to the approximate location of the true maxillary os.

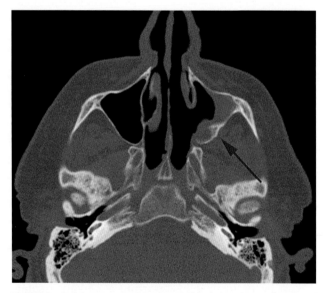

Fig. 21.2. Axial computed tomographic image revealing focal bony hyperostosis *(arrow)*, which suggests the attachment site of an inverted papilloma.

Radiographic Considerations

- All patients should undergo computed tomography (CT) imaging. In patients with inverted papilloma, this is very helpful in determining the site of attachment since hyperostosis (Fig. 21.2) has been reported to be associated with the origin of the tumor.[8] The CT scan should also be examined for any focal bony

erosion, as this is concerning for malignant transformation of the tumor. All boundaries of the sinus must be inspected for tumor.

- Magnetic resonance imaging (MRI) helps the surgeon distinguish tumor from inspissated secretions or polypoid mucoperiosteal thickening and reveals the status of extranasal tissue when sinus bone is eroded.
- CT showed the highest sensitivity for the site of attachment of inverted papillomas, while MRI showed greater specificity.[9] Preoperative CT plus MRI may provide more useful information than CT or MRI alone if the site of surgical attachment may change the planned operative approach.
- Stereotactic image guidance can be helpful to ensure that all regions of the maxillary sinus are addressed (Fig. 21.3).

INSTRUMENTATION

- 0-, 30-, and 70-degree telescopes
- Ball-tip probe
- Backbiting and downbiting punches (Fig. 21.4)
- Through-cutting punches (Fig. 21.5)
- Endoscopic scissors
- Tissue shaver with 15- and 70-degree drill attachments
- Curettes (Fig. 21.6)
- Ophthalmic crescent knife or keratome

PEARLS

- Meticulous preoperative analysis of CT and MRI scans and individual anatomy is essential for adequate surgery.
- The endoscopic technique can maintain key oncologic principles by performing complete resection of the tumor pedicle and allowing adequate margin control with the use of frozen sections intraoperatively.[10,11]
- Preserving a nasal floor mucosal flap aids in covering exposed bone after the case.
- Multiple expanded endoscopic techniques exist to reach the anterolateral aspects of the maxillary sinus, including the transseptal,[7] inferior meatal window approach,[12,13] endoscopic canine fossa puncture,[14] endoscopic anterior maxillotomy,[15] and the endoscopic Denker approach.[16]

POTENTIAL PITFALLS

- Knowledge of sinonasal anatomy is paramount as tumors such as inverted papillomas can often distort

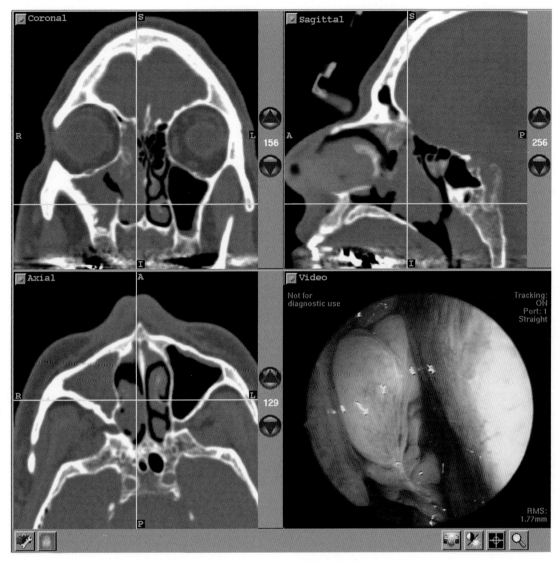

Fig. 21.3. Triplanar images are essential for completing an endoscopic medial maxillectomy. All portions of the maxillary and ethmoid sinuses must be examined for disease.

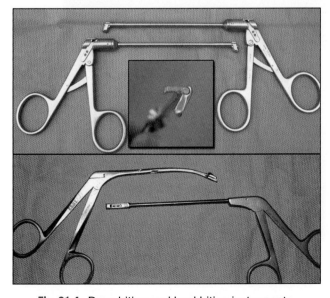

Fig. 21.4. Downbiting and backbiting instruments.

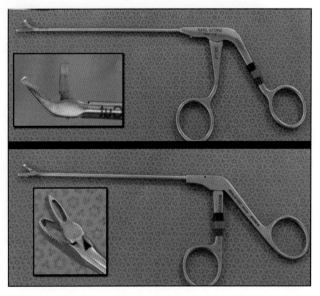

Fig. 21.5. Through-cutting instruments, straight and angled.

the normal anatomy and can lead to iatrogenic injuries to surrounding structures.

- Poor preoperative analysis of the CT and MRI scans can result in inadequate disease resection.
- Intraoperative injury to the lacrimal apparatus can cause postoperative epiphora and lead to dacryocystitis. A dacryocystorhinostomy should be performed at the time of resection if injury is suspected.
- Inadequate exposure can limit the use of instrumentation necessary for complete tumor resection and, furthermore, hinder postoperative surveillance of disease recurrence.
- Postoperative lateralization of the middle turbinate with synechiae formation can lead to inaccessibility of the mega-antrostomy for surveillance.

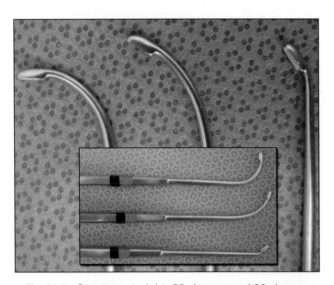

Fig. 21.6. Curettes: straight, 55-degree, and 90-degree.

- Endoscopic surgery has limitations, and the anterior recesses of the maxillary sinus are often inaccessible with an endoscopic medial maxillectomy alone. Reaching these areas requires an alternative or an adjunctive approach. This may come in the form of an external Caldwell-Luc approach or by use of the modified Denker approach.

SURGICAL STEPS

Step 1: Debulk the Tumor or Polyps

- Reflect the middle turbinate toward the septum and inspect the middle meatus. As the initial step, debulk any tumor with a tissue shaver to locate the site of attachment (Fig. 21.7). Take individual biopsies and collect all sinonasal contents in a suction trap.

Step 2: Remove the Uncinate Process and Identify the Natural Ostium

- Resect the uncinate process with a backbiting instrument and identify the natural os of the maxillary sinus using a 30-degree telescope (Fig. 21.8).
- Widen the natural ostium with through-cutting forceps or the microdébrider posteriorly and inferiorly (Fig. 21.9).

Step 3: Identify the Hasner Valve

- Once a wide antrostomy is performed, identify the Hasner valve in the inferior meatus (Fig. 21.10). The valve is located approximately 30 to 35 mm posterior to the limen nasi.
- If the tumor involves the nasolacrimal duct, sacrifice it and perform a dacryocystorhinostomy after the

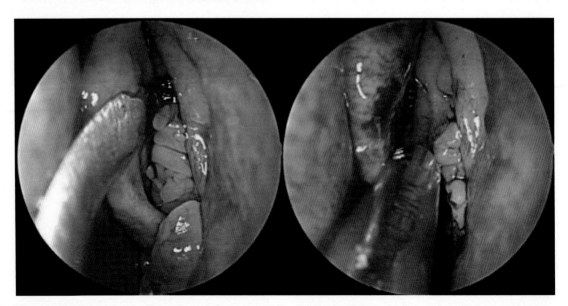

Fig. 21.7. The middle turbinate is reflected medially to reveal the contents of the middle meatus. Polyps and tumor can be debulked with instruments or the tissue shaver.

procedure to prevent epiphora. (Often, a clean transection of the lacrimal duct will result in a functional lacrimal apparatus.)

Step 4: Perform a Subtotal Inferior Turbinectomy

- Perform a subtotal inferior turbinectomy. Clamp the inferior turbinate with a hemostat at the junction of the anterior ⅓ and the posterior ⅔ of the inferior turbinate (Fig. 21.11).
- Incise the turbinate with endoscopic scissors along the crushed line toward the antrostomy, just posterior to the lacrimal duct or maxillary line (Fig. 21.12).

- After incising the inferior turbinate to the lateral nasal wall (Fig. 21.13A), continue incising the inferior turbinate until the medial pterygoid plate and posterior wall of the maxillary sinus is reached. Reflect the inferior turbinate superiorly or laterally (Fig. 21.13B), and then excise the inferior turbinate.
- Inspect the Hasner valve once more to ensure that it has not been damaged (Fig. 21.14).
- A suction Bovie or bipolar is often needed to cauterize the posterior stump of the inferior turbinate where a branch of the sphenopalatine artery enters. The anterior terminus of the inferior turbinate may also require electrocautery.

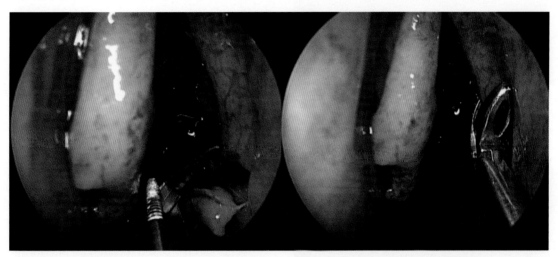

Fig. 21.8. The uncinate process is resected using a backbiter and a forceps.

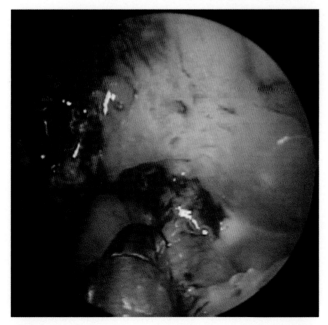

Fig. 21.9. The angled tissue shaver can be used to enlarge the antrostomy back to the pterygoid plates and down to the level of the inferior turbinate.

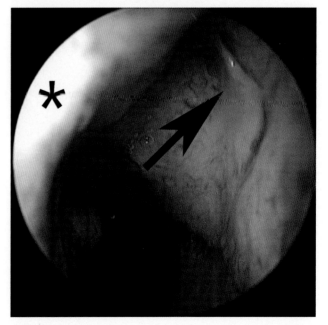

Fig. 21.10. The inferior turbinate (*) is elevated and the location of Hasner valve *(arrow)* is identified. The valve resembles a mucosal flap.

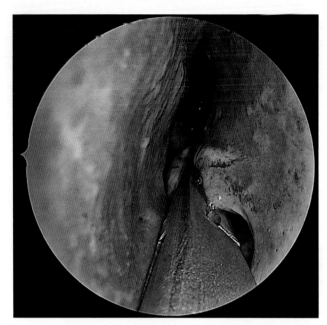

Fig. 21.11. The inferior turbinate is incised along the junction of the anterior ⅓ and posterior ⅔, just posterior to the Hasner valve.

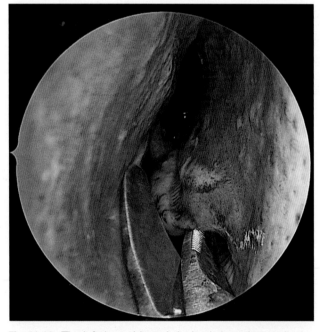

Fig. 21.12. The inferior turbinate is incised along the crushed line. The incision through the inferior turbinate is directed into the maxillary antrostomy, just posterior to the lacrimal canal.

Step 5: Create a Nasal Floor Mucosal Flap

- Incise the lateral nasal wall and the floor of the nasal cavity with an ophthalmic crescent knife or keratome at the posterior-most limit of the intended medial maxillectomy, which is near the pterygoid bone and the posterior wall of the maxillary sinus (Fig. 21.15).
- Design a similar lateral nasal wall and nasal floor incision at the anterior-most limit of the medial

maxillectomy, which is typically just posterior to the Hasner valve (Fig. 21.16).
- Incise the mucosa superiorly with a blade between the posterior and anterior lateral wall/floor incisions (Fig. 21.17).
- Elevate the mucosal flap (Fig. 21.18A) and drape the flap along the septum (Fig. 21.18B) to protect it from being injured during further medial maxillary wall resection.

Step 6: Mega-Antrostomy

- Using downbiting instruments and a high-speed irrigating drill, resect the medial maxillary wall until it is flush with the floor of the nasal cavity (Fig. 21.19).
- The Hasner valve is situated in the superior aspect of the inferior meatus. The Hasner valve and the distal aspect of the lacrimal duct may be sacrificed depending on the nature of the disease and/or the need for access. When the lacrimal apparatus is preserved, extend the resection of the medial maxillary wall inferior to the Hasner valve with a backbiting instrument (Fig. 21.20).

Step 7: Adjunctive Approaches: Inferior Meatal Window, Septal Window, Canine Fossa Puncture, Anterior Maxillotomy, and the Denker Approach

- Visualization with a 70-degree endoscope is performed through the mega-antrostomy while instruments can be passed through an inferior meatal window to access disease in the most anterior-lateral aspects of the maxillary sinus.[11,12]
- The concept of using 70-degree endoscopes and 90-degree or 120-degree currettes or microdébrider blades in the management of maxillary tumors is evolving to favor direct surgical access and the use of endoscopic drills to remove disease.
- Multiple factors affect the selection of adjunctive approaches, including the geometry and degree of pneumatization of the maxillary sinus, tumor extent into the anterior recesses of the antrum, and willingness of the surgeon and patient to perform an endoscopic dacryocystorhinostomy (DCR).
- If the tumor is known preoperatively or intraoperatively to involve the anterior-lateral maxillary wall, these regions can be addressed endoscopically through a septal window (Fig. 21.21).[7] A septal window allows for the utilization of 0-degree endoscopes and 15-degree drills in most cases but requires anterior septal reconstruction.[7]
- Alternatively, surgical access can be improved via an endoscopically created canine fossa puncture.[14] The infraorbital nerve can be protected by making the puncture at the intersection of the midpupillary line and the horizontal line through the floor of the nasal vestibule. A 1-cm sublabial mucosal incision

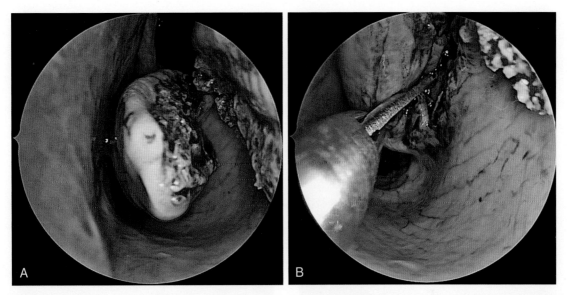

Fig. 21.13. The head of the inferior turbinate is separated from the anterior portion of the maxilloturbinal **(A)**, and the remaining portion of the inferior turbinate is excised with the endoscopic scissors **(B)**.

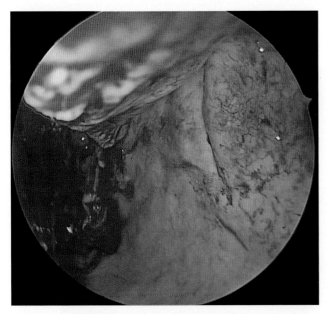

Fig. 21.14. Hasner valve is identified again prior to making incisions in the lateral nasal wall mucosa.

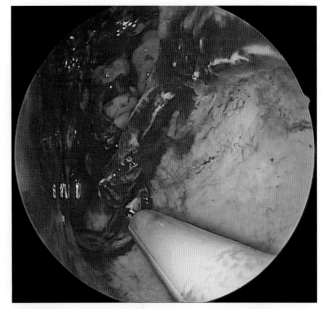

Fig. 21.15. An angled Beaver blade or keratome is used to make an incision in the posterior portion of the lateral nasal wall mucosa and extended along the floor of the nasal cavity.

is made approximately 1 cm above the gingival margin, a suction Freer elevator is used to elevate the soft tissue in the subperiosteal plane, and a trephine is made in the maxilla using an osteotome or a drill. This trephine can then be used to introduce an instrument while visualization is obtained through the maxillary antrostomy or, conversely, a scope can be introduced while an instrument is placed through the antrostomy. While this procedure is less invasive than maxillotomy approaches and involves less risk to the nasolacrimal duct

compared to the Denker approach, it does not provide as much access to the anterolateral aspect of the sinus due to the remaining bone.[7] The location of the tumor is also an important consideration, as the trephine may come through the tumor in its approach.[7] Moreover, this approach may lead to labial swelling and injury to the anterosuperior alveolar nerve. It also creates a temporary communication between the sinus and the oral cavity, with the risk of contamination with oral flora and an oroantral fistula.

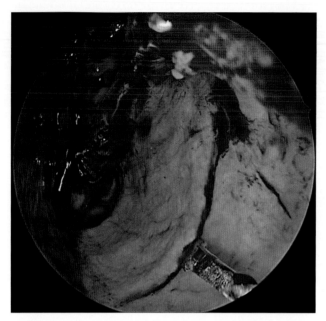

Fig. 21.16. The angled Beaver blade or keratome is then used to make a similar incision through the mucosa of the anterior lateral nasal wall and floor, just posterior to Hasner valve.

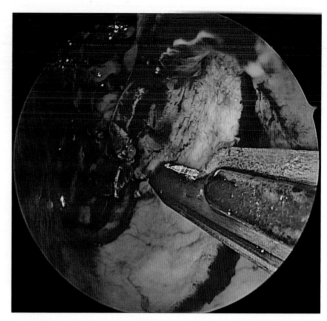

Fig. 21.17. A blade is used to incise the mucosal just inferior to the maxilloturbinal strut to connect the previously made posterior and anterior lateral nasal wall mucosal incisions.

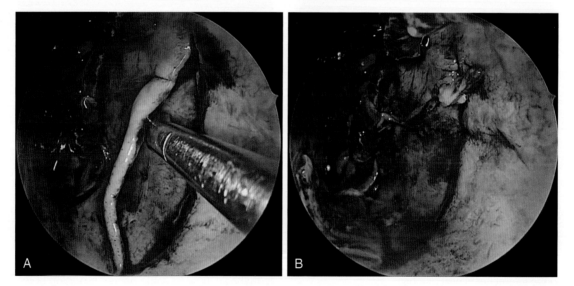

Fig. 21.18. An elevator is used to perform a subperiosteal dissection **(A)** to raise the lateral nasal wall/floor flap **(B)**, which is draped along the septum.

- More invasive than a canine fossa puncture and less invasive than an endoscopic Denker approach is an endoscopic anterior maxillotomy. The edge of the piriform aperture is palpated just anterior to the head of the inferior turbinate, and the mucosa is incised. A subperiosteal dissection is performed using a suction Freer elevator to expose the anterior maxilla, being careful to avoid transecting the infraorbital nerve branches. A window is created in the anterior wall of the maxilla using a 15-degree high-speed drill, being sure to stay inferior to the infraorbital nerve foramen and to preserve the main branches of the nerve. The size of the window varies based on need and can be mapped using an image guidance probe or suction.[15] The combination of an endonasal anterior maxillotomy and an endoscopic medial maxillectomy also allows for exposure of the infratemporal fossa. However, the additional dissection leads to risk to the infraorbital nerve and the possibility of cheek swelling and pain.

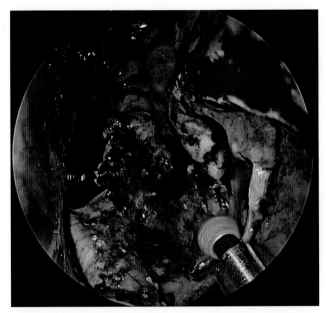

Fig. 21.19. A high-speed drill with continuous suction and irrigation is used to remove the lateral nasal wall/medial maxillary wall until the nasal floor is flush with the maxillary sinus cavity.

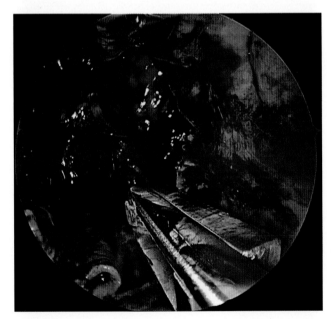

Fig. 21.20. A back-biting instrument may be used to extend the mega-antrostomy in an anterior direction. Care must be taken to avoid Hasner valve and remove bone and mucosa inferior to the valve.

- Alternatively, an endoscopic Denker maxillotomy approach can provide similar access as a septal window.[16] This procedure involves removal of the medial buttress with preservation of the lacrimal apparatus and is covered in detail in Chapter 22. However, the loss of the piriform ridge may lead to alar collapse.

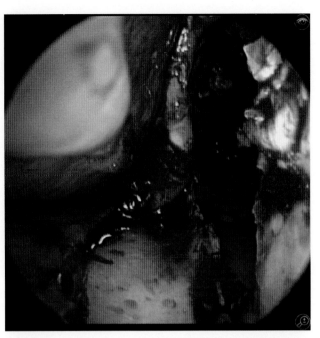

Fig. 21.21. A septal window is created in order to access the anterior and lateral maxillary sinus walls as needed. (Figure courtesy of Dr. Richard Harvey, Sydney ENT Clinic.)

- A study by Prosser et al. found that, compared to a maxillary antrostomy, a medial maxillectomy increased the exposure by 18.5 degrees, on average, and a 1-cm Denker approach provided an additional 33.5 degrees of exposure and access to the entire posterolateral wall in 54% of cases.[17] Equivalent access was obtained via a contralateral approach with a septotomy at approximately 1.56 cm from the columella.[17]

Step 8: Removal of the Tumor Pedicle
- Inverted papilloma may infiltrate the underlying bone at the site of attachment and harbor occult tumor; therefore, this bone must be removed. A high-speed suction–irrigation diamond bur is used to thin the bone along the attachment site of the tumor in order to address these histologic nests (Fig. 21.22).
- Upon completion, the mucosal flap is replaced and draped into the maxillary defect (Fig. 21.23).

Step 9: Ethmoid Involvement
- Ethmoid involvement is addressed simultaneously during this approach; this represents the superior-most aspect of the resection.
- If the tumor is attached to any degree to the lamina papyracea, the site is resected along with the bone itself to expose the periorbital. Bone may be removed with hand instruments or drilled down with the suction–irrigation bur.

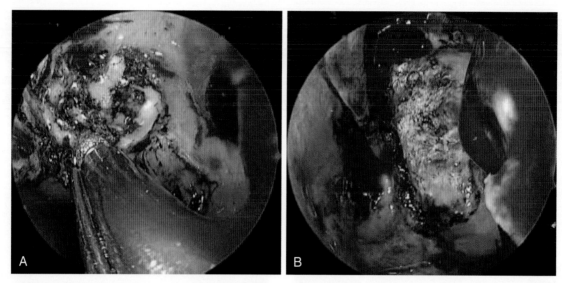

Fig. 21.22. Endoscopic images showing removal of the tumor pedicle. **(A)** The pedicle is resected and the surrounding bone drilled away to remove nests of tumor within the bone. **(B)** The area of attachment has been drilled down.

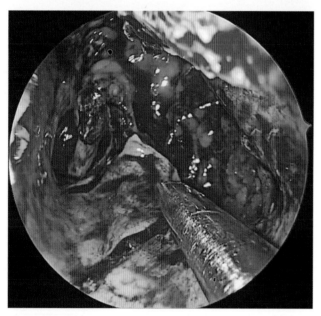

Fig. 21.23. At the termination of the procedure, the nasal floor flap is draped over the denuded bone of the medial maxillary/lateral nasal wall and floor to help with postoperative healing and to prevent excessive crusting.

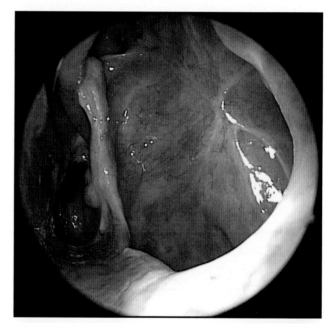

Fig. 21.24. Once healed, a well-designed medial maxillectomy cavity allows sufficient endoscopic evaluation of the tumor origin and surgical site for multiple years of surveillance.

Step 10: Endoscopic Dacryocystorhinostomy (When Necessary)

- When the nasolacrimal duct is transected, a DCR is advised to prevent postoperative nasolacrimal duct stenosis.
- The steps in DCR are described in Chapter 17 and include removing the remainder of the lacrimal bone, cannulating the nasolacrimal duct, and vertically incising the duct with eversion of the duct mucosa.
- In formal DCR, Crawford tubes are placed to stent the open duct, but this step is often unnecessary.

POSTOPERATIVE CONSIDERATIONS

- Postoperative care of the patient involves irrigation with saline solution to remove clots and crusts, followed by serial in-office débridements.[18]
- Long-term surveillance for inverted papilloma recurrence or for any malignant transformation is indicated in these patients (Fig. 21.24).

REFERENCES

Access the reference list online at ExpertConsult.com.

Endoscopic Denker Approach for Anterior Maxilla Tumors

Jivianne T. Lee and Alexander G. Chiu

INTRODUCTION

- Despite recent advances in endoscopic techniques, tumors involving the anterior maxilla remain difficult to reach through a purely endonasal approach.
- Even with cross-court procedures, lesions involving the anteroinferior and anterolateral corners of the maxillary sinus may be inaccessible endoscopically.[1,2]
- Sublabial incisions with canine fossa puncture or a Caldwell-Luc approach are often still necessary for surgical removal of anteriorly based maxillary pathology.[3,4]
- The endoscopic Denker approach is a technique that involves creation of an endonasal anterior maxillotomy without the need for a separate sublabial incision.[2,5]
- With this technique, complete exposure of the anterior maxilla is attained as well as the entire lateral and posterior walls of the maxillary sinus, enabling direct access to both the pterygopalatine and infratemporal fossae.

GENERAL PRINCIPLES

- The anteromedial maxillectomy was first described by Alfred Denker in 1906.[6] It involved removal of the ethmoids, lateral nasal wall, and middle and inferior turbinates through a gingivobuccal sulcus incision that was extended medially to the frenulum.
- In 1908, Sturmann and Canfield introduced an endonasal procedure to expose the anterior maxilla.[7,8]
  - An intranasal incision was made posterior to the vestibule.
  - Subperiosteal elevation was then performed laterally over the pyriform aperture into the canine fossa to access the anterior wall of the maxillary sinus.

- The endoscopic Denker approach is somewhat of an amalgamation of these two techniques, with the added feature of being performed completely under endoscopic visualization.[2,5] It has also been referred to as a total endoscopic anterior medial maxillectomy (TEAMM).
- A mucosal incision is initially made along the pyriform aperture followed by elevation of the soft tissues overlying the anterior maxilla in the subperiosteal plane.
- An endoscopic endonasal anterior maxillotomy is then created, taking care to preserve the anterosuperior alveolar and infraorbital nerves.[2]
- The size and position of the maxillotomy may then be adjusted according to the location and extent of the lesion.

SURGICAL TECHNIQUE

Step 1: Mucosal Cuts

- Under visualization with a 4-mm 0-degree rod-lens endoscope (Karl Storz Endoscopy, Tuttlingen, Germany), 1% lidocaine HCL with 1:100,000 epinephrine is first injected into the anticipated incision sites along the nasal floor, lateral nasal wall, and anterior to the head of the inferior turbinate (Fig. 22.1A).
- A unipolar electrocautery with a guarded needle tip (Megadyne, Draper, Utah) is used to incise the mucosa inferiorly at the junction of the nasal floor and lateral nasal wall, carrying the incision through the periosteum (Fig. 22.1B).
- A second mucosal incision is then made superiorly along the lateral nasal wall and carried anteroinferiorly to lie just in front of the anterior head of the inferior turbinate overlying the edge of the pyriform aperture (see Fig. 22.1B).

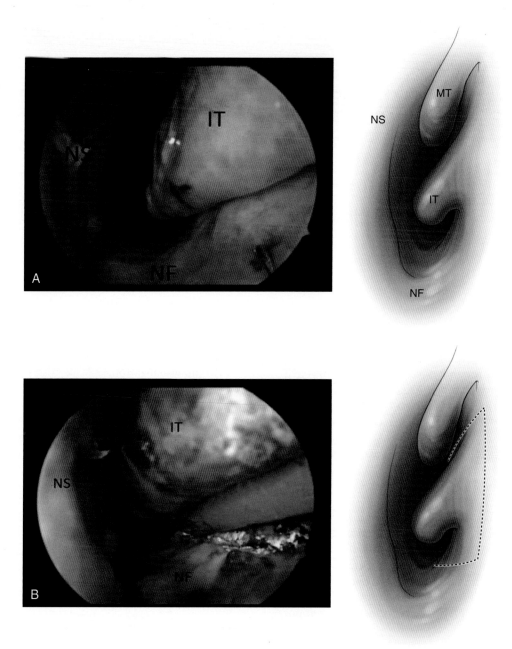

Fig. 22.1. (A) Anatomy of the left nasal cavity. **(B)** Intranasal incisions are made with cautery along the dotted lines and carried through the periosteum. Specifically, an inferior incision is made at the junction of the nasal floor and lateral nasal wall, followed by a superior incision along the lateral nasal wall and anteriorly overlying the pyriform aperture. *IT,* Inferior turbinate; *M,* middle turbinate; *NF,* nasal floor; *NS,* nasal septum.

Step 2: Soft Tissue Dissection Over the Maxilla

■ A subperiosteal dissection is performed with a suction Freer elevator to expose the anterior maxilla, the infraorbital foramen, and its neurovascular bundle as well as the lateral nasal wall (Figs. 22.2A and B).

Step 3: Bony Cuts to the Maxilla

■ A high-speed drill or osteotome is utilized to create a bony window into the anterior maxilla, taking care to stay inferior to the infraorbital nerve (ION) (Fig. 22.2C).

■ Burs or osteotomes are used to connect the window to the inferior bony cut of the medial maxillectomy, thereby allowing access to the anterior portion of the maxillary sinus.

■ In the accompanying video to this book, a recurrent inverted papilloma can be seen pedicled to the anteroinferior corner of the maxillary sinus.

■ Once the tumor is dissected free from the surrounding tissue and the site of attachment is identified, the remaining bony and mucosal cuts are

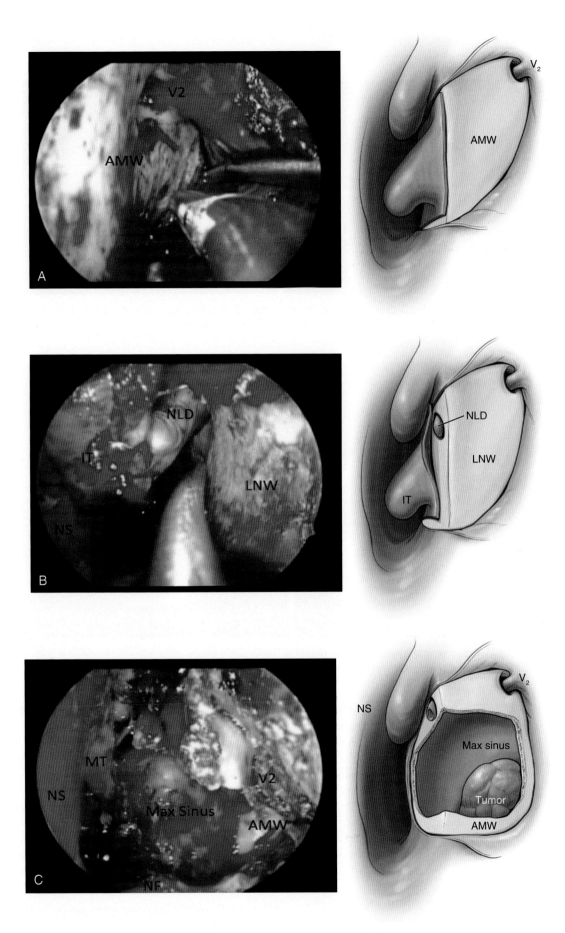

Fig. 22.2. **(A)** Elevating the mucosa off of the maxilla using a suction Freer. **(B)** Elevating the mucosa off of the lateral nasal wall. The nasolacrimal duct should be cut sharply once exposed. **(C)** Drilling is completed to expose the maxillary sinus. *AMW,* Anterior maxillary sinus wall; *IT,* inferior turbinate; *LNW,* lateral nasal wall; *NLD,* nasolacrimal duct; *NS,* nasal septum; *V2,* infraorbital nerve.

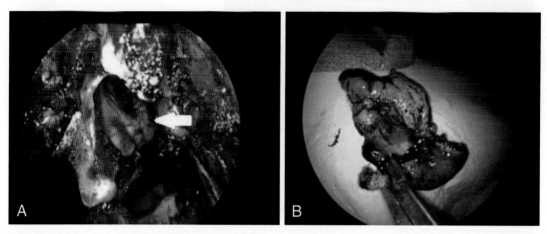

Fig. 22.3. (A) Intraoperative view with a 0-degree rigid nasal endoscope illustrating exposure of the inverted papilloma *(arrow)* and **(B)** en bloc resection of the lesion using the endoscopic Denker approach.

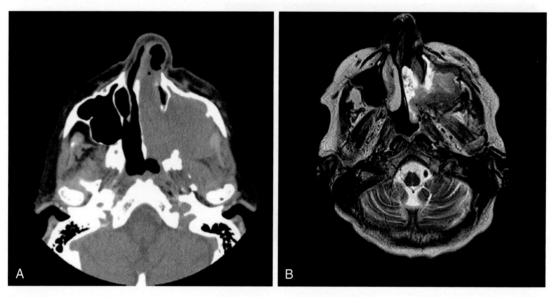

Fig. 22.4. (A) Axial computed tomography scan and **(B)** magnetic resonance image of an inverted papilloma with squamous cell carcinoma extending to the pterygopalatine and infratemporal fossae.

completed with burs, osteotomes, and endoscopic scissors, respectively. Specifically, a superior cut is made at the level of the roof of the maxillary sinus, an inferior cut at the junction of the nasal floor and medial maxillary wall, and a posterior cut along the posterior wall of the maxillary sinus. The lesion can then be resected en bloc along with its bony site of attachment, using straight instrumentation (Fig. 22.3).

- At the end of the procedure, the nasolacrimal duct is identified, preserved, and sharply cut at an oblique angle to prevent stenosis.
- Complete exposure of the posterior aspect of the maxillary sinus is also achieved, facilitating use of a 4-handed technique to remove tumors involving the pterygopalatine or infratemporal fossae if needed (Fig. 22.4A and B).

COMPARISON TO OTHER ENDOSCOPIC PROCEDURES

- A variety of endoscopic procedures have been recently described that provide incremental increase in access to the anterolateral portion of the maxillary sinus.
- Modified and total endoscopic medial maxillectomies (MEMM and TEMM, respectively) augment exposure of the maxillary sinus over standard antrostomy, with TEMM conferring an additional 12 degrees of anterolateral reach beyond MEMM.

"Cross-Court"/Transseptal Approaches

- These approaches have been introduced to capitalize on the additional access gained from passing instruments through the contralateral nostril.

- Robinson et al. reported on the use of nonopposing septal incisions to facilitate endoscopic tumor resection.[3]
- Harvey et al. presented an anterior transseptal technique to access anterolateral maxillary lesions in a cadaveric study[1] (Fig. 22.5A and B).
  - An inferiorly based U-shaped septal flap is elevated on the ipsilateral side and a large posteriorly based flap on the opposite side.
  - A cartilaginous septal window is created, through which an endoscope and instruments can be passed from the contralateral nostril.
  - This technique expanded surgical access by 14.7 degrees compared to ipsilateral procedures, with access to the area lateral to the ION and anterior maxilla improving from 63% to 98% and 25% to 95%, respectively.
  - Disadvantages
    - Patients with scarring from prior septal surgery or trauma may not be candidates for transseptal procedures.[1]
    - Transseptal approaches typically require use of angled telescopes, which may be technically difficult to maneuver, and the corresponding curved instruments may not have the precise size and angle needed to reach the specific area of interest.
- Septal dislocation: Ramakrishnan et al. proposed the use of septal dislocation to increase access to the anterolateral maxillary sinus[9] (Figs. 22.6 and 22.7).
  - The cartilaginous septum is detached inferiorly from the maxillary crest and posteriorly at the bony-cartilaginous junction, allowing lateral mobilization of the septum to the opposite side.
  - Minimally angled endoscopes and instruments can then be passed through the ipsilateral nostril to reach the anterolateral maxillary sinus and infratemporal fossa.
  - Overall, septal dislocation added another 20 degrees of anterolateral reach compared to TEMM; and only straight instrumentation was needed to access the anterior maxillary sinus. The additional space created by septal displacement also facilitates 4-handed surgery using the same nostril.
  - Disadvantages: Septal dislocation may be restricted by variations in the concavity of the anterior maxilla and the degree of protrusion of the contralateral pyriform ridge.[9]
- Canine fossa trephination (CFT): Robinson et al. supported the use of CFT as a port of entry to access maxillary sinus pathology.[10]
  - With this technique, a trocar is placed through the canine fossa, allowing insertion of an endoscope and/or instruments through the anterior maxilla.

- Seiberling et al. presented a series of 97 patients with severe maxillary nasal polyposis successfully cleared with CFT.[11]
- Disadvantages: For lesions pedicled to the anterior wall, CFT would not enhance surgical access and potentially come through the tumor itself. In addition, CFT carries the risk of neurologic complications, with possible injury to the anterior superior alveolar and infraorbital nerves.[4,10] Neuralgia, cheek swelling, and lip paresthesias have all been reported with this procedure.[4,10,11]

ADVANTAGES OF THE ENDOSCOPIC DENKER APPROACH

- The entire anterior maxilla and prelacrimal, anterior, inferior, and lateral recesses of the maxillary sinus can be directly accessed without the need for a sublabial or transseptal incision.[5]
- The entire posterior wall of the maxillary sinus is exposed, allowing straight entry into the pterygopalatine and infratemporal fossae.[5]
- For tumors pedicled to the lateral wall, the site of attachment can be drilled without the need for angled instrumentation.
- For tumors involving the anterior wall, the lesion can be resected together with the underlying bone without going through the tumor itself.[5]
- Curved instruments are rarely necessary due to the straight trajectory of the approach.
- Current techniques for endoscopic tumor resection involve countertraction, debulking, sharp dissection, and drilling, all of which are more easily performed with straight instrumentation.
- Unlike cross-court procedures, the endoscopic Denker procedure is not limited by the concavity of the anterior maxilla nor is it dependent on the use of angled scopes.
- The anterosuperior alveolar and infraorbital nerves are better visualized, facilitating preservation of these neural structures. Higher maxillotomy placement also reduces potential injury to the alveolar plexus.
- The absence of a gingivobuccal sulcus incision prevents potential contamination of the sinus cavity with oral flora and possible development of an oroantral fistula.

COMPLICATIONS

- Cheek pain and swelling may occur, similar to sublabial maxillotomy.[2]
- Caution must also be taken to avoid damage to the infraorbital and anterosuperior alveolar nerves during creation of the antral window.

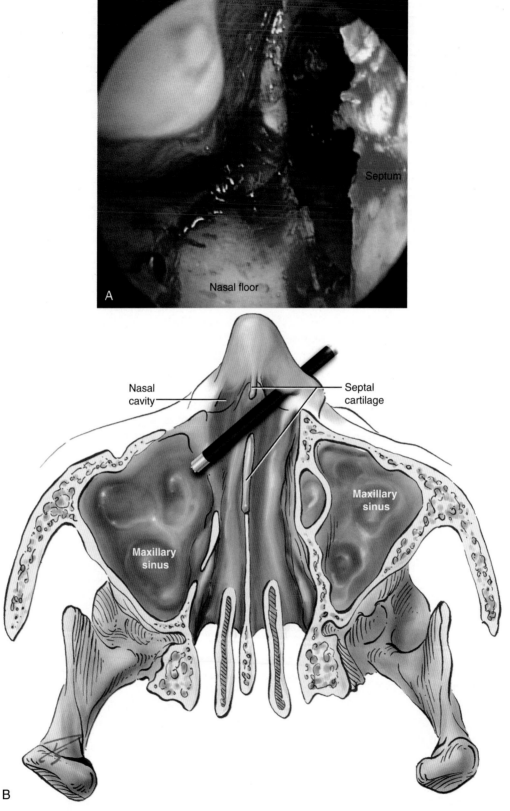

Fig. 22.5. **(A)** Endoscopic view after a septal window was created to access the anterior and lateral maxillary sinus. **(B)** Drawing in axial view showing the anterolateral access afforded by the septal window technique.

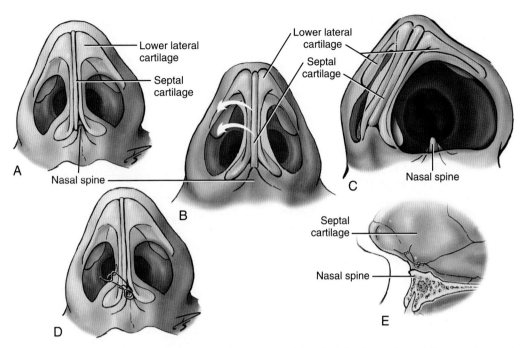

Fig. 22.6. Drawings illustrating septal translocation. **(A)** A hemitransfixion incision is made and the anterior septum is freed from the maxillary spine. **(B)** The septum and alar cartilages are dislocated. **(C)** A septal flap is raised for further posterior access. **(D, E)** Closure is obtained using a figure-eight suture.

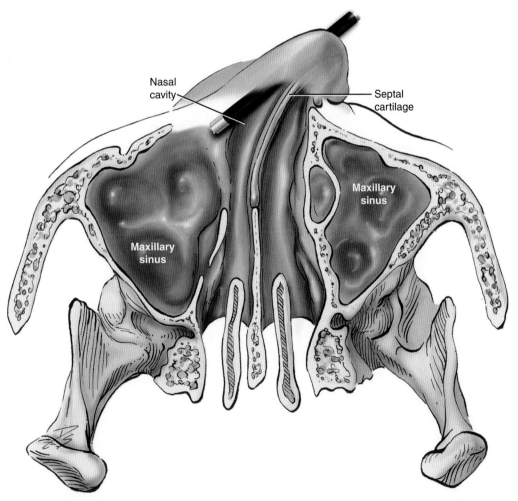

Fig. 22.7. Drawing in axial view showing the lateral-anterior access provided by the septal translocation technique. Septal translocation and septal window creation achieve the same objectives.

- Alar collapse secondary to loss of the pyriform ridge has also been reported.[12]
- Nasolacrimal duct stenosis may ensue, requiring possible dacryocystorhinostomy.

SURGICAL INDICATIONS

- As the endoscopic Denker technique essentially provides the same port of entry into the maxillary sinus as the Caldwell-Luc approach, similar surgical indications can be used for both procedures.
- Indications include:
  - Benign (i.e., inverted papilloma) or malignant tumors pedicled to the prelacrimal, anterior, inferior, or lateral recesses of the maxillary sinus
  - Lesions involving the pterygopalatine or infratemporal fossae
  - Odontogenic pathology
  - Refractory chronic rhinosinusitis with or without nasal polyposis

CONCLUSIONS

- The endoscopic Denker technique offers an innovative approach for resection of lesions involving the anterior portion of the maxillary sinus.
- Direct endonasal access to the prelacrimal, anterior, inferior, and lateral recesses of the maxillary sinus can be achieved, as well as to the pterygopalatine and infratemporal fossae.
- Adjunctive sublabial or transseptal incisions can be avoided, as well as the need for angled endoscopes and instrumentation.
- However, given the vast repertoire of endoscopic procedures currently available, choice of operative technique will ultimately depend on surgeon preference,

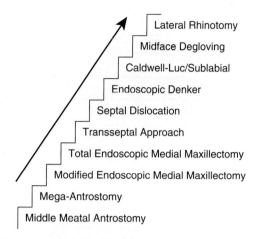

Fig. 22.8. Stepwise algorithm for surgical management of maxillary sinus lesions. Each successive procedure provides an incremental increase in access to the anterior recesses of the maxillary sinus and infratemporal fossa.

tumor extent, resection margins, and individual anatomy.
- Adoption of a stepwise algorithm for surgical management of maxillary sinus lesions is recommended. Beginning with a standard middle meatal antrostomy, one may progress to MEMM, TEMM with nasolacrimal duct resection, cross-court approaches, endoscopic Denker, and so on, in a graduated fashion, so that each successive procedure provides incremental increase in access to the anterior recesses of the maxillary sinus (Fig. 22.8).

REFERENCES

Access the reference list online at ExpertConsult.com.

Endoscopic Vidian Neurectomy

Raymond Sacks and Rahuram Sivasubramaniam

INTRODUCTION

- Vidian neurectomy has been performed to relieve the symptoms of vasomotor rhinitis since the 1960s after being introduced by Golding-Wood as a transantral procedure.[1]
- Transnasal endoscopic vidian neurectomy was introduced by Kamel and Zaher[2] and later refined by many, including El Shazly,[3] El-Guindy,[4] and Robinson and Wormald.[5]
- Better understanding of the anatomy with improving imaging modalities and better visualization of the operative field has led to decreasing complication rates and improving outcomes with endoscopic vidian neurectomies for vasomotor and allergic rhinitis.

ANATOMY

- Understanding the anatomy of the vidian canal is a key element to the approach and thus the success of the procedure (Fig. 23.1).
- The vidian nerve is formed by the confluence of the greater superficial petrosal and deep petrosal nerves and travels in the pterygoid canal carrying the parasympathetic fibers, which synapse in the pterygopalatine ganglion, and the postganglionic fibers are distributed with the branches of the maxillary nerve.
- Computed tomography (CT) scans allow for more precise appreciation of the location of the vidian nerve to the sphenoid sinus (type 1 and type 2 lying above or on the sphenoid sinus floor and type 3 canal being more embedded and deep).[6]
- The opening of the vidian canal into the pterygopalatine fossa is found at the junction of the medial pterygoid plate and the floor of the sphenoid sinus and is lateral to the smaller palatovaginal canal that houses the pharyngeal nerve, which runs in a medial to lateral direction.
- Understanding the relationship of the vidian canal and the palatovaginal canal (lies inferomedial to the

vidian canal transmitting the pharyngeal branches of the maxillary artery and pterygopalatine ganglion and is often mistaken for the vidian canal) is therefore vital for a successful outcome.

PREOPERATIVE CONSIDERATIONS

- The main indication is for refractory vasomotor rhinitis in which topical measures have failed to give adequate relief for the patient or when the patient does not tolerate or is unwilling to continue with topical treatment, such as intranasal anticholinergic sprays.
- Increasing evidence for the use of vidian neurectomy in both allergic and nonallergic rhinitis for control of watery rhinorrhea.[7]

INSTRUMENTATION

- 0-degree endoscope
- Sickle knife or a scalpel with a No. 11 blade
- Freer or Cottle dissector
- Lusk 90-degree ball probe
- 2-mm upbiting Kerrison rongeur
- Bipolar forceps
- Bone wax (Ethicon, Somerville, New Jersey)
- Surgicel (Ethicon, Somerville, New Jersey)

PEARLS AND POTENTIAL PITFALLS

- The most common error and cause of failure relates to incorrect identification of the medially placed pharyngeal nerve and therefore incorrect neurectomy.
- Relapse of symptoms at 12 to 24 months relates to neural reanastomosis and is avoided by plugging bone wax into the canal postneurectomy.
- Dry eye is a sequela rather than a complication, but while the Schirmer test always remains reduced, symptomatic dry eye typically resolves within 1 month.

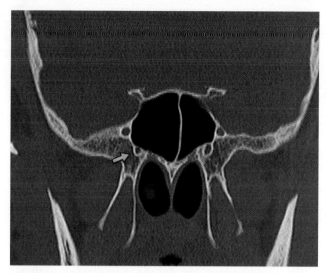

Fig. 23.1. Computed tomography (CT) scan of the paranasal sinus in coronal views with the *arrow* showing the vidian canal.

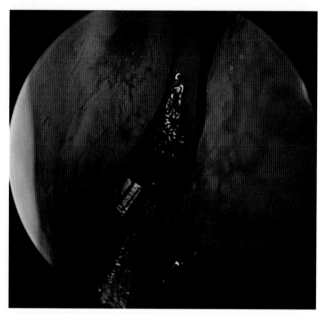

Fig. 23.2. Endoscopic image showing the uncinectomy with a backbiting instrument.

SURGICAL PROCEDURE

Step 1: Perform a Wide Maxillary Antrostomy

- Start with an uncinectomy and identify the maxillary ostium with a ostial seeker (Fig. 23.2).
- Perform maxillary antrostomy and open to the posterior wall of the maxillary sinus.

Step 2: Raise a Mucosal Flap and Ligate the Sphenopalatine Artery

- Once the maxillary antrostomy is performed, identify the posterior wall and raise a mucosal flap on the lateral nasal wall posteriorly (Fig. 23.3).

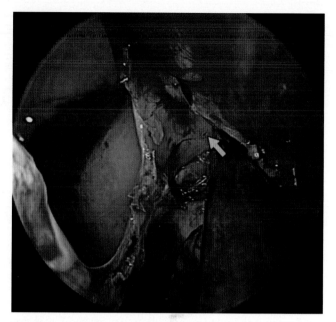

Fig. 23.3. Posterior elevation of the flap and the arrow showing the crista ethmoidalis *(arrow)*.

- The crista ethmoidalis should be identified and removed along with the posterior wall of the maxillary sinus using the 2-mm upbiting Kerrison rongeur to expose the fat of the pterygopalatine fossa along with the sphenopalatine artery.
- The artery (and adjacent branches) needs to be bipolar cauterized and transected with sickle knife or scissors (Fig. 23.4).
- The flap is then continued posteriorly.

Step 3: Identify the Pharyngeal Nerves and the Vidian Nerve

- Posterior dissection leads to the pharyngeal nerve and the vidian nerve tethering the pterygopalatine contents and preventing them from mobilizing laterally.
- The pharyngeal nerve runs laterally and thus sits at almost right angles to the vidian nerve.
- Both nerves are divided using a sickle knife.
- The artery of the vidian canal will need to be cauterized at this stage as well.
- The pterygopalatine contents can now be mobilized laterally to visualize the stumps of both structures (Fig. 23.5).
- The entire bony rim of the vidian canal should be identified to ensure that complete neural transection has occurred.

Step 4: Apply Bone Wax

- Bone wax is applied to the proximal stump of the nerve using a Freer elevator and is pushed down the canal (Fig. 23.6).
- This assists in preventing the reanastomosis between the proximal and distal stumps of the nerve.

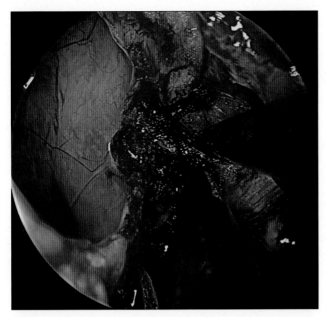

Fig. 23.4. Bipolar cauterization of the sphenopalatine artery after removing the crista ethmoidalis and partially removing the posterior wall of the maxillary sinus.

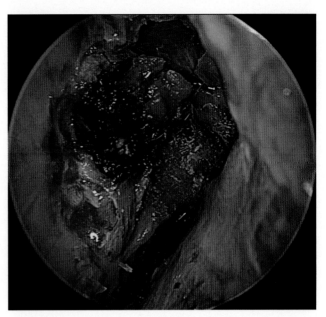

Fig. 23.6. Bone wax being applied to the proximal stumps prior to replacing the mucosal flaps.

Step 5: Replace the Mucosal Flap and Dressing

■ Hemostasis is reconfirmed and the mucosal flap can be repositioned laterally.
■ A small strip of Surgicel is placed over the flap as a dressing.

POSTOPERATIVE CONSIDERATIONS

■ Saline irrigations needs to begin on day 1 postoperatively in order to prevent crust formation.
■ Artificial tears should be used twice daily for 30 days to prevent dry eye symptoms.

REFERENCES

Access the reference list online at ExpertConsult.com.

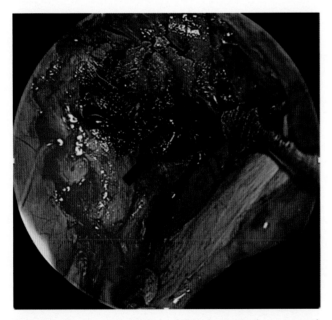

Fig. 23.5. Bipolar and dividing of the pharyngeal nerves and the vidian nerve. The pterygopalatine contents are retracted laterally, showing the proximal stumps of those nerves. The *solid arrow* shows the vidian nerve, and the *hollow arrow* shows the pharyngeal nerve.

Pterygopalatine/Pterygomaxillary Space Approaches, Maxillary Artery Ligation, and Approach to Juvenile Nasopharyngeal Angiofibroma

Edward C. Kuan, Rakesh Chandra, Bert W. O'Malley, Jr., and Nithin D. Adappa

INTRODUCTION

■ Pterygopalatine/pterygomaxillary space (PPS) approaches are used to treat lesions in areas posterior to the maxillary sinus, including the pterygopalatine fossa and lateral recess of the sphenoid sinus (LSR).[1–3] Pathologic processes within the PPS are rare; the most common ones are juvenile nasopharyngeal angiofibroma (JNA),[4–8] neurogenic tumors such as schwannoma,[9–12] and perineural extension of sinonasal malignancy.[13] A characteristic lesion found within the LSR is the encephalocele, which is commonly associated with idiopathic intracranial hypertension (IIH).[14–17]

■ Endoscopic, endonasal PPS approaches have paved the way for minimally invasive treatment of these lesions, providing excellent visualization and instrument accessibility, as well as reduced morbidity. In contrast, surgeons have traditionally used open transfacial approaches (e.g., midfacial degloving, lateral rhinotomy) with medial maxillectomy and/or subtemporal craniotomy to treat these lesions. Compared with these options, a PPS approach may obviate the need for open incisions, although at times an adjunctive canine fossa incision is a useful complement to the endoscopic approach, especially for posterolateral access.

■ Exposure of the pterygopalatine fossa through a PPS approach allows maxillary artery ligation both for management of refractory/recurrent epistaxis[18,19] and for arterial control during resection of tumors, such as JNA.

ANATOMY

■ The PPS is bounded by the posterior wall of the maxillary sinus (anterior), perpendicular plate of the palatine bone (medial), pterygoid process of the sphenoid bone (posterior), and body of the sphenoid bone (superior). Inferiorly, it is in continuity with the greater palatine canal. Laterally, it connects with the infratemporal fossa (Fig. 24.1).[20]

■ Several foramina provide passageways for neurovascular structures residing in the PPS and thus form the path of least resistance to the orbit, palate, skull base, infratemporal fossa, and nasal cavity for pathologic processes.

■ The vascular and neural structures are located anteroinferiorly and posterosuperiorly, respectively, within the PPS. The sphenopalatine artery, a terminal branch of the maxillary artery, is found between the sphenoid and palatine bones and enters the nasal cavity at the sphenopalatine foramen. If access posterior to the artery is necessary (e.g., LSR), then once the artery is identified it can sometimes be retracted down. However, it will often need to be divided and ligated, as simple retraction may increase the risk of arterial avulsion and subsequent hemorrhage.

■ The maxillary artery is a terminal branch of the external carotid system. In traditional anatomic nomenclature, it has been referred to as the internal maxillary artery.

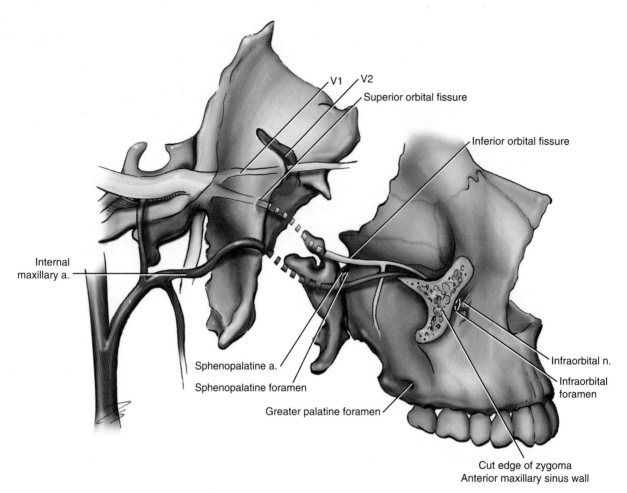

Fig. 24.1. Anatomic drawing showing the relationship of the pterygopalatine space to the adjacent sphenoid, maxillary, and palatine bones. Note the course of the maxillary artery and V_2 through the potential space, which can be enlarged by pathologic processes. *a.*, Artery; *n.*, nerve.

- The maxillary division of the trigeminal nerve (V_2) and the vidian nerve emanate from the posterior wall of the space, from the foramen rotundum (superomedial) and the pterygoid canal (inferolateral), respectively. They form the pterygopalatine ganglion and branch into the infraorbital nerve exiting through the inferior orbital fissure and the greater and lesser palatine nerves passing through the correspondingly named foramina. Through these terminal branches, the maxillary nerve provides sensation to the cheek skin, lower eyelid, upper lip, nasal sidewall, and hard and soft palate. The vidian contributors traveling with the maxillary branches produce secretory function of the lacrimal, nasal, and palatal glands. The vidian canal is found within the floor of the sphenoid sinus and can often be identified by elevating the mucosa overlying the anterior face of the sphenoid sinus off the bone in an inferolateral direction.
- Posterior to the PPS, pneumatization of the lateral portion of the sphenoid bone can result, forming a lateral sphenoid recess. This is observed in up to 25% to 48% of patients; the bone is extensively pneumatized in 8% of cases.[21] The roof of this space can lie directly beneath the temporal lobe in the middle cranial fossa and is a common location for middle cranial fossa encephaloceles.

PREOPERATIVE CONSIDERATIONS

- The need for transfusion should be anticipated given the proximity to the maxillary arterial system and pterygoid venous plexus, especially for vascular lesions such as a JNA. Preoperative angiography and embolization may be necessary with certain pathologic processes such as JNA.[22–24]
- Neurosurgical consultation should be strongly considered, particularly in the setting of an encephalocele or cerebrospinal fluid (CSF) leak, or if there is intracranial extension of pathology.
- Magnetic resonance imaging (MRI) and computed tomography (CT) should both be performed; image-guided

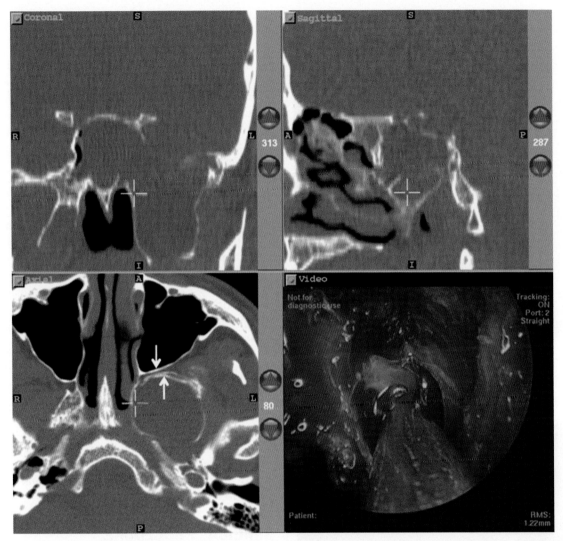

Fig. 24.2. Triplanar computed tomography (CT) images showing a large, complex lateral sphenoid recess meningoencephalocele splaying the pterygoid plates. The endoscopic view *(lower right)* reveals the fluorescein-stained sac, which has been exposed by removal of the posterior wall of the maxillary sinus and bone of the pterygoid root. These bony layers are indicated by *white arrows* on the axial CT image *(lower left)*.

surgical navigation is useful intraoperatively. When an LSR encephalocele is being addressed, intrathecal administration of diluted fluorescein may be necessary to identify or confirm the site of the leak intraoperatively (Fig. 24.2).

- Whether a nasoseptal flap will be necessary for skull base reconstruction should be determined. The flap may be raised at the beginning of surgery and tucked posterolaterally (i.e., in the nasopharynx) for the remainder of the procedure to avoid trauma to the flap while the approach is performed.

- The patient should be counseled on the possible sequelae of PPS approaches, including ipsilateral palatal or cheek numbness or dry eye.

Radiographic Considerations

- High-resolution CT images should be obtained using a stereotactic navigational protocol (1-mm axial slices). Neurogenic tumors in the PPS will characteristically enlarge the bony openings as they pass through foramina, which is often visible on CT imaging studies (Fig. 24.3).[25]

- MRI will better define soft tissue structures, including perineural spread of a sinonasal or skull base neoplasm (Fig. 24.4). Adenoid cystic carcinoma is notorious for spreading into neural foramina, and perineural invasion may proceed intracranially. The palatine branch of the maxillary nerve innervates the mucosa of the hard palate, which contains minor salivary glands and can also harbor neoplasms.

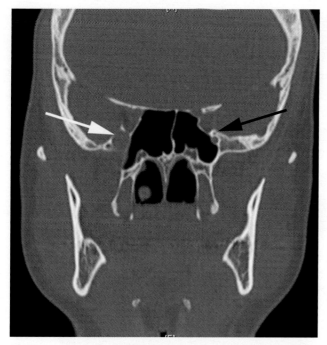

Fig. 24.3. Coronal computed tomography (CT) sinus scan showing a right schwannoma involving the enlarged foramen rotundum *(white arrow)*. The *black arrow* denotes a normal-appearing foramen rotundum.

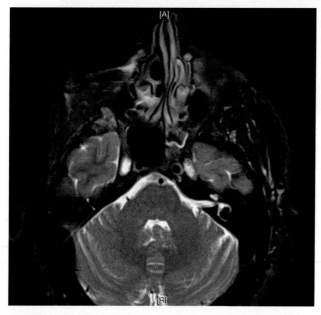

Fig. 24.4. Axial T2-weighted magnetic resonance image (MRI) showing a right-sided adenoid cystic carcinoma involving V_2 *(arrow)* and traversing through inferior orbital fissure.

INSTRUMENTATION

- 0-degree and 30-degree endoscopes
- Standard endoscopic sinus surgical tray
- 4-mm diamond choanal atresia bur or 15-degree angled diamond bur

- Extended-length Kerrison rongeurs
- Through-cutting instruments
- Endoscopic clip applier
- Suction monopolar cautery or endoscopic bipolar cautery, to have available for small branches of the maxillary artery
- Endoscopic microscissors
- Blunt dissecting instrument, such as curette or ball-tip probe
- Image-guided surgical navigation system

PEARLS AND POTENTIAL PITFALLS

- A wide maxillary antrostomy allows appropriate exposure of the PPS and provides fixed anatomic landmarks for dissection. For large lesions, consideration should be given to a medial maxillectomy for exposure.
- Use of image guidance is important.
- Specific surgical landmarks of the palatine bone (orbital, pterygoid roots) should be identified.
- A drill should be used when necessary to remove the dense bone of the pterygoid process.
- One should be prepared to extend the approach with a Caldwell-Luc procedure or endoscopic Denker approach (see Chapter 22) for expanded access lateral to the infraorbital nerve.
- Any branches of the maxillary artery encountered must be identified and cauterized. They may go into spasm and can cause profuse bleeding postoperatively.

SURGICAL PROCEDURE

- Undertake the usual preparations for endoscopic sinus surgery:
  - Topically vasoconstrict and anesthetize the nasal cavities with pledgets soaked in 4% cocaine, oxymetazoline, or 1:1000 epinephrine.
  - Inject 1% lidocaine with 1:100,000 epinephrine into the axilla of the middle turbinate and the region of the sphenopalatine foramen. Intraoral injection of the greater palatine foramen can be performed as well.
- Maxillary artery ligation is often performed as part of pterygopalatine fossa surgery for both access and preemptive vascular control.

Step 1: Wide Maxillary Antrostomy and Sphenoidotomy

- A wide antrostomy is the first key to the procedure. After performing the uncinectomy and the middle meatal antrostomy to enter through the natural ostium, enlarge posteriorly through the region of the posterior fontanelle using through-cutting forceps

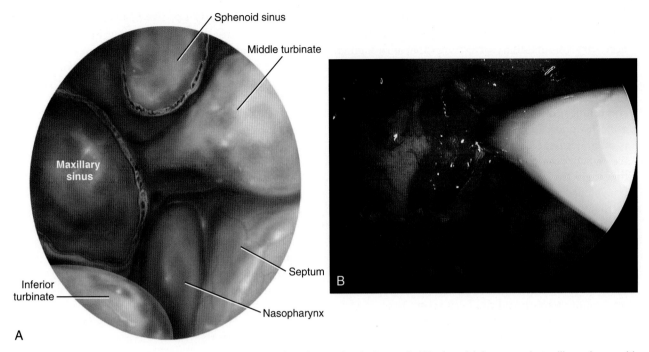

A

Fig. 24.5. Artist's depiction in endoscopic view **(A)** and endoscopic photograph **(B)** of a widely opened maxillary sinus, with attachment of the middle turbinate posteriorly. The medial wall of the maxillary sinus should be resected to the orbital process of the palatine bone.

and a microdébrider. This will expose the orbital process of the palatine bone (Fig. 24.5).

- It is important to take the posterior fontanelle flush to the posterior wall of the maxillary sinus.
  - Be prepared for bleeding from this maneuver, as branches of the sphenopalatine and descending palatine arteries may be transected. This can typically be controlled with suction monopolar cautery.
- For extended lesions, anterior and posterior ethmoidectomy may be required with identification of the skull base starting in the posterior ethmoid cavity.
- After maxillary antrostomy has been performed, create a wide sphenoidotomy toward the floor of the sphenoid sinus. During this maneuver, it is often necessary to control the posterior septal branch of the sphenopalatine artery, which courses within the mucosal tissues along the anterior face of the sphenoid sinus, inferior to the sphenoid os.

Step 2: Elevation of Mucosa of the Posterior Wall of the Maxillary Sinus and Drilling

- Elevate the mucosa in a submucoperiosteal plane.
- Using a diamond bur and Kerrison forceps, remove the ascending process of the palatine bone and the bone from the posterior wall of the maxillary sinus, thus opening the anteromedial wall of the PPS (Fig. 24.6).

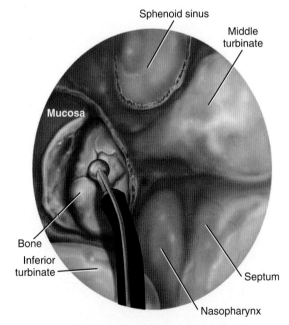

Fig. 24.6. Artist's depiction (in endoscopic view) of reflection of the mucosa of the posterior wall of the maxillary sinus and use of a suction irrigation drill to thin the wall. The posterior wall of the maxillary sinus is thinned until the fascia of the pterygopalatine fossa is encountered.

- For maxillary artery ligation alone, generally only the posterior wall of the maxillary sinus needs to be taken down.

Step 3: Enlargement of the Window Into the PPS

- The step of enlarging the window into the PPS is not necessary for maxillary artery ligation, although it is often helpful to follow the sphenopalatine artery back to the maxillary artery.
- Enlarge the sphenoidotomy laterally and bring it into communication with the soft tissue of the sphenopalatine foramen and medial pterygopalatine space. It is often necessary to cauterize the sphenopalatine artery where it exits its foramen during this step. Note that there may be several branches.
- Using a drill, Blakesley forceps, and Kerrison forceps, further enlarge the opening into the posterior wall of the maxillary sinus laterally to expose the soft tissue of the PPS.
- Make sure to open widely to prevent complications. Take great care not to perforate the fascia until the bone is widely removed. The contents of the PPS are often under tension and can herniate into the nose; if the artery is damaged, control of the artery is difficult.

Step 4: Incision of the Anterior Pterygopalatine Fossa Periosteum

- Incise the anterior pterygopalatine fossa periosteum with either a sickle knife or a suction monopolar cautery applied at a low setting (Fig. 24.7).
- Once the periosteum is cut, use blunt instruments, such as a J-curette or ball-tip probe, to widely open the remainder of the periosteum.

Step 5: Identification of the Maxillary Artery

- The maxillary artery is generally buried within the pterygopalatine fat and traveling from lateral to medial through the posterior wall of the maxillary sinus.
- Often, pulsations can be visualized to identify the location of the vessel.
- Tease the artery out of the fascia with a blunt instrument, such as a ball-tip probe (Fig. 24.8).

Step 6: Ligation of the Maxillary Artery

- Once the maxillary artery has been isolated, place endoscopic clips at the midpoint of exposure (Fig. 24.9).
- Take care not to initially attempt clip application too laterally because a vessel may tear and the subsequent hemorrhage is difficult to control.
- The authors usually apply two clips laterally and one clip medially, then transect in between with endoscopic microscissors.
- After clip application, additional hemostasis can be achieved with the use of suction monopolar cautery or endoscopic bipolar cautery.

Step 7: Removal of the Disease Process in the PPS

- A 3- or 4-hand, 2-surgeon approach may be useful here and may be augmented through a Caldwell-Luc procedure (Fig. 24.10).

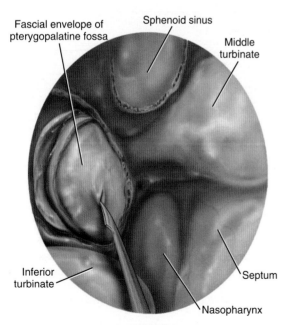

Fig. 24.7. Artist's depiction of incision of the fascia of the pterygopalatine fossa in endoscopic view. Great care should be used when incising the fascia, because the maxillary artery can be easily injured.

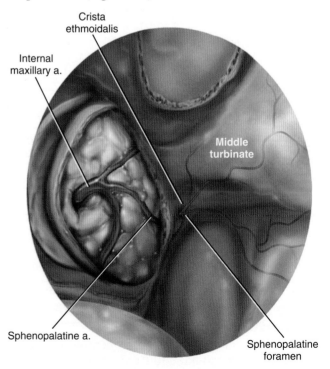

Fig. 24.8. Artist's depiction of the exposed maxillary artery in endoscopic view. Gentle monopolar or bipolar cautery can be used to reduce the fat and provide better visualization of the artery. *a.,* Artery.

- Perform dissection with endoscopic instruments (e.g., Blakesley forceps, microdébrider, radiofrequency ablation) to debulk exophytic portions of the lesion.
- For more meticulous dissection, use endoscopic microscissors to tease through the fat of the PPS to dissect vascular branches away from the area of the lesion, which can be confirmed with image guidance.

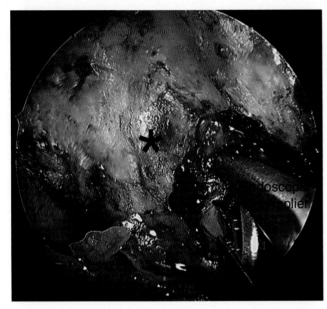

Fig. 24.9. Endoscopic view of the posterior maxillary wall *(asterisk)*. The dashed line indicates the course of the maxillary artery. An endoscopic clip applier can be used to ligate the vessel.

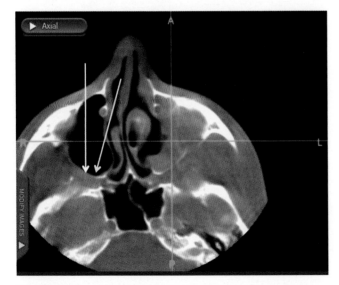

Fig. 24.10. Axial computed tomography (CT) scan showing the trajectories of the transmaxillary approach to the pterygomaxillary space via the transnasal *(yellow arrow)* and canine fossa *(white arrow)* routes.

- Bipolar cautery can be used to cauterize the fat of the PPS to allow better identification of the neurovascular structures.
- Identify branches of the maxillary artery in the PPS and control bleeding using electrocautery and/or surgical clips. Recall that vascular structures (the maxillary artery and its branches) are found inferomedially in the PPS, whereas neural structures (V_2, sphenopalatine ganglion) are situated posterosuperiorly.
- Proceed with dissection from inferomedial to superolateral until the foramen rotundum is encountered. Identify the nerve within the foramen rotundum (Fig. 24.11). Using an elevator, continue to dissect in a subperiosteal plane along the uppermost aspect of the pterygoid root. If further dissection is necessary, use a diamond drill to remove the bone along the medial hemisphere of the foramen rotundum, which allows dissection of the nerve along the body of the LSR to the point of the cavernous sinus.

Step 8: Access of the LSR

- For certain cases, access to the LSR may be achieved by blunt dissection in the area posteromedial to the foramen rotundum. Retraction of the PPS contents inferolaterally may further facilitate exposure.
- A key maneuver in LSR access is extending the sphenoidotomy as laterally as possible to connect it to the transpterygoid dissection.
- LSR encephaloceles or CSF leaks may then be directly visualized with angled scopes.

Step 9: Closure

- Repair any CSF leakage and skull base defects as described in other chapters.
- Treat the resection bed with topical hemostatic matrix. Commercially available collagen or gelatin matrix mixed with thrombin is effective. Follow this with a layer of gelatin foam pledgets and a nonabsorbable packing.
- Exposed fat or bone may be covered with a free mucosal graft or biocompatible allograft.

APPROACH TO JUVENILE NASOPHARYNGEAL ANGIOFIBROMA

Introduction

- JNA is a well-vascularized benign neoplasm typically occurring in adolescent males and with clinical symptoms of epistaxis and/or nasal obstruction.
- Although pathologically benign, they often behave in a locally invasive manner.

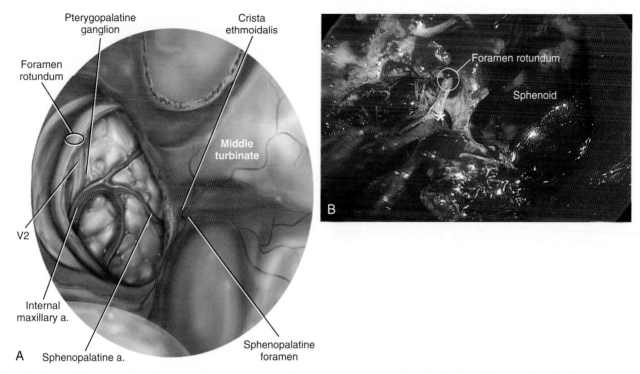

Fig. 24.11. Artist's depiction **(A)** and endoscopic image **(B)** showing the operative field before **(A)** and after **(B)** the contents of the pterygopalatine fossa have been cleared. Note that the pterygopalatine fossa is a small space until a pathologic process enlarges it. In **(B)**, fat in the pterygopalatine/pterygomaxillary space has been dissected to expose the foramen rotundum and V_2 *(asterisk)*.

- Surgical resection is considered first-line therapy. Primary or adjuvant radiation is generally reserved for extensive lesions or recurrent tumors in which high morbidity would preclude surgical intervention.[26]
- Reported alternative treatment options include cryotherapy, chemotherapy, and hormonal manipulation.
- Classic resection involved an open approach; currently, JNA is often resected endoscopically.

Anatomy

- Typically, JNA originates from the pterygopalatine fossa.
- The pterygopalatine fossa lies just posterior to the posterior wall of the maxillary sinus.
- Just lateral to the pterygopalatine fossa is the infratemporal fossa. The maxillary nerve sits at the junction of the infratemporal fossa and the orbit.
- The pterygopalatine fossa is covered by periosteum and contains fat and neurovascular structures. The maxillary artery and subsequent branches, including the sphenopalatine artery, lie anteromedial to the underlying nerves of the V_2.
- JNAs arise in close proximity to the sphenopalatine artery, along the lateral nasal wall.

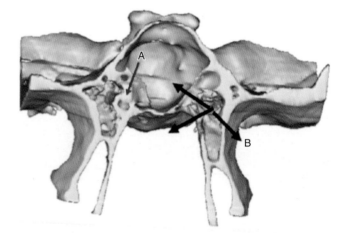

Fig. 24.12. Routes of potential spread of JNA, including the vidian canal (A, *red arrow*), infratemporal fossa (B), inferior orbital fissure, and sphenopalatine foramen (*black arrows*). Note the widened vidian canal from posterior extension.

- The tumor can extend into nasopharynx, through the sphenopalatine foramen or inferior orbital fissure, eventually extending into the infratemporal fossa and subsequently intracranially (Fig. 24.12).[27]

TABLE 24.1 Andrews et al. Juvenile Nasopharyngeal Angiofibroma Staging System

	Andrews Stage
I	Tumor limited to the nasal cavity and nasopharynx
II	Tumor extension into the pterygopalatine fossa, maxillary, sphenoid, or ethmoid sinuses
IIIa	Extension into the orbit or infratemporal fossa without intracranial extension
IIIb	Stage IIIa with small extradural intracranial (parasellar) involvement
IVa	Large extradural intracranial or intradural extension
IVb	Extension into cavernous sinus, pituitary, or optic chiasm

From Andrews JC, Fisch U, Valavanis A, Aeppli U, Makek MS. The surgical management of extensive nasopharyngeal angiofibromas with the infratemporal fossa approach. *Laryngoscope.* 1989;99:429–437.

Preoperative Considerations

- Surgical resection can be performed endoscopically or through an open approach. Most tumors with an Andrews stage I, II, and select IIIa can be resected endoscopically (Table 24.1).[28] For the purpose of this chapter, we will focus on endoscopic resection techniques.
- Although en bloc resection is preferable, if the JNA is large and obstructing visualization at the level of the nasopharynx, it may be necessary to divide and resect the anterior portion prior to complete resection or debulk it prior to identifying sites of attachment.
- Given the vascularity of JNAs, full preparation for significant blood loss should be anticipated, including two large-bore intravenous lines, an arterial line, and additional blood products on hold.

Radiographic Considerations

- Evaluate both axial and coronal CT and MRI (Fig. 24.13).
- JNAs, which frequently involve the pterygopalatine fossa, typically present with anterior bowing of the posterior wall of the maxillary sinus as seen on axial CT or MRI. This is known as the Holman-Miller sign.
- Special attention should be paid to lateral extension into the pterygomaxillary space and/or infratemporal fossa, vidian canal involvement (Fig. 24.14), and posterior extension involving the superior and inferior pterygoid plates.

- Preoperative embolization is generally advocated to reduce intraoperative bleeding (Fig. 24.15).
- Embolization is performed by angiographic study evaluating bilateral carotid arteries, specifically looking at vessels supplying the tumor.
- Most common feeding vessels include the distal branches of the maxillary artery, ascending pharyngeal artery, vidian artery, accessory meningeal artery, mandibular artery, and the facial artery.[29]
- Embolization should be performed within 24 hours of surgery. Prolonged duration can lead to the development of significant collateral blood supply and subsequent revascularization of the tumor. This is also the reason why revision JNA cases in which previous embolization has been performed increases the difficulty of the case.
- Embolization may also have the favorable effect of shrinking the tumor burden.

Additional Instrumentation

- Curved and straight beaver blades
- Suction Freer
- Adenoid bipolar (Fig. 24.16)

Pearls and Potential Pitfalls

- Wide exposure, including opening of all adjacent sinuses, is critical prior to addressing the actual tumor. This creates drip spaces and working room for instrumentation.
- A posterior septectomy may be necessary if the tumor is adherent to the septum.
- For large tumors, we often utilize a 3- or 4-hand, 2-surgeon technique. In this situation, we develop a partial septectomy for a binostril approach. When performed, the authors will have the second surgeon in the contralateral nostril applying countertraction to the mass as the primary surgeon dissects the tumor free from surrounding structures.
- Despite embolization, if the maxillary artery is not adequately ligated intraoperatively, significant blood loss is possible due to recanalization following embolization.
- The posterior extent of the JNA often extends into the nasopharynx; resection of this posterior margin can be difficult at times.
  - On large JNAs, we will consider resecting the posterior aspect transorally prior to resection of the remainder of the tumor.
- Judicious use of frozen-section pathology is used intraoperatively to confirm negative tumor margins.

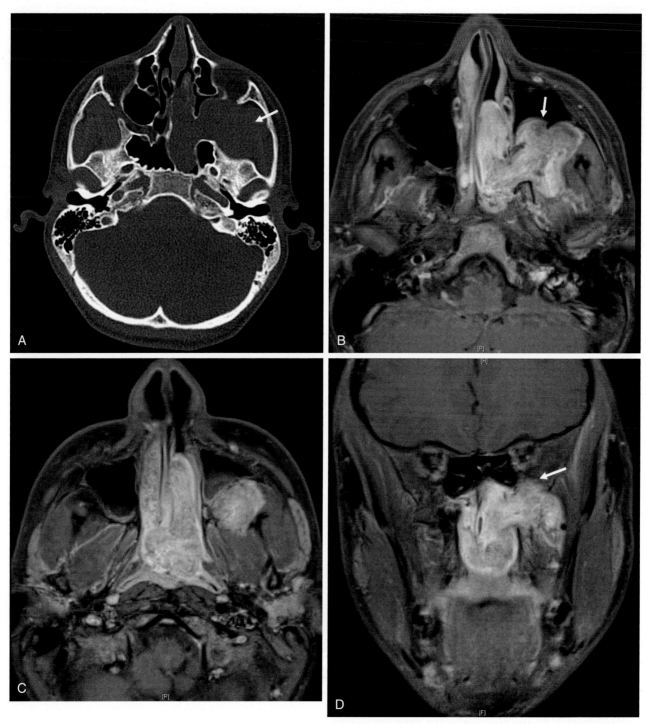

Fig. 24.13. (A) Axial computed tomography (CT) image revealing a massive juvenile nasopharyngeal angiofibroma within the widened left pterygopalatine fossa with lateral extension into the infratemporal fossa (abutting muscles of mastication, *solid arrow*), anteriorly expanding into the left nasal cavity and posteriorly along the medial pterygoid plates into the sphenoid sinus. Note that there is a significant mass effect of the tumor against the nasal septum. **(B)** Axial T1-weighted magnetic resonance (MR) image confirming relationships of the tumor indicated in Fig. 24.2A. The *solid arrow* demonstrates a pronounced case of anterior bowing of the posterior wall of the maxillary sinus, also known as the Holman-Miller sign. **(C)** Axial T1-weighted MR image of the same tumor at a lower level demonstrates gross extension into the nasopharynx through the posterior nasal septum. **(D)** Coronal T1-weighted MR image of the same tumor showing its posterior relationships. In this view, the tumor can be seen extending superiorly into the left inferior orbital fissure *(solid arrow)*.

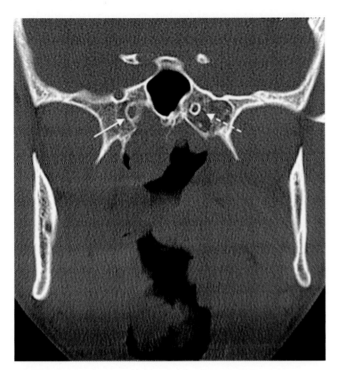

Fig. 24.14. Coronal computed tomography (CT) image showing a different right-sided JNA with sclerotic changes along the pterygoid process. Note the widened vidian canal *(solid arrow)* and the normal contralateral canal *(dashed arrow)*.

SURGICAL STEPS

Step 1: Perform a Wide Maxillary Antrostomy, Ethmoidectomy, and Sphenoidotomy

- JNAs tend to be bulky tumors that challenge the surgeon's ability to access the tumor boundaries within the confines of the nasal cavity (Fig. 24.17). Thus, early wide access is key.
- See Chapters 6, 7, and 8 for description of procedures.
- The sphenoidotomy may only be necessary if the JNA extends posteriorly into the sinus. This is essential for improved control of the posterior extension of the lesion along the vidian canal and allows for clear delineation of the JNA from critical structures, such as the optic nerve, internal carotid artery, and middle cranial fossa.
- Some surgeons will also perform an inferior and/or middle turbinectomy on the side of the lesion to improve exposure. With large tumors, a medial maxillectomy may be necessary.

Step 2: Expose the Sphenopalatine and/or Maxillary Artery

- Resect the bony posterior maxillary wall with either a high-speed drill or Kerrison rongeurs.
- Identify the feeding artery lateral to the tumor.
  - If the tumor has significant lateral extension, a Caldwell-Luc procedure or endoscopic Denker approach may be necessary to adequately isolate the artery.

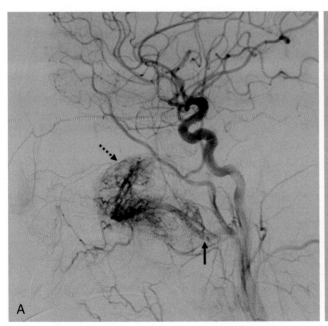
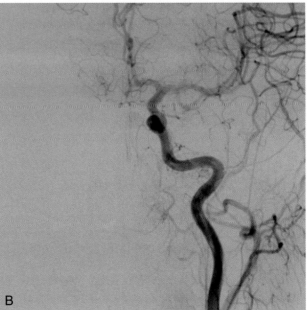

Fig. 24.15. **(A)** Preembolization image of the left-sided juvenile nasopharyngeal angiofibroma (JNA) *(dashed arrow* represents tumor blush). Note that the majority of blood flow is coming from the maxillary artery *(solid arrow)*. **(B)** Postembolization demonstrates no further uptake of tumor contrast.

Step 3: Perform a Sphenopalatine or Maxillary Artery Ligation

- See Chapter 3 for complete description.
- The authors use an endoscopic clip applier for ligation (Fig. 24.18).

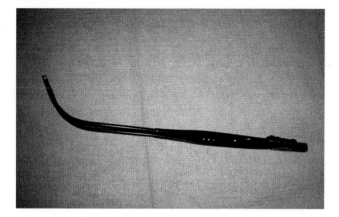

Fig. 24.16. Adenoid bipolar. Its curved end can be placed transorally to address the nasopharyngeal component of tumor.

- Vascularity is often further decreased after clip ligation despite previous embolization (Fig. 24.19).

Step 4: Dissect the Posterior Nasopharyngeal Component Free From Surrounding Tissues

- The authors use a curved adenotome bipolar (Fig. 24.16) transorally and visualize cautery either using an angled scope placed transorally or transnasally to free up this portion of the tumor.

Step 5: Dissect the Intranasal Portions of the Tumor From the Surrounding Tissues

- If the tumor is attached or invading the posterior septum, then a posterior septectomy may be required to ensure complete resection (Fig. 24.20).
  - We use a combination of a curved beaver blade and suction monopolar cautery.
  - This should be considered early in the surgery to improve access, and further consideration should be given to cauterization of the contralateral posterior septal branch of the sphenopalatine artery to decrease septal vascular supply.

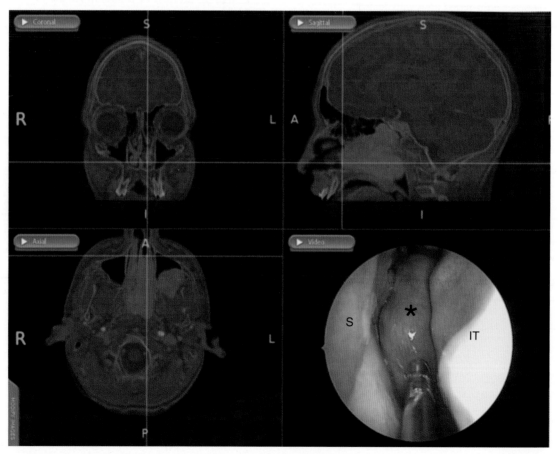

Fig. 24.17. Triplanar computed tomography (CT) image guidance display and endoscopic view demonstrating the same left-sided tumor *(asterisk)* at the time of surgery, nearly filling the entire left nasal cavity. Crosshairs in CT represent the distal end of the image-guidance probe. *IT,* Inferior turbinate; *S,* septum.

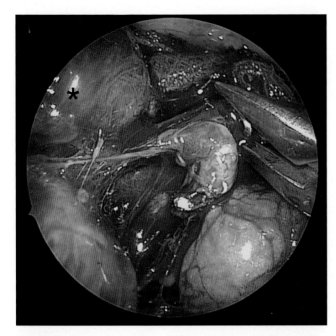

Fig. 24.18. Endoscopic view of the posterior maxillary wall with the exposed tumor *(asterisk),* with an endoscopic clip applier over the left maxillary artery.

■ Proceed to dissect along the subperiosteal plane to free the mass from the lateral nasal wall. We utilize a bipolar cautery to remove the tumor off the lateral nasal wall and medial pterygoid plate (Fig. 24.21).

Step 6: Remove the Tumor Either Transnasally or Transorally Depending on Its Size
■ Larger JNAs require a transoral approach, especially in younger patients (Fig. 24.22).

Step 7: Evaluate the Pterygoid Processes and Vidian Canal
■ If the tumor invades the pterygoid process or the vidian canal, the bone should be drilled down with a 15-degree diamond bur until clear margins are achieved. Bipolar cautery (and possibly bone wax) is used to control bleeding in the vidian canal (Fig. 24.23).

Step 8: Cover the Surgical Defect
■ Exposed fat and/or bone over the pterygopalatine fossa can be covered with a free mucosal graft or biocompatible allograft to promote healing.

Postoperative Considerations
■ If nasal packing is placed, the patient should receive broad-spectrum antibiotics while the packing is in

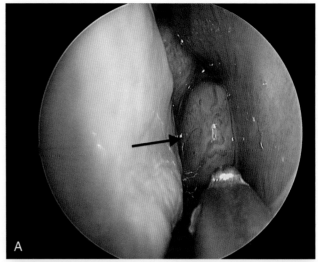

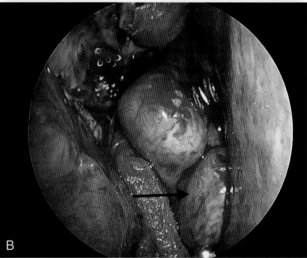

Fig. 24.19. **(A)** Endoscopic view of a juvenile nasopharyngeal angiofibroma (JNA) *(arrow)* prior to ligation of the maxillary artery. **(B)** Endoscopic view of JNA *(arrow)* following maxillary artery ligation (note the decreased vascular prominence and fullness of the tumor).

place and while there is still significant crusting in the cavity.
■ The packing is débrided 4 to 7 days postoperatively. If no skull base repair was required, the patient performs saline irrigations and makes serial office visits for débridement.
■ If clear margins are not possible in JNA resection, one can consider adjunctive radiation therapy versus close observation.
■ Postoperative surveillance of JNA includes endoscopic examination and radiographic evaluation. Recurrence tends to appear submucosally; thus, contrast-enhanced CT or MRI is suitable for monitoring.

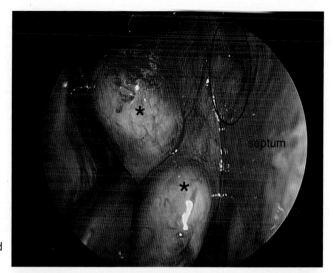

Fig. 24.20. Endoscopic view showing a tumor *(asterisk)* attached to the right nasal septum *(oval)*.

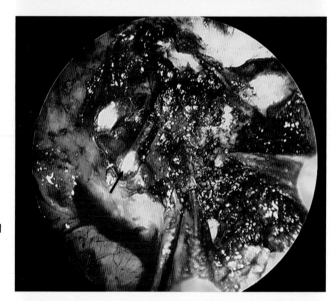

Fig. 24.21. Endoscopic resection of a juvenile nasopharyngeal angiofibroma attached to the pterygoid process with bipolar cautery. Note the removal of the tumor directly off the bony pterygoid process. The previously applied vascular clip can be clearly seen *(arrow)*.

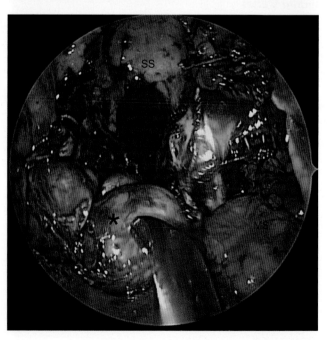

Fig. 24.22. Final endoscopic view of wide access for a 6-cm juvenile nasopharyngeal angiofibroma (JNA). Note the posterior septectomy, wide left maxillary antrostomy (with inferior turbinate resection), complete left ethmoidectomy, and bilateral sphenoidotomy. Tumor *(asterisk)* is being delivered through the nasopharynx and will be removed transorally. *MS,* Maxillary sinus; *SS,* sphenoid sinus.

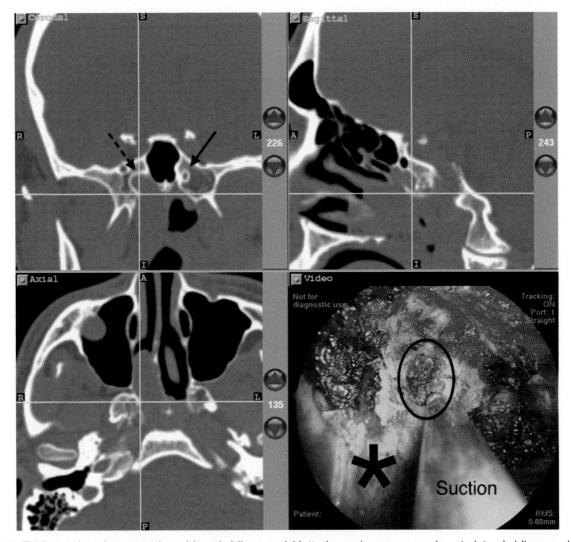

Fig. 24.23. Triplanar view demonstrating widened vidian canal *(dotted arrow)* versus normal contralateral vidian canal *(solid arrow)*. On the endoscopic view, the circle indicates the corresponding widened vidian canal *(asterisk)* medial pterygoid plate. The enlarged canal must be drilled down to resect the entire invading tumor.

CONCLUSION

- PPS approaches are useful for the treatment of lesions within the LSR and PPS, as well as for treatment of JNA.
- Control of the sphenopalatine and maxillary arteries is necessary for successful surgery.
- Access to and identification of sites of attachment for JNAs are critical for complete resection.

REFERENCES

Access the reference list online at ExpertConsult.com.

Endoscopic Craniofacial Resection

Elisabeth H. Ference, Vijay R. Ramakrishnan, and Jeffrey D. Suh

INTRODUCTION

- Endoscopic craniofacial resection (CFR) has emerged as an alternative to the traditional CFR originally credited to Ketcham in 1963.[1]
- The standard craniofacial approach for tumor resection combines a transfacial approach via a lateral rhinotomy or midface degloving to gain access for removal of the sinus component of the tumor with a transcranial approach to remove the skull base and intracranial portion of the tumor. The most common indications for CFR are tumors arising from the nasal cavity, frontal sinuses, or ethmoid sinuses extending to or through the anterior skull base.
- The major reason for selecting endoscopic CFR is to avoid the morbidity associated with open CFR.
- The rates of complication associated with open CFR as reported in the literature vary considerably.
  - In the largest study to date evaluating open CFRs, Ganly et al. reported an overall complication rate of 36.3% and a mortality rate of 4.7%.[2]
  - The rate of CSF fistula after major CFR may be as high as 20%.[3]
  - The rate of meningitis after CFR is reported in the literature to be 5% to 7.7%.[4]
- Despite the wide exposure afforded by the open CFR, the close proximity of the orbit, brain, and other critical neurovascular structures often prevents surgeons from taking large margins without causing significant morbidity. In fact, one multicenter study looking at outcomes of open CFRs reported a 30% incidence of positive margins.[1]
- It has been suggested that the magnified view provided by the endoscope can also make tumor mapping more precise, especially in deep areas such as the pterygopalatine fossa and sphenoid sinus, where visualization and illumination can be difficult in an open procedure. Furthermore, for some tumors, unilateral endoscopic resection is possible, thus preserving smell on the contralateral side.[5]
- A major criticism of endoscopic CFR is that the tumors are removed piecemeal. Traditional teaching is that tumors should be removed en bloc to ensure maximal survival.[6-8] This principle is founded on the concept that surgical violation of the tumor predisposes to spread of the cancer through lymphatic or vascular channels, thereby increasing the risk of local, regional, and distant tumor spread. Furthermore, there is concern that tumor removal is more likely to be incomplete with a piecemeal as opposed to an en bloc resection.[9] However, data from transoral laser microsurgery[10] and transoral robotic surgery,[11] as well as more recent data from endoscopic CFRs,[9,12] show that this is not the case. The most important surgical variable affecting survival, regardless of the method used, is achieving complete tumor resection with negative margins.
- A study comparing endoscopic versus open craniofacial resection found no significant differences in survival, metastatic rates, or complication rates between the two groups.[13] The endoscopic group had shorter hospital stays and the added benefit of a better cosmetic outcome.[14] However, comparison of oncologic outcomes between the groups was limited by discrepancy in histologic grade and clinical stage between the two retrospective, nonrandomized groups.[13,14]

ANATOMY

- Surgery of the skull base is complex because of its proximity to the dura, brain, and orbit. Tumors will be adjacent to or involve one or more of these structures during endoscopic CFR.
- Sphenoid sinus anatomy deserves special mention. The optic nerve and cavernous sinus are located

along the lateral wall, whereas the sella turcica is located posteriorly and centrally.

- Refer to the appropriate chapters in this text for more detailed anatomic descriptions of the sphenoid sinus, ethmoid roof, and frontal sinus.

PREOPERATIVE CONSIDERATIONS

- Endoscopic CFR may be considered in the management of benign and malignant tumors of the paranasal sinuses involving the skull base.
- This chapter focuses on the treatment of esthesioneuroblastoma, which is one of the more common tumors approached by this method. However, this technique can be applied to the majority of benign and malignant tumors involving the anterior skull base.
- Preoperative images should be thoroughly analyzed; the findings will ultimately determine tumor resectability and critical anatomic constraints.
- A multidisciplinary approach—including, when pertinent, specialists in neurosurgery, ophthalmology, medical oncology, and radiation oncology—is critical.
- A definitive tissue biopsy is necessary preoperatively, especially when critical anatomic structures such as the orbit, dura, or neurovascular regions are involved.
- *Indications* include any benign or malignant tumor of the nasal cavity and/or paranasal sinuses that involves the anterior skull base.
- *Contraindications* include poor surgical candidacy because of comorbidities, involvement of skin or brain parenchyma, and bilateral orbital involvement.
- *Relative contraindications* include extension into the cavernous sinus, orbit, and lacrimal system, as well as massive tumors with unfavorable histologic features. Another contraindication to the approach is the inability to reconstruct the skull base due to factors such as previous surgery, radiation exposure, or defect size.

Workup and Staging

- Esthesioneuroblastoma, first described by Berger and Luc in 1924, arises from the olfactory epithelium and accounts for approximately 3% to 6% of malignancies of the nasal cavity and paranasal sinus.[15]
- Tumor staging is an important guide for prognosis and therapy. The most common staging systems are the Kadish staging system (Table 25.1),[16] the University of California at Los Angeles–Dulguerov and Calcaterra staging system (Table 25.2),[17] and the Hyams histopathologic grading system (Table 25.3).[18] In a 1993 study by Morita et al.[19] examining prognostic factors, Hyams histopathologic grade was found to be the most significant prognostic factor, with a 5-year survival rate of 80% for

TABLE 25.1 Kadish Staging System

Stage	Characteristics
A	Disease confined to nasal cavity
B	Disease in nasal cavity and one or more paranasal sinuses
C	Disease extending beyond the nasal cavity and paranasal sinuses

TABLE 25.2 UCLA–Dulguerov and Calcaterra TNM Staging

Stage	Characteristics
T1	Tumor involving the nasal cavity and/or paranasal sinuses (excluding sphenoid), sparing the most superior ethmoid cells
T2	Tumor involving the nasal cavity and/or paranasal sinuses (including the sphenoid) with extension to or erosion of the cribriform plate
T3	Tumor extending into the orbit or protruding into the anterior cranial fossa, without dural invasion
T4	Tumor involving the brain
N0	No cervical lymph node metastasis
N1	Any form of cervical lymph node metastasis
M0	No metastases
M1	Distant metastasis

TNM, Tumor, node, metastases; *UCLA,* University of California at Los Angeles.

32 patients with low-grade tumors and 40% for 15 patients with high-grade tumors.

Radiographic Considerations

- Before endoscopic CFR, the primary tumor site must be examined using magnetic resonance imaging (MRI) and computed tomography (CT). The scans should be analyzed closely for involvement of the eye, dura, brain, and neurovascular structures (Fig. 25.1). As with any oncologic surgery, the goal of endoscopic CFR is to achieve clear margins. If this goal cannot be achieved, then other approaches should be used. For advanced-stage sinonasal malignancies, a workup for metastasis should include examination of the neck and lungs. Consideration can be given to performing positron emission tomography instead of neck and chest CT.[20]
- The extent of the tumor should be identified radiographically. Ideally, an additional layer of tissue should be included in the resection to obtain a margin; that is, if the tumor extends to the skull base, an additional dural margin should be taken once the involved skull base is resected.

TABLE 25.3 Hyams Histopathologic Grading

Grade	Lobular Architecture Preservation	Mitotic Index	Nuclear Polymorphism	Fibrillary Matrix	Rosettes	Necrosis
I	+	None	None	Prominent	HW rosettes	None
II	+	Low	Moderate	Present	HW rosettes	None
III	+/−	Moderate	Prominent	Low	FW rosettes	Rare
IV	+/−	High	Marked	Absent	None	Frequent

FW, Flexner-Wintersteiner; *HW,* Homer Wright.

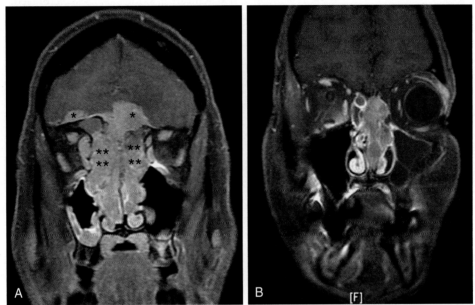

Fig. 25.1. Tumor extent is the main determinant of the feasibility of performing an endoscopic craniofacial resection (CFR) with successful complete tumor resection. **(A)** Coronal T1-weighted contrast-enhanced magnetic resonance image (MRI) of a sinonasal mass with massive intracranial extension *(single asterisks)* and periorbital involvement *(double asterisks)*. This tumor, with its wide dural involvement, would be better treated using an open craniotomy approach. **(B)** Coronal MRI of a different paranasal mass. Note that this mass also invades the periorbita as well as the dura but still may be amenable to endoscopic CFR.

INSTRUMENTATION

Many of the instruments employed in endoscopic CFR are the same as those used in simple functional endoscopic sinus surgery. The following are the extra instruments specific to the endoscopic CFR procedure:

- 0-, 30-, and 70-degree endoscopes
- Reverse endoscopes are preferred when working at the skull base. These endoscopes are designed to have the light cord directed upward, which frees up the area below the endoscope for the instruments.
- Endoscopic bipolar forceps
- Suction coagulator (suction Bovie)
- Straight and angled endoscopic drills
- Straight and angled microdébrider burs
- Carotid Doppler ultrasound device

- Image guidance system with possible MRI/CT fusion to better delineate tumor margins

PEARLS AND POTENTIAL PITFALLS

- Consideration should be given to placement of a lumbar drain at the onset of surgery.
- A two-surgeon, four-handed, two-nostril technique is preferred for fine dissection at the skull base.
- Endoscopic bipolar forceps and clip appliers are helpful for arterial ligation.
- A complete set of skull base instruments is invaluable.
- The size of the defect and available local reconstructive options should be continuously reevaluated as the tumor dissection proceeds.
- A skilled pathologist is essential to assess the frozen-section margins.

SURGICAL PROCEDURE

Step 1

- Place the patient in a supine position and apply and calibrate the image guidance system.
- Fix the patient's head with a Mayfield clamp if needed.
- If reconstruction using extranasal tissue is possible, obtain appropriate consent and prepare the patient's abdomen and leg for possible harvest of a fat graft and/or fascia lata graft, respectively.

Step 2

- Inspect the nasal cavity (Fig. 25.2) and decongest it with pledgets soaked in oxymetazoline. Perform surgical preparation of the nares and nearby facial structures.
- Consider placing the patient in a slight reverse Trendelenburg position (approximately 20 degrees). This reduces cardiac output and can improve visualization during surgery.
- The pterygopalatine fossa can also be infiltrated with vasoconstrictor solutions through the greater palatine foramen, which has been demonstrated to significantly reduce intraoperative bleeding.[21]

Step 3

- Debulk the tumor and remove it in piecemeal fashion using a microdébrider. In addition to debulking, the goal is to identify the site of tumor attachment to the skull base (Figs. 25.3 and 25.4).

Step 4

- Once the site of attachment is identified, perform a complete sphenoethmoidectomy with modified Lothrop procedure. Excise the middle turbinates as well. This fully exposes the skull base and medial orbital walls, and opens the frontal, sphenoid, and maxillary sinuses to prevent postoperative stenosis with resultant retention of secretions (Figs. 25.5 and 25.6).

Step 5

- Once the skull base is skeletonized, identify the anterior and posterior ethmoid arteries and cauterize them with bipolar cautery (Fig. 25.7). The arteries can also be clipped using the endoscopic clip applier prior to being bipolared at the distal end.

Step 6

- After the tumor is debulked to the skull base and the tumor removed, obtain margins from the nasal septum, posterior and anterior skull base, and both medial orbital walls (Fig. 25.8).

Step 7

- Clearly delineate the site of tumor origin (Figs. 25.9A and B). With tumors in the midline or those that erode through the nasal septum, skeletonize the entire skull base so that the septum is removed and all superior ethmoid bony partitions are removed (Fig. 25.9C).

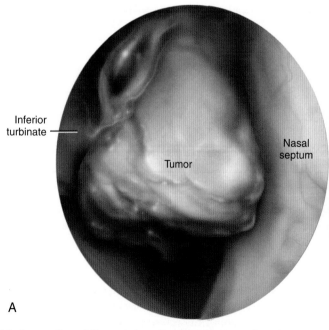

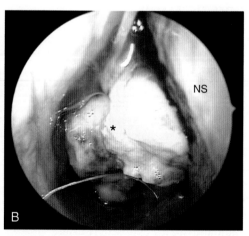

Fig. 25.2. Inspection of the nasal cavity after decongestion. Artist's depiction **(A)** and endoscopic image **(B)** showing a large tumor filling the right nasal cavity. The asterisk in **(B)** indicates tumor. *NS,* Nasal septum.

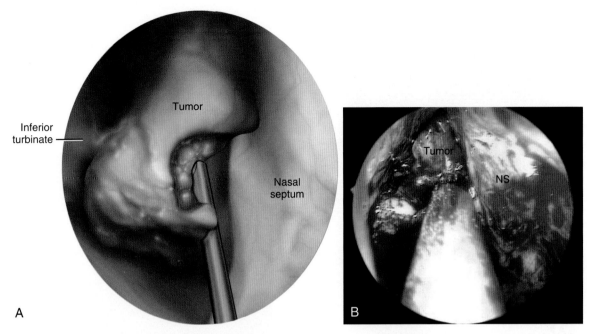

Fig. 25.3. Artist's depiction **(A)** and endoscopic image **(B)** of tumor debulking. It is critical that the surgeon evaluate for the site of tumor attachment as the tumor is removed. In these views, the microdébrider is in a plane between the nasal septum *(NS)* and tumor.

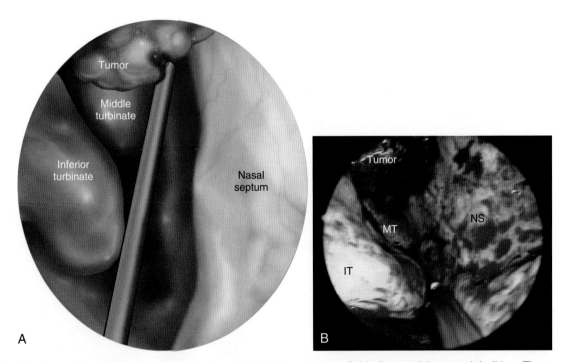

Fig. 25.4. Artist's depiction **(A)** and endoscopic image **(B)** of the operative field after partial tumor debulking. The nasal septum *(NS)*, right inferior turbinate *(IT)*, and middle turbinate *(MT)* are seen and noted to be grossly uninvolved with tumor.

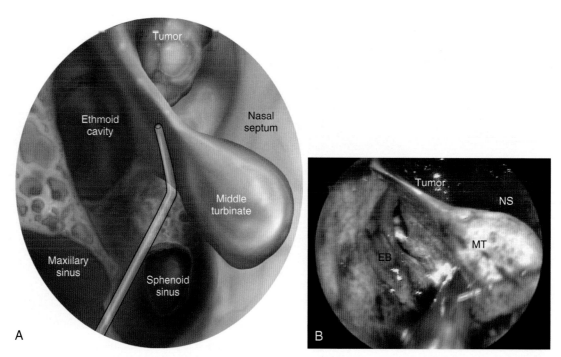

Fig. 25.5. Artist's depiction **(A)** and endoscopic image **(B)** showing medialization of the right middle turbinate *(MT)* after tumor is debulked to the skull base. The right middle turbinate is resected to perform standard functional endoscopic sinus surgery dissection. Note that the mucosa lateral to the middle turbinate appears to be uninvolved with tumor. *EB,* Ethmoid bulla; *NS,* nasal septum.

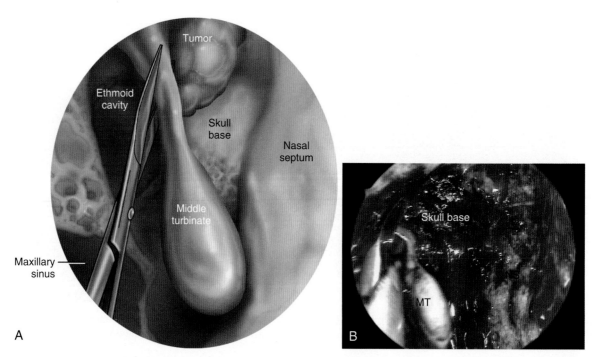

Fig. 25.6. Artist's depiction **(A)** and endoscopic image **(B)** showing resection of the middle turbinate *(MT)* to the skull base with curved endoscopic scissors. This maneuver provides more access to the skull base for tumor resection and achievement of wide margins. *NS,* Nasal septum.

Step 8

- Remove the anterior skull base with a drill, starting 1 cm posterior and anterior to the attachment of the tumor. This commonly requires the drilling of the skull base from the posterior frontal recess to the posterior ethmoid roof and from the medial orbital wall to the contralateral medial orbital wall for an esthesioneuroblastoma that has crossed the midline (Fig. 25.10). Drilling is best performed using a high-speed, angled diamond bur.

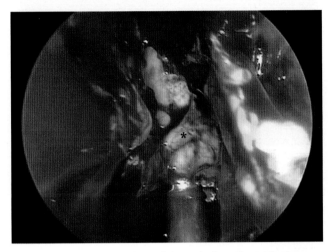

Fig. 25.7. Endoscopic view of the anterior ethmoid artery *(asterisk)* seen along the skull base in the left nasal cavity.

Step 9

- Expose the dura, cauterize it with a bipolar cautery, and resect it for either a dural margin or for intracranial entry to remove extension of tumor into the brain. This is best performed in tandem with a neurosurgeon skilled in endoscopic techniques (Figs. 25.11 and 25.12).

Step 10

- Repair the dura and reconstruct the skull base (Figs. 25.13 and 25.14) in multiple layers. When possible, use pedicled mucosal flaps in patients who will receive postoperative radiation therapy. When the tumor involves the nasal septum, posterior ethmoids, or pterygopalatine fossa, it is better to use free fascia and mucosal grafts taken well away from the tumor site. Further discussion of skull base reconstruction can be found in Chapters 26, 27, and 31.

Step 11

- Use nasal packing to support the skull base defect. Rolled thin Silastic stents of 0.25 mm thickness can be used to help support the packing and prevent the grafts from moving. These stents can be placed in the frontal sinus and then pushed back along the skull base, covering the graft and initial packing layer. The packing and stents are often left in place for 14 to 21 days. Place nasal trumpets in the nasal cavity

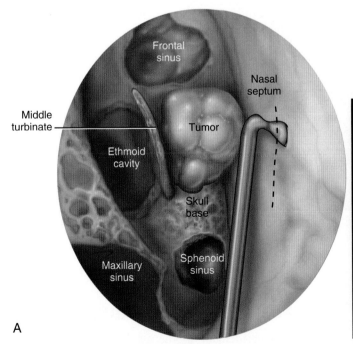

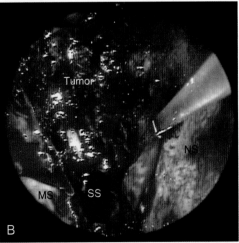

Fig. 25.8. Artist's depiction **(A)** and endoscopic image **(B)** showing excision of the septal margin with a curved blade *(dashed line* in A). Wide margins are obtained around the tumor. Frozen sections are examined to confirm negative margins. *MS,* Maxillary sinus; *NS,* nasal septum; *SS,* sphenoid sinus.

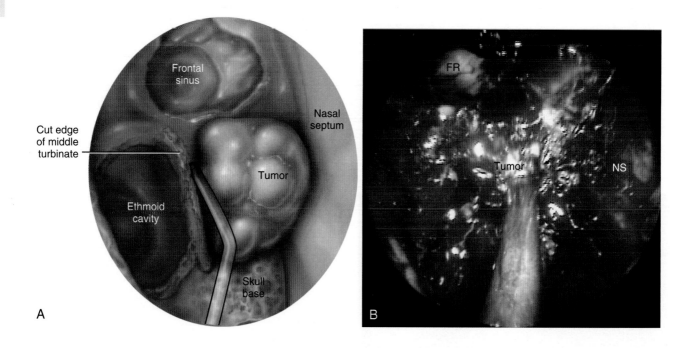

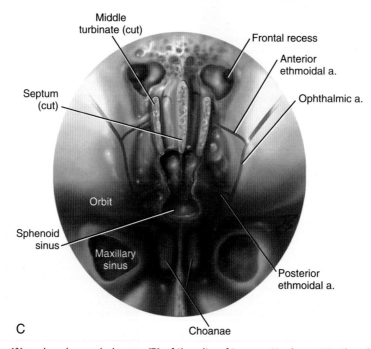

Fig. 25.9. Artist's depiction **(A)** and endoscopic image **(B)** of the site of tumor attachment to the skull base along the superior ethmoid roof, posterior to the right frontal recess *(FR)*. **(C)** Artist's depiction of the endoscopic view of a skeletonized skull base with the superior nasal septum and middle turbinates removed. *a.,* Artery; *NS,* nasal septum.

and sew them in place across the nasal septum in the septocolumellar junction. The trumpets are kept in place for 48 to 72 hours postoperatively. The trumpets divert air away from the skull base defect and prevent postoperative pneumocephalus.

POSTOPERATIVE CONSIDERATIONS

- Débridement in the area of the skull base repair should be avoided in the period immediately after surgery (2 weeks).

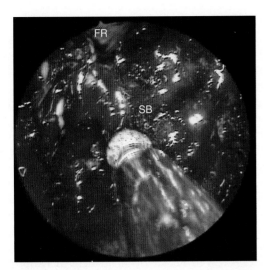

Fig. 25.10. Endoscopic view of removal of the skull base *(SB)* with an angled drill. An angled diamond bur is used to avoid inadvertent injury to the dura or brain. *FR,* Frontal recess.

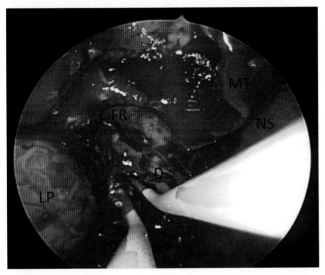

Fig. 25.11. Endoscopic view of cauterization of the dura (D) with a bipolar cautery before resection. *FR,* Frontal recess; *LP,* lamina papyracea; *MT,* middle turbinate; *NS,* nasal septum.

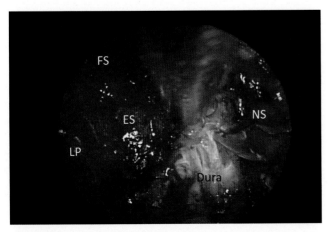

Fig. 25.12. Endoscopic image showing resection of the dura with a sickle knife. *ES,* Ethmoid sinus; *FS,* frontal sinus; *LP,* lamina papyracea; *NS,* Nasal septum.

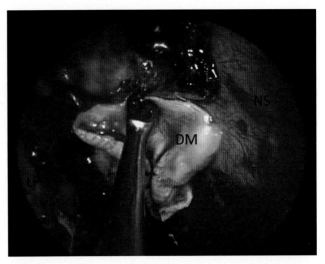

Fig. 25.13. Endoscopic image showing a dural defect filled with a synthetic dural matrix *(DM)* to close a cerebrospinal fluid leak. The dural matrix is preferably tucked inside the cut edges of the dura. For large defects, a second intracranial layer (fascia or bone) is often tucked extradural and intracranial to repair the skull base. *LP,* Lamina papyracea; *NS,* nasal septum.

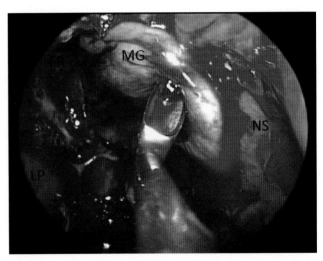

Fig. 25.14. Endoscopic image showing placement of a free mucosal graft *(MG)* over the bony skull base defect as an overlay graft. *FR,* Frontal recess; *LP,* lamina papyracea; *NS,* nasal septum.

- After this time, patients will often need frequent débridements of crusting secondary to exposed bone of the skull base and nasal septum.
- Patients should be told to avoid nose blowing, heavy lifting, and straining until the primary site has healed.
- Consultations for radiation therapy and possible chemotherapy should be initiated when indicated.

SPECIAL CONSIDERATIONS

- Many of the complications of open skull base surgery can also occur when the endoscopic approach is used. Some of the more common sequelae of endoscopic skull base surgery are nasal crusting, impaired olfaction, palatal numbness, and epistaxis.

- Surgical morbidity is more likely to occur if there is significant drilling, leaving exposed bone, dissection near the olfactory cleft, or resection of the neurovascular structures in the pterygopalatine fossa. In most cases, the symptoms are temporary and resolve with time and careful postoperative management.

- A study by a group at the University of Pittsburgh examining morbidity after endoscopic skull base surgery found that nasal crusting was present for an average of 101 days and slightly longer for more complex approaches. Remucosalization of the nasal septum after nasoseptal flap creation usually occurred by 3 months.[22]

- Despite nonsterile conditions in the nasal cavity and sinuses, infectious complications after endoscopic skull base surgery are rare. The incidence of meningitis after traditional transsphenoidal surgery ranges from 0.7% to 3.1%.[4,23]

- The rate of postoperative cerebrospinal fluid leak, another potential complication after endoscopic CFR, is usually below 10%.[9,12,24] Most cerebrospinal fistulas can be successfully managed with lumbar drainage or endoscopic repair.

- Pneumocephalus is also a rare, but potentially catastrophic, complication of endoscopic skull base surgery. Tension pneumocephalus is a medical emergency and requires immediate attention to prevent fatal complications. If left untreated, tension pneumocephalus can lead to progressive brain compression, resulting in changes in mental status, headache, displaced ventricles, brainstem herniation, and death. The incidence of clinically significant pneumocephalus in patients undergoing anterior skull base procedures is 0% to 12%.[25] Management of symptomatic pneumocephalus usually includes decompression and aspiration of the air, administration of 100% oxygen, temporary tracheotomy, administration of antibiotics, cessation of lumbar drainage, and closure of the skull base defect.

REFERENCES

Access the reference list online at ExpertConsult.com.

Skull Base Reconstruction

Repair of Cerebrospinal Fluid Leak and Encephalocele of the Cribriform Plate

Avinash V. Mantravadi and Kevin C. Welch

INTRODUCTION

- Cerebrospinal fluid (CSF) rhinorrhea originating near the cribriform plate results from the breakdown of barriers separating the subarachnoid space and the paranasal sinuses. This may result from traumatic, iatrogenic, neoplastic, congenital, and inflammatory processes.[1,2]
- A CSF leak in the cribriform region may also be spontaneous in nature and may present with a meningoencephalocele, which is the herniation of the anterior cranial fossa soft tissue through the skull base.
- Although conservative management may be used to treat cribriform CSF leaks after blunt force trauma, surgical intervention is generally required for closure of other forms to prevent serious complications, including meningitis and abscess formation.[2]
- Open intracranial approaches for CSF leak repair involving frontal craniotomy, first described by Dandy in the 1920s, were limited by significant morbidity, including anosmia, intracerebral hemorrhage, frontal lobe deficits, extended hospital stay, and higher recurrence rates.[2-11]
- The endoscopic approach for repair of cribriform CSF leaks occurring during endoscopic ethmoidectomy was first described by Wigand and Stankiewicz in the 1980s and further detailed by many others.[11-16]
- Today, transnasal endoscopic approaches for repair of cribriform CSF leaks and encephaloceles are the mainstay of surgical therapy, with success rates as high as 98%, low complication and recurrence rates, and decreased morbidity.[2,17]

ANATOMY

- The ethmoid labyrinth forms the bulk of the anterior skull base, with the cribriform plate being the lowest portion of the anterior skull base in the midline. The cribriform plate is suspended bilaterally by the lateral cribriform lamellae, which thicken as they extend laterally into the fovea ethmoidalis. Therefore, when performing an ethmoid skull base dissection, the surgeon is, in fact, operating above the lowest level of the anterior cranial fossa.
- The depth of the cribriform plate is dictated by the length of the lateral cribriform lamellae, as classified by Keros[18] (Fig. 26.1):
  - Keros type 1: The cribriform plate is located 1 to 3 mm below the roof of the ethmoid, resulting in a short lateral cribriform lamella.
  - Keros type 2: The cribriform plate is located 4 to 7 mm below the roof of the ethmoid.
  - Keros type 3: The cribriform plate is located 8 to 16 mm below the roof of the ethmoid, resulting in a long vertical lamella.
- The cribriform plate is perforated by numerous olfactory fibers (Fig. 26.2). Despite these perforations, the cribriform plate itself is fairly thick.
- The anterior ethmoidal artery originates from the ophthalmic artery and passes through the anterior ethmoidal foramen near the frontoethmoidal suture. Its bony canal may be partially or completely dehiscent in 40% of cases.[19] The artery crosses the skull base until it gives rise to meningeal branches at the cribriform plate.

PREOPERATIVE CONSIDERATIONS

- Preoperative intrathecal injection of fluorescein is frequently used to localize the source of CSF leakage. Although neurologic complications—including seizures, headaches, and cranial nerve deficits—have been reported, a concentration of 0.1 mL of 10%

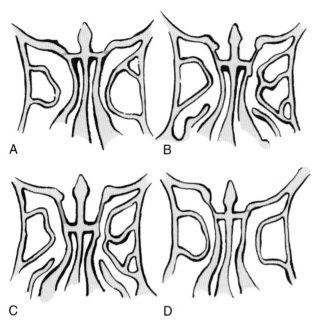

Fig. 26.1. Illustration depiction of computed tomography scans showing the Keros classification. **(A)** Keros Class I; **(B)** Keros Class II; **(C)** Keros Class III; **(D)** asymmetric skull base.

fluorescein mixed with 10 mL of CSF injected slowly has been shown to be of low risk.[20,21]

- The utility of lumbar drainage in the early management of cribriform CSF leak repair is controversial. When used, they can be conduits for fluorescein administration and are deployed to divert CSF for 2 to 5 days.
- The routine use of perioperative prophylactic antibiotics in patients undergoing cribriform CSF leak repairs is also controversial, albeit reasonable.

Radiographic Considerations

- Patients with cribriform CSF leaks should be evaluated with high-resolution computed tomography (CT) scanning with coronal, axial, and sagittal views to clarify the location of the skull base defect and the anatomy of the skull base itself (asymmetry, low-lying, and so on; Fig. 26.3). Coronal views are best to evaluate defects of the cribriform plate and fovea ethmoidalis.
- Patients presenting with spontaneous CSF rhinorrhea should be evaluated with magnetic resonance imaging (MRI) with axial, coronal, and sagittal views to evaluate for the presence of a meningoencephalocele if a soft tissue mass is identified near a skull base defect on CT imaging (Fig. 26.4).
- Stereotactic image-guidance CT imaging is helpful for intraoperative localization of the skull base defect but is neither required nor is the standard of care (Fig. 26.5).

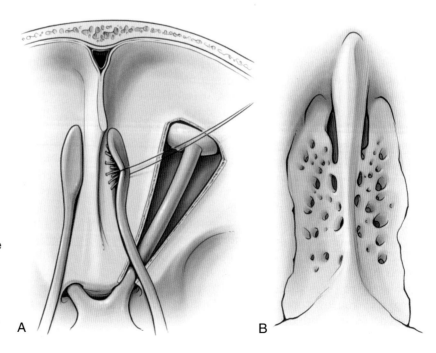

Fig. 26.2. Illustration of the intracranial view of the floor of the anterior cranial fossa, with the olfactory tracts traversing the floor **(A)**. Note the thin cribriform plate and lateral lamella medially and thicker fovea ethmoidalis (ethmoid roof) laterally **(B)**. (Adapted from Logan BM, Reynolds, PA, Hutchings RT, eds. *McMinn's Color Atlas of Head and Neck Anatomy.* 3rd ed. St. Louis: Mosby; 2003.)

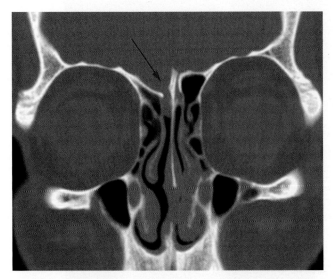

Fig. 26.3. Preoperative computed tomography scan of the anterior skull base with attention to the cribriform region. The skull base is notably asymmetric and there is a dehiscence along the right cribriform *(red arrow)* with soft tissue opacification of the olfactory cleft suggesting a meningoencephalocele.

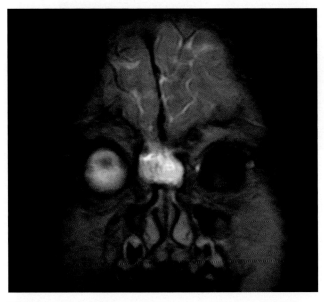

Fig. 26.4. Preoperative magnetic resonance image (MRI) of a child who presented with soft tissue fullness in the prenasal space. The MRI revealed a meningoencephalocele based on the right anterior skull base involving the cribriform region.

INSTRUMENTATION

- Hand-held conventional and powered endoscopic sinus instruments
- Instrumentation for obtaining extranasal graft tissue
- Stereotactic image-guidance surgical system

- Electrocautery, including needle-tip monopolar, bipolar, and/or radiofrequency or cold ablation device
- Subarachnoid drain and/or 10% injectable (nonophthalmic) fluorescein
- Fibrin glue/sealant
- Absorbable packing materials (e.g., GelFoam or GelFilm)
- Nonabsorbable packing materials (e.g., nasal sponge)
- Hemostatic agents (e.g., Floseal)

PEARLS AND POTENTIAL PITFALLS

- 10% fluorescein is not approved by the US Food and Drug Administration for intrathecal administration, and full informed consent is recommended. Administration, however, can greatly aid in identification of leaks intraoperatively (Fig. 26.6).
- Small or very-low-flow leaks may require a blue light filter for identification.
- Stereotactic image-guidance equipment assists in intraoperative identification of the skull base defect. Its use during endoscopic repair of cribriform CSF leaks is supported by the American Academy of Otolaryngology—Head and Neck Surgery (http://www.entnet.org/Practice/policyIntraOperativeSurgery.cfm).
- A rigid underlay graft (e.g., bone, cartilage) is generally preferred in cases of encephalocele to mitigate the effects of elevated intracranial pressure, while cribriform CSF leaks without encephalocele may be repaired safely without rigid graft material (e.g., mucosa, fat).
- Numerous grafting materials and tissue sealants exist. The choice of which one to use is dependent on surgeon preference and the size of the defect. A brief algorithm for skull base reconstruction strategies is presented in Fig. 26.7.
- Mucosal grafts should always be oriented and placed with the mucosal surface toward the nasal cavity to prevent subsequent mucocele formation.
- Extubation should be performed deeply to prevent increases in intracranial pressure related to patient agitation and coughing. Bag-mask ventilation should be avoided, as this can result in postoperative pneumocephalus.

SURGICAL PROCEDURE

- The repair of cribriform CSF leaks is performed under general anesthesia using totally intravenous anesthesia with remifentanyl and propofol, with the head of bed elevated to 10 to 15 degrees.
- If desired, an intrathecal injection of fluorescein (0.1 mL of 10% injectable fluorescein, diluted in 10 mL of preservative-free or bacteriostatic saline or the patient's own CSF) is performed prior to initiation of surgery with or without a lumbar drain.

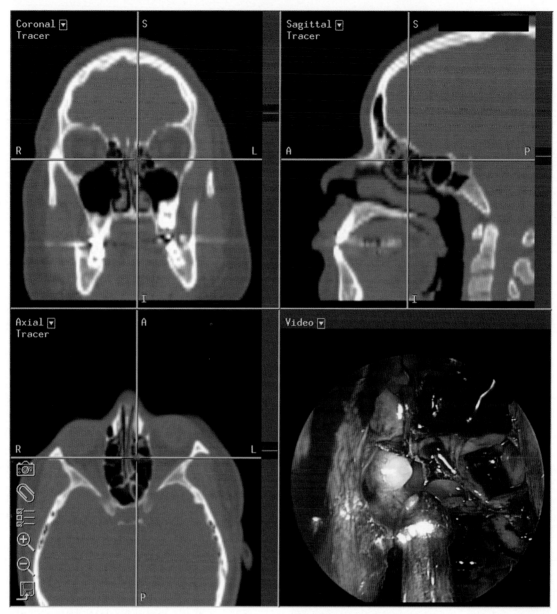

Fig. 26.5. While not essential, stereotactic navigation can be useful intraoperatively for localizing the cribriform defect and assessing intraoperatively the size of the defect.

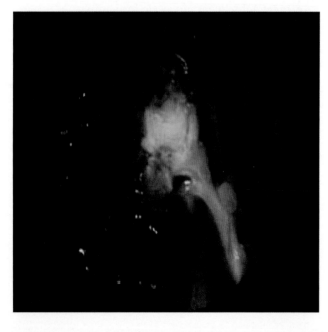

Fig. 26.6. The administration of intrathecal fluorescein aided greatly to the identification of a small encephalocele in this patient with a left cribriform-related cerebrospinal fluid leak.

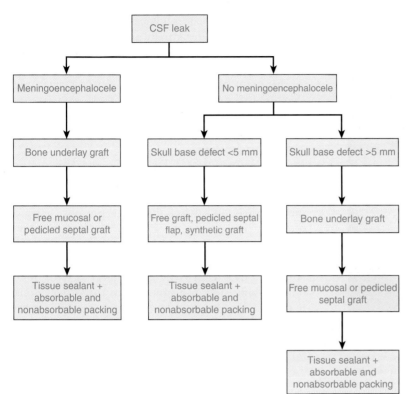

Fig. 26.7. Although meta-analysis has suggested that successful repair of cribriform cerebrospinal fluid leaks can be accomplished with multiple grafting techniques, the corresponding author (KCW) presents a proposed algorithm for anterior skull base reconstruction that has worked well for these leaks.

- Cottonoids soaked in 1:1000 epinephrine solution are placed atraumatically in the nasal cavities to allow for proper decongestion and hemostatic effects.
- The stereotactic image guidance system is properly calibrated and ensured to be in proper working order.
- Endoscopic examination of the region of concern is undertaken, with attention to any regions of meningoencephalocele formation (Fig. 26.8) or notable for yellow-green fluorescein (Fig. 26.9).
- A complete maxillary antrostomy, sphenoethmoidectomy, and—if necessary—frontal sinusotomy are performed to completely expose the defect and surrounding tissue. If necessary, the middle turbinate is resected (Fig. 26.10) to expose the entirety of the cribriform plate and lateral cribriform lamella where a CSF leak or meningoencephalocele may hide. Turbinate mucosa and bone should be saved for grafting material.
- Stereotactic navigation is used to confirm the site of the leak and its proximity to vital structures.
- Often, cribriform region CSF leaks will involve olfactory fila (Fig. 26.11).
- Bipolar cautery is used to reduce the meningoencephalocele and to fulgurate any nests of mucosa that surround the defect (Fig. 26.12).

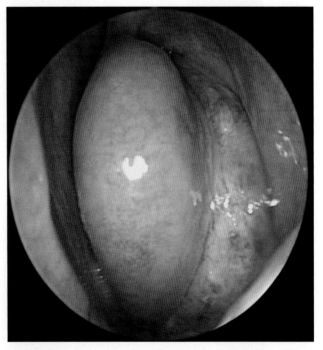

Fig. 26.8. Initial inspection of the left nasal cavity reveals a very large meningocele in the middle meatus that corresponds to a left cribriform/lateral cribriform lamella defect.

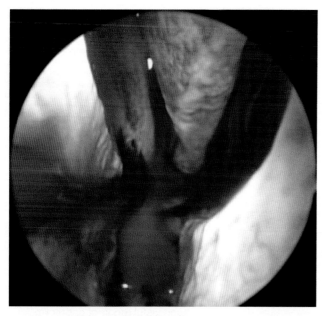

Fig. 26.9. Initial inspection of the left nasal cavity reveals fluorescein in the nasopharynx, confirming the presence of a cerebrospinal fluid leak. In this case, a septoplasty has been performed to assist with access to the left cribriform region.

- If a large meningoencephalocele is present, it should be exposed circumferentially and bipolar electrocautery or coblation is applied directly to the encephalocele until it is reduced intracranially.
- At this point, the size of the bony defect is measured (Fig. 26.13).
- Any bleeding around the defect is controlled with bipolar cautery. Char is removed to create a smooth surface for grafting.
- In our algorithm (see Fig. 26.7), the size of the defect and surgeon preference dictate the choice of reconstructive material. If a larger defect (>5 mm) and/or an encephalocele is present, a rigid underlay or composite graft may be necessary. Composite (mucosa and bone) graft may be harvested from the excised middle turbinate, which is split in half to provide graft material with bone only on one side and mucosa on the other. Bone may also be obtained from the posterior septum or mastoid tip.
- An overlay mucosal graft may be obtained using septal, middle turbinate, or nasal floor mucosa. These are considered free grafts and should be of sufficient

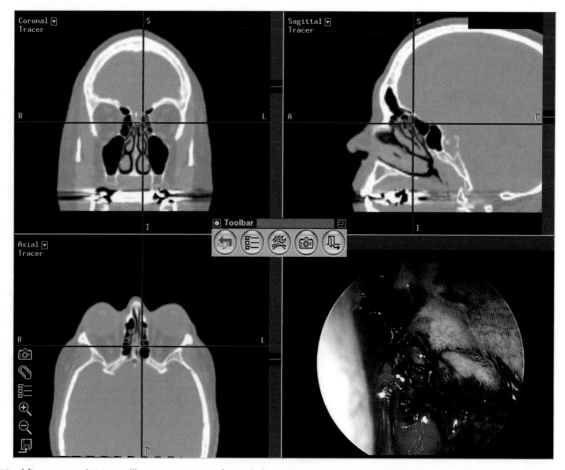

Fig. 26.10. After a complete maxillary antrostomy, frontal sinusotomy, and sphenoethmoidectomy have been performed, it may be necessary to remove the middle turbinate to provide adequate access to the cribriform region. The middle turbinate is removed with endoscopic scissors and the tissue is saved as potential grafting material.

size to cover the entire defect as well as surrounding, denuded sinus bone (Fig. 26.14).

■ If a nasoseptal mucosal flap is to be utilized, needle-tip electrocautery is used to make an incision at the inferior aspect of the bony septum at the level of the maxillary crest until the mucocutaneous junction is encountered. A vertical incision is carried at the

anterior end of the septum superiorly, stopping at least 5 mm below the skull base to preserve the olfactory fibers in this region.

■ The mucoperichondrial flap is elevated in a manner similar to septoplasty. Since the flap is based on the

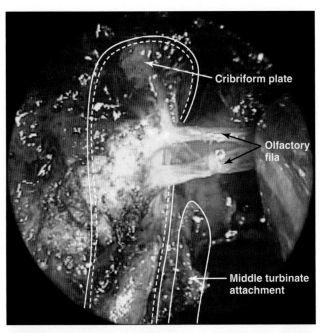

Fig. 26.11. Cribriform defects may involve the olfactory fila, shown here in this intraoperative photograph.

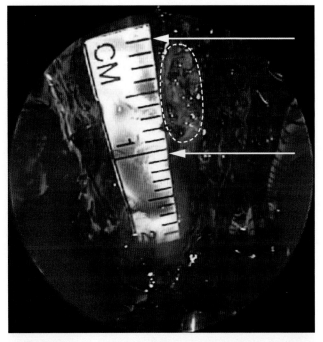

Fig. 26.13. The defect *(dotted oval)* is sized using a ruler.

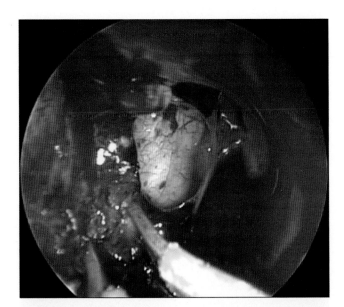

Fig. 26.12. Small meningoencephaloceles can be reduced with bipolar cautery. After reduction, the surrounding mucosa is fulgurated with bipolar cautery to achieve hemostasis and prepare the recipient bed for grafting.

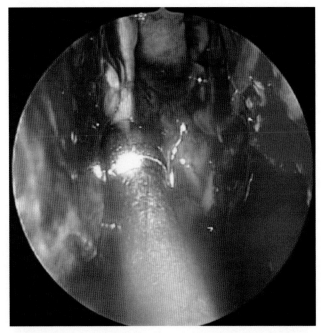

Fig. 26.14. In this situation, a free mucosal graft harvested from the septum was used to cover the defect in overlay fashion. It is important to ensure that there is adequate coverage of the defect.

septal branch of the sphenopalatine artery, flap elevation stops at the choana until the mucosa containing the septal branch is isolated and elevated off the face of the sphenoid sinus.

- The vascularized pedicled mucosal flap may then be rotated up to the cribriform region or fovea ethmoidalis for use as a graft (Fig. 26.15).

- At this point, no additional fluorescein or CSF should be visible from the defect. A Valsalva maneuver is performed to ensure water-tight closure.

- The repair is then coated with fibrin sealant. A frontal sinus stent is placed to ensure that graft or flap swelling does not obstruct the frontal sinus outflow (Fig. 26.16).

- A hemostatic agent is the placed over the site to ensure a dry field and to promote scarring in the region (Fig. 26.17). GelFoam (Pfizer, New York, NY) is then applied over the repair to serve as a smooth barrier to removable packing that will be placed to bolster the repair.

- A Merocel (Medtronic, Mystic, Connecticut) sponge is then secured inside a nonlatex glove finger, and the pack is placed against the repair (Fig. 26.18).

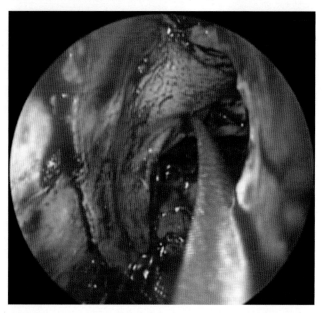

Fig. 26.15. The pedicled septal flap is transposed over the cribriform defect and secured with fibrin glue (tissue sealant).

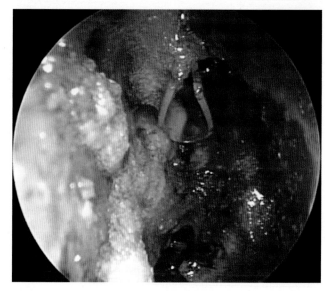

Fig. 26.17. A hemostatic agent is placed around the graft to assist with bleeding as well as promote scar tissue formation.

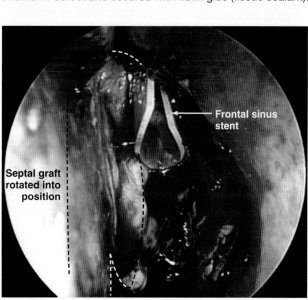

Fig. 26.16. In order to overcome the flap or graft edema around the frontal sinus, a frontal sinus stent (in this case, rolled silicone sheeting) is placed.

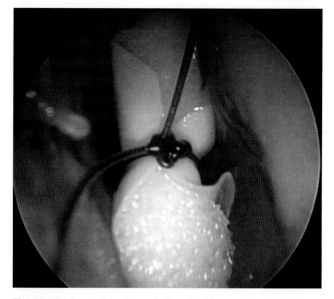

Fig. 26.18. A combination of absorbable and nonabsorbable packing is placed against the graft.

- Unilateral or bilateral nasal trumpets may be placed to divert airflow from the repair to the nasopharynx, with care taken to prevent excessive pressure on the alar rim that can result in skin necrosis.
- Close communication should exist with the involved anesthesia team to coordinate a deep extubation in order to prevent bucking or coughing that can increase intracranial pressure. Positive pressure ventilation (via bag-mask) should be avoided at all costs to prevent postoperative pneumocephalus.

POSTOPERATIVE CONSIDERATIONS

- Neurologic status is followed closely, specifically with regard to clinical suspicion of pneumocephalus or meningitis. In some institutions, this may require admission to an intensive care unit.
- A head CT is advisable for the detection of surgery-related bleeding and/or pneumocephalus (Fig. 26.19).
- Nonabsorbable packs are left in place for a minimum of 5 days postoperatively.
- In the absence of clinical evidence of meningitis, oral antibiotics with adequate staphylococcal coverage are continued as long as packs are in place.
- If there is no evidence of persistent CSF rhinorrhea after pack removal, the patient is started on saline nasal sprays 4 to 6 times daily, to be continued until seen in follow-up.

SPECIAL CONSIDERATIONS

- If a lumbar drain is utilized, the patient is maintained in the supine position and the drain is used judiciously, removing 10 to 15 mL/hour for 2 to 5 days. The drain is then clamped and the patient monitored for evidence of recurrent CSF leak or change in neurologic status. If the patient remains clinically stable, the drain is removed.
- The patient should have long-term follow-up, especially in the cases of spontaneous cribriform CSF leaks or meningoencephaloceles. Graft sites can be monitored with endoscopic procedures in the clinic (Fig. 26.20).

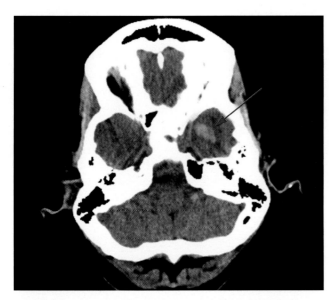

Fig. 26.19. It is reasonable to obtain a head computed tomography scan after performing cerebrospinal fluid (CSF) leak repairs. In this example, a patient who underwent a transpterygoid CSF leak repair had intraoperative bleeding *(red arrow)* into the temporal lobe that resulted in seizure activity that was present during emergence from anesthesia.

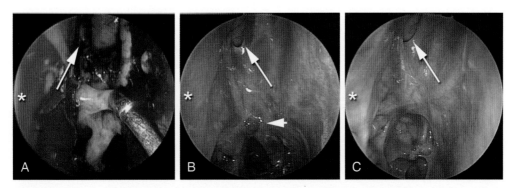

Fig. 26.20. The appearance of a cribriform cerebrospinal fluid leak repair intraoperatively **(A)** as well as 2 months postoperatively **(B)** and 6 months postoperatively **(C)**. Granulation along the skull base *(arrowhead)* is present at 2 months. The frontal sinus *(arrow)* remains patent.

REFERENCES

Access the reference list online at ExpertConsult.com.

Sphenoid Sinus Cerebrospinal Fluid Leak and Encephalocele Repair

Benjamin S. Bleier and Rodney Schlosser

INTRODUCTION

- Dandy, in 1926, was the first to report a transcranial technique for the closure of a cerebrospinal fluid (CSF) leak using a fascia lata graft.[1]
- Open approaches were associated with morbidities, including seizures, memory deficits, and intracranial hemorrhage.[2-4]
- Dohlman pioneered an extracranial technique in 1948 with success rates approaching 80%.[5]
- The first transeptal and fully endonasal approaches were introduced by Hirsch and by Vrabec, respectively.[6]
- The first endoscopic CSF leak repair was reported by Papay et al. in 1989.[7]
- The importance of the lateral extension of the sphenoid sinus with respect to CSF rhinorrhea was recognized as early as 1965 by Morley and Wortzman.[8]

ANATOMY

- The majority of the sphenoid bone is formed from the endochondral ossification of five discrete ossification centers beginning in the thirteenth week of development.[9]
- Incomplete fusion of the greater wing can result in persistence of a lateral craniopharyngeal canal, which was first described by Sternberg[10] in 1888 and may be seen in up to 4% of patients.[11]
- A role for the Sternberg canal in the pathogenesis of lateral sphenoid CSF leaks is doubtful.
- The degree of pneumatization may be quite variable and when assessed in the sagittal plane may progress from a relative lack of aeration or "conchal" pattern (5%–10%), through a presellar pattern

(25%–30%), and ultimately to a postsellar pattern in which pneumatization extends posteriorly to the level of the clivus (65%).

- When viewed in the coronal plane, lateral pneumatization into the pterygoid plates is evident in 35.3% of subjects and is bilateral in 17.4%.[11]
- Tomazic and Stammberger reported a series of five sphenoid CSF leaks, noting that 100% were associated with a patent canal.[12] Conversely, Bernal-Sprekelsen et al.[13] found that among 25 patients with lateral sphenoid leaks, 24 were lateral to the foramen rotundum, which suggests no association with a Sternberg canal.
- A more accepted etiologic factor in these spontaneous lateral sphenoid lesions is chronic benign intracranial hypertension (BIH).
- Although lateral sphenoid CSF leaks most commonly occur spontaneously, central leaks tend to result from iatrogenic causes, often in the setting of prior transsphenoidal pituitary surgery.[6]
- The vidian canal and its associated neurovascular bundle is a key anatomic landmark in the management of these lesions because it may be used to orient the surgeon in both the approach and the localization of critical intracranial structures adjacent to the defect.
- The vidian nerve can serve as an important landmark in this region because it can reliably be traced to the lateral surface of the anterior genu of the petrous carotid artery.[14]
- In the midline, the sella contains the pituitary gland, which is surrounded by its associated dural reflections, hypophyseal arteries, optic chiasm, and superior and inferior intercavernous sinuses (Fig. 27.1).

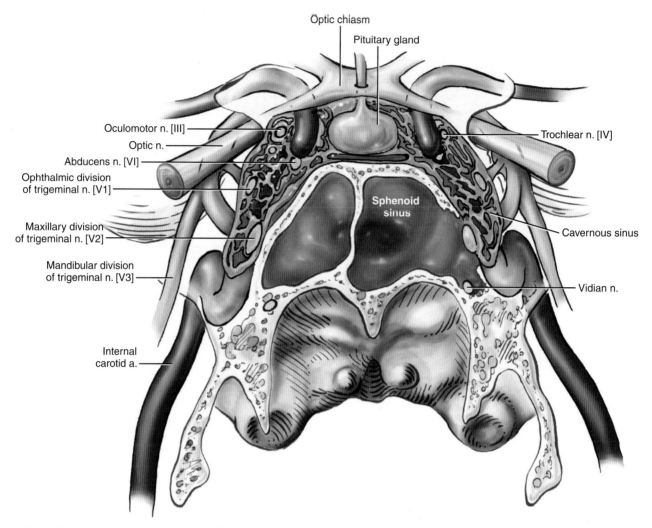

Fig. 27.1. Drawing of a coronal cross-section through the sphenoid sinus and associated structures. Note that loss of bone is depicted over the patient's left cavernous sinus, V2, vidian nerve, and carotid artery as can often present with encephaloceles. *a.,* Artery; *n.,* nerve.

PREOPERATIVE CONSIDERATIONS

Patient History

- Clinical symptoms may include CSF rhinorrhea (85%), chronic headache (77%), and a history of meningitis (15%).[9] Patients with spontaneous leaks often have increased body mass index with its associated comorbidities, including hypertension, sleep apnea, and BIH.
- Any history of trauma, inflammatory rhinologic disorders, or prior surgeries (particularly transsphenoidal pituitary procedures) should be elicited.

Clinical Diagnosis

- Confirmation of CSF rhinorrhea may be performed by testing the fluid for the presence of β_2-transferrin. Samples collected by the patient will remain stable for β_2-transferrin testing for up to 1 week at room temperature.[15]
- Nasal endoscopy may reveal fluid or a meningoencephalocele sac emanating from the sphenoethmoid recess; however, negative examination findings do not preclude the presence of a pathologic process.

- The cavernous sinus proper lies immediately lateral to the pituitary fossa and transmits multiple cranial nerves as well as the cavernous (or C4) segment of the internal carotid artery.
- With extensive pneumatization, the sphenoid may continue laterally to the foramen rotundum beneath the floor of the middle cranial fossa. Inferiorly, this pneumatization pattern may extend into the pterygoid plates inferolateral to the vidian canal.

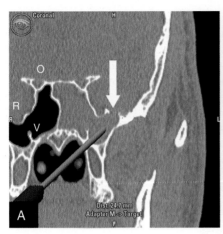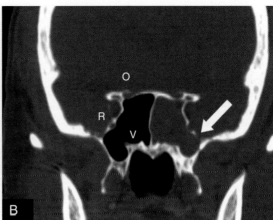

Fig. 27.2. Noncontrast coronal computed tomography (CT) images from patients with lateral sphenoid meningoencephaloceles *(white arrows)*. The patient in **(A)** has a more significantly pneumatized lateral recess than the patient in **(B)**. Note the significant amount of right middle fossa arachnoid pitting seen in **(B)**. The relative positions of the optic nerve *(O)*, foramen rotundum *(R)*, and vidian canal *(V)* are shown.

- Pneumatic otoscopy should also be performed in these patients to exclude the presence of middle ear fluid, which raises concern for a primary or synchronous temporal bone CSF leak.

Intrathecal Fluorescein Administration

- Intrathecal fluorescein administration is a useful adjunct in the management of these lesions. The most common dose is 0.1 mL of 10% sodium fluorescein mixed with 10 mL of the patient's own CSF or sterile saline and injected over a 10-minute period.
- Patients must be counseled that this represents an off-label use and that seizures and other neurologic complications have been reported with the use of fluorescein at higher doses.
- Excitation of the fluorescein with blue light leads to emission of green wavelengths and, when used in conjunction with a blue light–blocking filter, helps to maximize visualization of even small volumes of stained CSF.[4]
- Placement of a lumbar drain also provides an opportunity for the measurement of opening pressures, which may help to guide postoperative management.

Radiographic Considerations

Computed Tomography

- Fine-cut, noncontrast, maxillofacial computed tomography (CT) scans should be obtained for any patient with a suspected sphenoid CSF leak or meningoencephalocele.
- The use of image guidance may be quite helpful; if this is planned, the CT images can be ordered using the available institutional image guidance protocol.

- The pneumatization pattern and status of the skull base should be assessed in all three planes. The site of the lesion may be indicated by a focal attenuation of the middle fossa bone or frank dehiscence with soft tissue prolapse.
- The presence of any Onodi cells, laterally based partitions, or dehiscence of the optic nerves or internal carotid arteries should be noted. The location of the vidian canal and foramen rotundum should be identified and the site of abnormalities relative to these structures noted.
- In the setting of BIH, the CT may reveal several additional stigmata, including an empty sella, arachnoid pitting in the middle cranial fossa, and thinning of the tegmen (Fig. 27.2).
- The location of the lesion relative to the foramen rotundum should be determined because this will dictate whether a medial, transethmoid, or transpterygoid approach will be required to gain adequate surgical access.

Magnetic Resonance Imaging

- Use of T1- (with and without gadolinium) and T2-weighted magnetic resonance imaging (MRI) allows for soft tissue characterization, which helps to differentiate between a CSF leak, encephalocele, and meningoencephalocele.
- The MRI scan provides additional information on the relationship between the various segments of the internal carotid artery and the site of the defect. Although it is uncommon, the MRI may also provide evidence for any prolapsed intracranial vasculature associated with the defect. If this is a concern, magnetic resonance or interventional angiography should be performed to further characterize these vessels.

- An empty sella resulting from prolapse of the suprasellar arachnoid cistern into the sellar cavity is also easily seen on a sagittal T1-weighted MRI scan and provides confirmatory evidence for the presence of elevated intracranial pressures.
- The MRI may be overlaid with the CT data to provide simultaneous intraoperative information on the local bony and soft tissue anatomy.

Adjunctive Imaging

- The use of angiography, CT/MRI cisternography, and radioactive tracer studies in the workup of these lesions has been previously described. Their use has declined with the increasing popularity of β_2-transferrin and intrathecal fluorescein confirmatory testing.

INSTRUMENTATION

- Adequate exposure of sphenoid CSF leak and meningoencephalocele sites should allow the use of primarily straight instrumentation. The intermittent use of angled endoscopes and instruments with distal angulations may occasionally be required (Fig. 27.3).
  - 0- and 45-degree endoscopes
  - J-curette and ball-tip probe
  - 15-degree diamond drill
  - Straight and curved suction devices
  - Upbiting and downbiting 2-mm Kerrison punches
  - Straight Blakesley forceps
  - Endoscopic clip applier
  - Bipolar cautery

PEARLS AND POTENTIAL PITFALLS

Pearls

- The choice of approach will be dictated by how lateral the lesion is. Increased lateral access will be gained by migrating from a medial to transethmoid and finally a transpterygoid approach.
- Lesions within a highly pneumatized lateral sphenoid recess will virtually always require a transpterygoid approach.

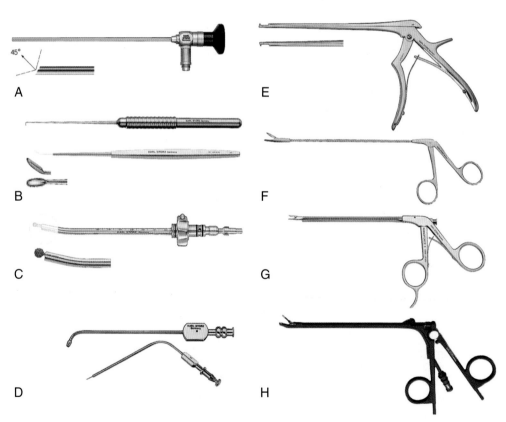

Fig. 27.3. Photograph of instruments commonly used in the repair of sphenoid sinus cerebrospinal fluid leaks and meningoencephaloceles. **(A)** 45-degree Hopkins Rod Endoscope; **(B)** right-angle probe and spoon curette; **(C)** 15-degree diamond bur; **(D)** straight and curved suction catheters; **(E)** upbiting and downbiting Kerrison punches; **(F)** straight-through punch; **(G)** endoscopic clip applier; **(H)** endoscopic bipolar cautery. (©2017 Photo Courtesy of Karl Storz Endoscopy-America, Inc.)

- During the initial sphenoidotomy, resection of the inferior third of the superior turbinate will greatly enhance access to the sphenoid face without sacrificing postoperative olfactory function.
- The sphenoidotomy may be maximally expanded in the inferior dimension without requiring sacrifice of the posterior septal branch provided the mucosa is dissected off the bone in the subperiosteal plane. A relaxing incision along the vomer will facilitate this maneuver.
- If a nasoseptal flap will be used in the reconstruction, it should be elevated at the start of the operation and stored in the nasopharynx to prevent inadvertent sacrifice of the pedicle later in the procedure.
- When a transpterygoid approach is used, the posterior maxillary sinus mucosa should be elevated before the bone is removed because it may be laid back in place at the conclusion of the surgery to aid in wound healing.

Potential Pitfalls

- Failure to obtain adequate exposure of the defect during the approach will greatly prolong the procedure because the surgeon will struggle to manipulate the instruments through a limited sphenoidotomy.
- After removal of the posterior maxillary wall during a transpterygoid approach, a bipolar cautery should be used on all fat before manipulation. Multiple small vessels permeate the tissue that will otherwise tend to bleed throughout the procedure, greatly impeding visualization.
- Before a pneumatized lateral recess is entered, the foramen rotundum and vidian canal should be identified; failure to do so may result in inadvertent injury to their respective neurovascular bundles.

SURGICAL PROCEDURE

- Even in the setting of a laterally based lesion, perform an ipsilateral transethmoid sphenoidotomy to aid in surgical manipulation and postoperative sinus drainage. What follows describes a transethmoid approach and a transpterygoid approach.
- If a lumbar drain is being placed for intrathecal fluorescein instillation, do this up to 1 hour before the start of the procedure. Place the patient in the Trendelenburg position to aid in circulation of the fluorescein.
- Once the patient is anesthetized, perform routine sinus injections using 1% lidocaine with 1:100,000 epinephrine. If a nasoseptal flap will be raised, inject the flap with at least 3 mL of local anesthetic. Then, pack the nose with pledgets containing a topical

vasoconstrictor. The use of high-dose epinephrine (1:1000) is limited, because the dissection approaches the skull base, particularly when there is an active CSF leak. Place pledgets medial, lateral, and anterior to the middle turbinate.
- If a nasoseptal flap is to be used, raise the flap and place it in the nasopharynx at the start of the surgery. Cover the pedicle with a pledget to protect it as the surgery proceeds.

Step 1

- Begin the transethmoid approach by performing an uncinectomy, maxillary antrostomy, anterior ethmoidectomy, and posterior ethmoidectomy as described in previous chapters.

Step 2

- Once the posterior ethmoids have been dissected, identify the cleavage plane between the middle and superior turbinates by manipulating the middle turbinate and looking for the medial portion that does not move. Identification of the superior turbinate may require further removal of the inferomedial quadrant of the vertical portion of the basal lamella. Once it has been identified, use straight, through-cutting forceps to resect the inferior third of the superior turbinate.

Step 3

- After superior turbinate resection, identify the natural os of the sphenoid. Use a J-curette to dilate the os in an inferomedial direction. Once the sphenoid lumen is visualized, use an upbiting and downbiting 2-mm Kerrison punch to remove the sphenoid face superiorly to the skull base, inferiorly to the sphenoid floor, and laterally to the orbital apex (Fig. 27.4).
- For medially based lesions, repair the defect through this transethmoid access. For lateral lesions, proceed to the transpterygoid approach.

Step 4

- As the initial step for the transpterygoid approach, laterally elevate and preserve the posterior maxillary mucosa. Then, place a Kerrison punch into the sphenoethmoid foramen and remove the posterior maxillary wall. This maneuver will expose the sphenopalatine artery and pterygopalatine ganglion (Fig. 27.5).

Step 5

- Elevate and incise the pterygopalatine fossa periosteum, exposing the fat (Fig. 27.6). Branches of the internal maxillary artery may also be visible at this point. Use bipolar forceps to cauterize the fat. The fat should continue to be cauterized posteriorly toward the pterygoid plates.

- Palpate the pterygoid plates with a J-curette and elevate the periosteum medially and laterally. Pneumatization of the lateral recess may lend a translucent, bluish hue to the pterygoid process, which will aid in directing the point of entry.

Step 6

- Use the J-curette to fracture the face of the lateral recess to enter the lumen. A diamond drill may also be used to enter this region if the bone is too thick to fracture. Then, use a Kerrison punch to expand this opening superolaterally. At the conclusion of this approach, a medial bridge of soft tissue transmitting the vidian and infraorbital nerves should remain intact (Fig. 27.7).

Step 7

- When an encephalocele or meningoencephalocele is present, carefully cauterize the prolapsed soft tissue with bipolar cautery and reduce it to the level of the bony defect. Although this neural tissue is nonfunctional, it may contain vessels that can retract intracranially; therefore, maintain meticulous hemostasis at all times.
- Regardless of the type of lesion, completely strip the mucosa adjacent to the defect to prepare the site for repair.

Step 8

- Proceed with the repair in a multilayered fashion. The choice of graft materials is largely based on preference. Some surgeons prefer to place a collagen-based dural graft matrix in an underlay fashion into the defect. If possible, this is followed by placement of an underlay bone graft harvested from the thin perpendicular plate of the ethmoid bone (Fig. 27.8).

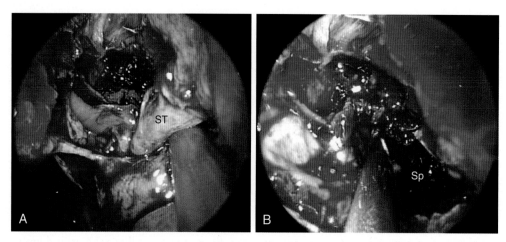

Fig. 27.4. (A) Endoscopic image showing identification and lateral reflection of the right superior turbinate *(ST)* using a straight Frazier suction catheter in anticipation of resection of the inferior third. **(B)** Endoscopic image showing wide exposure of the sphenoid sinus lumen *(Sp)* after resection of the sphenoid face using a Kerrison punch.

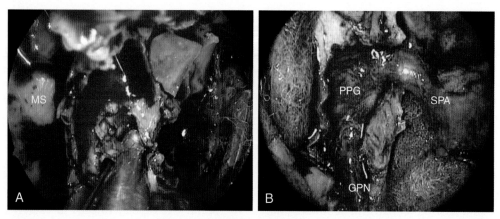

Fig. 27.5. (A) Endoscopic image showing resection of the perpendicular plate of the palatine bone and posterior right maxillary wall using a Kerrison punch. A wide maxillary antrostomy has already been performed exposing the maxillary sinus *(MS)* lumen. **(B)** Endoscopic view after removal of the medial aspect of the posterior maxillary wall. The greater palatine nerve *(GPN)*, pterygopalatine ganglion *(PPG)*, and sphenopalatine artery *(SPA)* are easily visualized.

- Remain acutely aware of the intracranial structures adjacent to the defect to avoid extensive manipulation around the internal carotid artery.

Step 9

- After placement of the underlay materials, place an additional small piece of dural graft matrix extracranially, followed by a mucosal overlay graft. When using a free mucosal graft, ink the mucosal

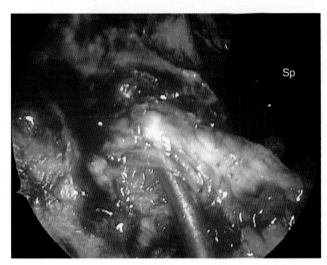

Fig. 27.6. Endoscopic image showing controlled elevation and incision of the periosteum using a ball-tip probe following removal of the posterior maxillary wall. This prevents inadvertent injury to arborizations of the internal maxillary artery lying immediately posterior to this periosteal layer. The sphenoid sinus *(Sp)* has been widely opened and is seen posteromedial to the tip of the probe.

side using a marking pen to prevent inadvertent inset of the graft in an inverted position.

- If a nasoseptal flap has been elevated, rotate it into position (Fig. 27.9). In some instances, the lateral recess is not large enough to accommodate multiple graft layers even when maximal access has been achieved. In these cases, simply pack the cavity with dural graft matrix after mucosal stripping.

- After completing the repair, pack the sphenoid with an absorbable gelatin sponge (Gelfoam) and apply tissue glue to the area. Then, place the preserved maxillary sinus mucosa over the pterygopalatine fossa to aid in postoperative remucosalization.

- Using a nonlatex glove finger to serve as a middle meatal spacer, place it in the operated side, and suture it to the septum using a 2-0 polypropylene (Prolene) suture.

POSTOPERATIVE CONSIDERATIONS

Packing

- Previous series have reported the use of packing for up to 4 to 7 days postoperatively.[13,16] However, it is preferred that the middle meatal spacers be removed within the first postoperative week.

Antibiotics

- Although the evidence supporting a correlation between packing and toxic shock syndrome is weak, it is recommended that all patients receive antibiotics for 7 to 14 days, which is consistent with reported practice.[16]

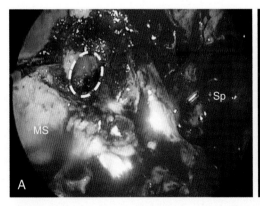
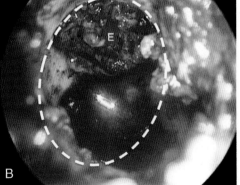

Fig. 27.7. **(A)** Endoscopic view of transpterygoid access to the lateral sphenoid recess *(dashed oval)* after bipolar cauterizing and clearing of the intervening fat. The maxillary sinus *(MS)* and medial sphenoid sinus *(Sp)* are both widely opened and are seen anterolateral and posteromedial to the lateral recess, respectively. Note the preservation of the neurovascular structures between the lateral recess and the medial aspect of the sphenoid sinus. **(B)** Magnified endoscopic view through the transpterygoid osteotomy *(dashed oval)* showing the reduced encephalocele *(E)* sac flush with the bony defect in the floor of the middle cranial fossa.

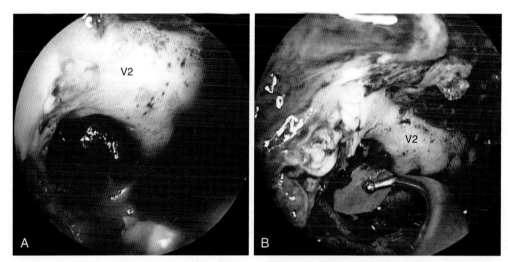

Fig. 27.8. (A) Endoscopic view of a sphenoid encephalocele following reduction and placement of a dural graft matrix in an underlay fashion. Note that the location of this defect is immediately inferior to the second division of the trigeminal nerve *(V2)* in a sinus with limited lateral pneumatization. This lesion was repaired using a strictly transethmoid approach. **(B)** Given the size of this defect, an underlay bone graft was placed into position using a ball-tip probe.

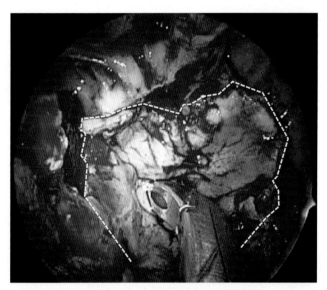

Fig. 27.9. Endoscopic image showing the insetting of a pedicled nasoseptal flap *(dashed white line)* into the sphenoid lumen in an overlay position.

Lumbar Drain

- The use of postoperative lumbar drainage as reported in the literature is highly variable, with groups describing usage rates ranging from 0% to 73%.[6] The recommendation is to restrict the use of lumbar drains to patients with obvious signs of BIH or persistent high-flow intraoperative CSF leaks.
- When the surgeon elects to use a lumbar drain, the patient must be placed in an inpatient unit with knowledgeable nursing staff. This will help reduce the risk of severe drain-associated complications, including spinal headache, overdrainage with potential cerebellar herniation, pneumocephalus, infection, and catheter tip retention.

Acetazolamide

- Acetazolamide is a carbonic anhydrase inhibitor that can reduce intracranial pressure.[6] Patients with BIH may benefit from long-term postoperative use of acetazolamide to help prevent recurrence or the development of a second leak. It is recommended that acetazolamide be used in all patients with suspected BIH or high opening pressures on lumbar puncture.

SPECIAL CONSIDERATIONS

- Patients with BIH and spontaneous meningoencephalocele are at risk of recurrence or development of a second leak. Reported rates of postoperative CSF leak range from 0.5% to 9%. Such leaks may present up to 2 years postoperatively.[4,6,13] Consequently, patients at risk should be maintained on long-term acetazolamide therapy and should be routinely monitored for recurrence. Placement of a ventriculoperitoneal shunt should be considered in cases refractory to medical therapy.
- Patients with active CSF leaks are also at risk of developing ascending meningitis[13]; thus, symptoms of recurrent leak or meningismus should be evaluated promptly.

■ Patients in whom a transpterygoid approach was used are at risk of hypesthesia referable to the second trigeminal division (cheek and palate) and loss of reflex tearing.[17] Although this risk is low even if the vidian fibers are not deliberately preserved,[18] patients must be appropriately counseled of these additional risks during the informed consent process.

■ Sautter et al.[16] reported a 22.2% rate of transient postoperative diabetes insipidus in their series of nine patients undergoing endoscopic repair of sphenoid CSF leaks. Although this rate is not supported by other studies, the surgeon should be aware of this possibility.

REFERENCES

Access the reference list online at ExpertConsult.com.

Endoscopic Resection of Pituitary Tumors

Stephanie A. Joe

INTRODUCTION

- The endoscopic resection of sellar and suprasellar tumors involves access to the sella via dissection through the sphenoid sinus.[1–4]
- These procedures are often done in a combined operation with both a neurosurgeon and otolaryngologist and thus employ a two-surgeon technique.
- In this approach, the otolaryngology team provides the "pathway" and the neurosurgery team resects the tumor, with visualization provided by the otolaryngologist.
- A wide sphenoidotomy is performed transnasally while preserving nasal structures such as the middle and inferior turbinates.

ANATOMY[5]

- The sphenoid sinus originates from pneumatization of the sphenoid bone.
- There are left and right sinuses, with an intersinus septum.
  - Each may pneumatize to varying sizes.
  - The sphenoid intersinus septum also has an unpredictable course. It often attaches off midline adjacent to a carotid artery.
  - Additional incomplete septa may also be present.
  - The sinus may pneumatize laterally beyond the vidian canal and foramen rotundum, forming a lateral recess.
- A number of important structures are adjacent to the sphenoid sinus.
  - The sella often makes an impression to a variable extent along the posterior wall of the sphenoid sinus.
  - The optic nerves lie superolaterally.
  - The carotid arteries course lateral to the sinus bilaterally.
  - Both the optic nerves and carotid arteries may indent the sinus, either covered in thin bone or partially dehiscent.
  - The third, fourth, fifth, and sixth cranial nerves course in the cavernous sinuses situated lateral to the sinuses bilaterally.
  - The vidian nerve courses inferolaterally and may run within the sinus.
  - The size of the sella can affect the course of the carotid arteries; for example, a narrower sella is associated with more medially situated carotid arteries.
- The superior portion of the sphenoid sinus can be affected by pneumatization of the posterior ethmoid cells when they form Onodi cells.
- The degree of sphenoid pneumatization and the relationship of this pneumatization to the sella will affect the surgical time and amount of drilling required.
  - The postsellar configuration, the most common pattern, is characterized by pneumatization extending under the sella to its posterior portion (Fig. 28.1A).
  - Sphenoid pneumatization occurs to a lesser extent in the sellar configuration; thus, a smaller impression is seen along the posterior sphenoid wall (Fig. 28.1B).
  - In the presellar configuration, the sinus pneumatization does not reach the anterior wall of the sella (Fig. 28.1C).
  - The conchal pattern is the least common pattern, characterized by a lack of sphenoid pneumatization with solid bone anterior and inferior to the sella.

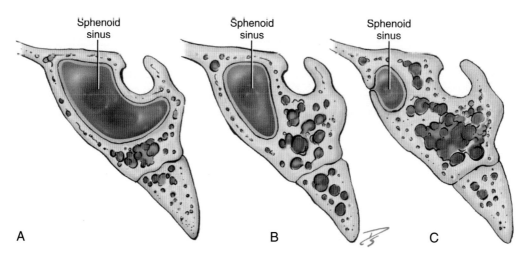

Fig. 28.1. Drawings illustrating configurations of the sella. **(A)** Postsellar. **(B)** Sellar. **(C)** Presellar.

PREOPERATIVE CONSIDERATIONS

- The neurosurgery service is usually the primary service and requests a consultation with the otolaryngology service after a decision for surgery has been made.

- An ophthalmologic evaluation is recommended and is often obtained preoperatively given the potential effect on the optic chiasm.

- If the patient is not already being seen by an endocrinologist, an endocrinology consultation is also often obtained to evaluate the hormonal functional status of the tumor.

- It is the role of the otolaryngologist to evaluate the sinonasal cavities for surgical planning and approach to the sella and parasellar regions.

- During the patient's preoperative visit, any history of sinonasal disease and/or previous surgery is elicited because this can impact the surgical approaches. Chronic rhinitis, rhinosinusitis, and sinonasal polyps should be controlled before surgery.

- Nasal endoscopy is performed.
  - The size of the nasal cavities and the shape and deviation of the septum are noted. A septoplasty is planned for deviations that could hinder exposure of the surgical site and implementation of the two-surgeon technique with its required use of both nasal cavities during surgery.
  - The status of the sphenoethmoid recess is evaluated. The surgeon notes the ability to visualize the sphenoid ostia.
  - The location of the sphenoid ostium is noted.

- Radiologic studies are obtained for surgical planning.
  - The presence of a tumor has usually already been diagnosed by magnetic resonance imaging (MRI).
  - A useful study for surgical planning is a computed tomography (CT) scan with an angiogram. It

is recommended that this be done using the image guidance protocol.
  - These images can be used on the image guidance planning station to view the operative area in three planes—axial, coronal, and sagittal—for preoperative evaluation and surgical planning.
  - In addition, image guidance is often used during surgery to aid in confirming location during the dissection.

- The teams must review a plan for reconstruction of the skull base once the tumor has been resected. This can often be accomplished with the use of free grafts (e.g., fascia or fat from the abdomen) in an underlay and/or overlay fashion. An additional option is the use of a nasoseptal flap, particularly in the presence of a cerebrospinal fluid (CSF) leak.

- When the surgery is discussed with the patient, the role of each service is described in detail.
  - The risks of surgery are outlined, including orbital injury, vision loss, intracranial injury, CSF leakage, septal perforation, and decreased sense of smell.

Radiographic Considerations

- The MRI best shows the tumor involvement and suprasellar extension as well as the relationship of the tumor to the pituitary gland and optic chiasm and involvement of the cavernous sinus and/or carotid arteries.

- A CT scan of the sinuses is imperative for evaluation of the sinuses and for surgical planning. As mentioned previously, an invaluable step is review of the images in three planes using the image guidance planning station.

- With these views, the sphenoid anatomy and pneumatization pattern are seen. The size of the sphenoid sinus on each side and the relationship of the sinus to the sella is evaluated.

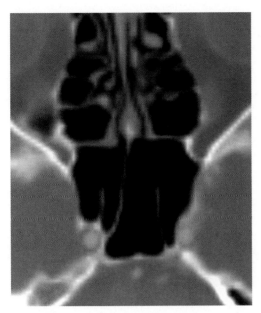

Fig. 28.2. Axial computed tomography scan through the sphenoid ostia. Note that the intersinus septum attaches adjacent to the right internal carotid artery. Additional incomplete septa are seen.

- The sella configuration—whether presellar, sellar, postsellar, or conchal—is easily seen in the sagittal views.
- The site of the sphenoid ostia is determined. This is best identified in the axial views (Fig. 28.2); then, the relationship of the ostia to the skull base is correlated in the sagittal views. This is an important anatomic landmark for orientation during the surgery. Ostia location is also crucial to identifying the location of the branch of the sphenopalatine artery when the plan is to use a nasoseptal flap for skull base reconstruction.
- As mentioned earlier, the intersinus septum rarely courses in the midline; rather, it usually attaches off the midline adjacent to the carotid artery.
- If the CT scans are done with angiography, the location and course of the carotid arteries are followed in all three planes. In particular, the relationship of the arteries to the sella is reviewed (Fig. 28.3). The presence of any bony dehiscences is also noted.
- The location of the optic nerves and their bony coverings is reviewed in the axial and coronal views. The presence of Onodi cells is recognized and planned for during surgery.
- The relationship of the tumor to the carotid arteries and optic nerves is noted for surgical planning and can be confirmed intraoperatively (Fig. 28.4).

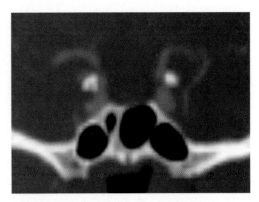

Fig. 28.3. Coronal computed tomography angiogram showing the carotid arteries outlining a sellar tumor.

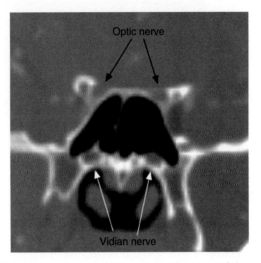

Fig. 28.4. Coronal computed tomography scan of the optic and vidian nerves.

INSTRUMENTATION (FIG. 28.5)

- 0-degree 2.7- and 4-mm endoscopes
- Lens washer, for example, Endo-Scrub (Medtronic ENT, Jacksonville, Florida)
- Straight 2.9- and 4.0-mm microdébrider blades
- Cottle and Freer elevators
- Straight-cutting and noncutting forceps
- Kerrison punches, mushroom punch
- Drill for thick bone (e.g., sphenoid rostrum)

SURGICAL PROCEDURE

- Fig. 28.6A shows the operating room setup with both surgeons on the right side of the patient. An alternative setup is to have the surgeons stand opposite each other with two monitors for visualization (Figs. 28.6B and 28.6C).
- Apply topical decongestants before the procedure for maximal mucosal decongestion.

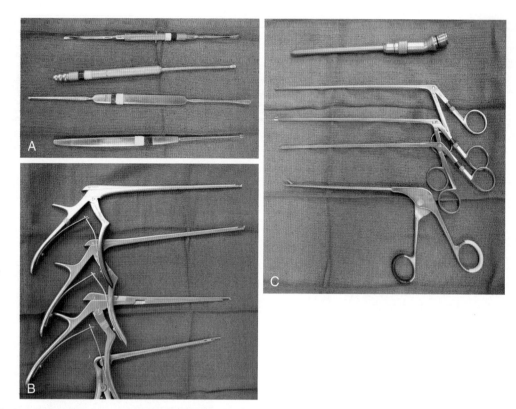

Fig. 28.5. Photographs of instruments used in the endoscopic resection of sellar and suprasellar tumors. **(A)** Freer elevator, suction Freer elevation, Cottle elevator, J-curette. **(B)** Kerrison rongeurs. **(C)** Long drill handpiece, straight-cutting instruments.

- As with all surgical procedures, exposure is the key element in proper surgical dissection. Take as much time as needed to achieve exposure of the anterior wall of the sphenoid sinus while preserving natural nasal structures. Occasionally, the middle or superior turbinates are partially resected in the setting of anatomically narrow nasal cavities. Otherwise, the nasal turbinates are lateralized.
- Hemostasis is achieved in multiple ways during surgery. Communicate frequently with the anesthesiologist throughout the procedure. The patient's blood pressure is maintained up to 20% below the patient's baseline pressure. Elevate the patient's head above the lower half of the body.

Step 1: Vasoconstriction
- At the beginning of the procedure, inject 1% lidocaine with 1:100,000 epinephrine into strategic points for vasoconstriction.
- Inject areas adjacent to the sphenopalatine artery with this mixture: for example, along the posterolateral nasal wall at the insertion of the middle turbinate and along the anterior wall of the sphenoid sinus.
- Cotton pledgets dampened with topical decongestant are used intermittently during the procedure. Hemostatic agents such as Surgicel, Gelfoam, and topical thrombin may also be used.

Step 2: Sphenoidotomy
- Locate the natural sphenoid ostium and perform a sphenoidotomy. Extend the sphenoidotomy 1 to 2 mm superiorly and laterally; avoid inferior dissection to preserve the arterial supply for a possible nasoseptal flap harvest. Use a Freer elevator to inferiorly retract the mucosa with the septal artery. The underlying bone can be removed to enlarge the opening into the sphenoid sinus (Fig. 28.7).
- If a nasoseptal flap is planned for reconstruction, develop the flap as shown in Fig. 28.8 and place it into the choana.

Step 3: Posterior Septectomy
- Once the location of the sphenoid sinuses is confirmed, begin a posterior septectomy just anterior to the anterior wall of the sphenoid sinuses. Resect the posterior septum for wide exposure of the sphenoid sinuses bilaterally. The posterior septectomy can be extended anteriorly to the level of the anterior heads of the middle turbinates as necessary for exposure and access (Figs. 28.9 and 28.10). It is important to try not to bring the septectomy too far forward, as it may cause prolonged septal crusting in the postoperative period.

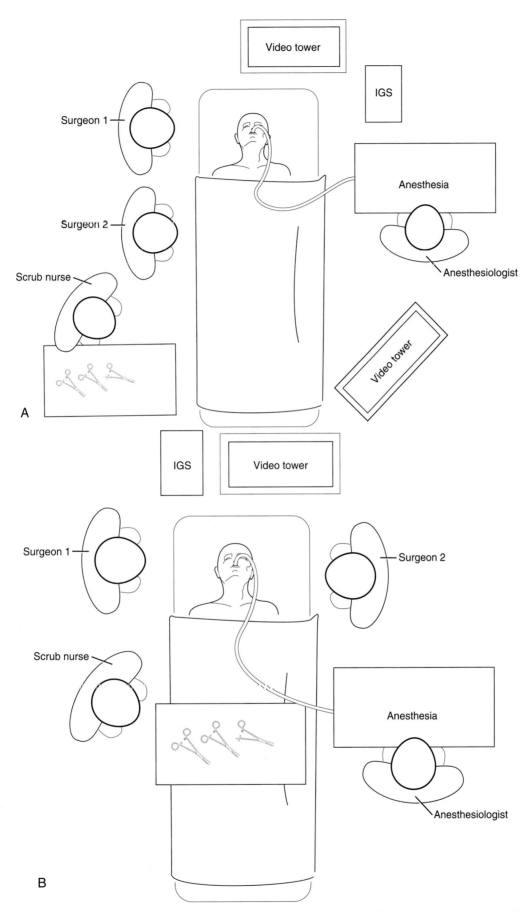

Fig. 28.6. (A–C) Schematic drawings showing three possible operating room setups for four-handed endoscopic skull base surgery. *IGS,* Image guidance system.

Continued

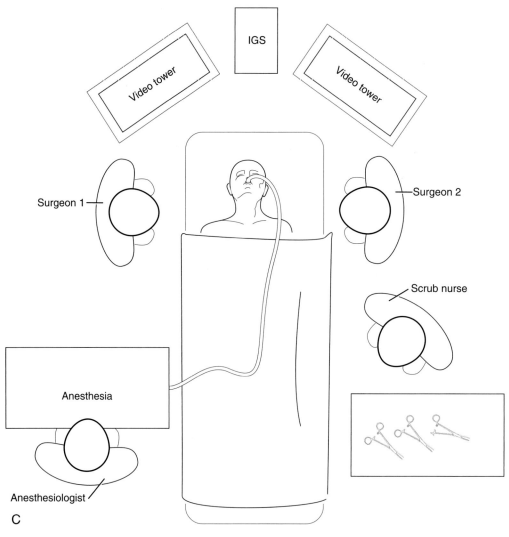

Fig. 28.6, cont'd.

Step 4: Anterior Sphenoid Resection
- Widely resect the anterior sphenoid wall bilaterally.
- Inferiorly, the rostrum is often thick and requires the use of a drill for removal.
- With resection of the anterior wall and wide exposure of the posterior wall, the outline of the sella is easily noted. Delineate the location of the skull base, carotid arteries, and optic nerves and confirm with image guidance.
- Oftentimes, the anterior sphenoid wall must be resected inferiorly to the sinus floor to gain exposure and access to the sella. A good rule is to resect the sphenoid face inferiorly to the point where a straight suction can be placed in the sphenoid sinus at a level just inferior to the floor of the sella.

Step 5: Removal of the Intersinus Septum
- Take down the intersinus septum with through-cutting instruments or a high-speed drill.

- Pay special attention to any intersinus septum that attaches to the bone adjacent to a carotid artery. In these cases, a high-speed drill is a better option to take down the intersinus septum because use of through-cutting instruments may inadvertently result in a carotid wall injury. Drill the bone overlying the dura at the face of the sphenoid until the dura is seen (Fig. 28.11).

Step 6: Neurosurgical Resection of the Tumor
- The otolaryngology team often provides endoscopic visualization and assistance with dissection during tumor resection.
- A two-surgeon, four-hand technique can be used.
- After the dura is identified, gently remove bone to expose the entire sella. Make the incision into the dura by first using bipolar cautery to outline the dural incision to prevent bleeding and then using a retractable blade to incise the dura itself (Fig. 28.12).

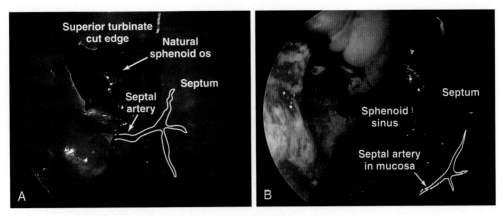

Fig. 28.7. (A) Endoscopic view of right sphenoid os after the inferior portion of the superior turbinate is resected. **(B)** Endoscopic view of the mucosa retracted off the inferior sphenoid face.

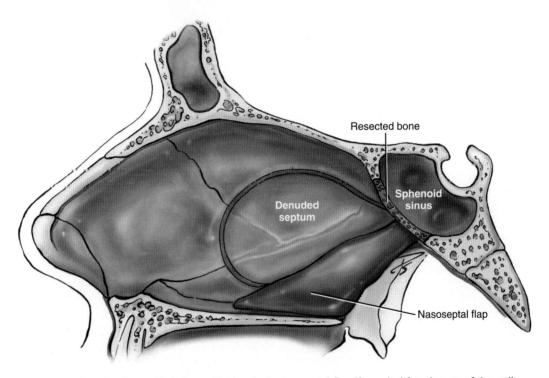

Fig. 28.8. Drawing in sagittal view of harvested nasoseptal flap if needed for closure of the sella.

- Once the dura is incised, use a combination of ring curettes and suction to gently remove the tumor. Take special care to avoid puncturing the diaphragm, if possible. Also, use angled scopes to ensure removal of all portions of tumor (Fig. 28.13).

Step 7: Repair of Cerebrospinal Fluid Leak (If Necessary)

- If a CSF leak occurs during tumor resection, repair it according to endoscopic principles using underlay and/or overlay techniques with free grafts. In addition, a nasoseptal flap can be harvested and rotated to cover the surgical defect. See Chapters 27 and 31 for a description of closure of the defect when a CSF leak occurs. If no leak is present, simply place Gelfoam or other dissolvable surgical packing over the defect and return the flaps.
- Tissue glue may be used if needed.

Step 8: Application of Absorbable Packing

- With either type of repair, place absorbable packing, such as small pieces of compressed Gelfoam, along the graft site and use it to pack the sphenoid sinus.
- FloSeal Hemostatic Matrix (Baxter Healthcare, Deerfield, Illinois) may also be used.
- Packing can be placed in the nasal cavity if needed.

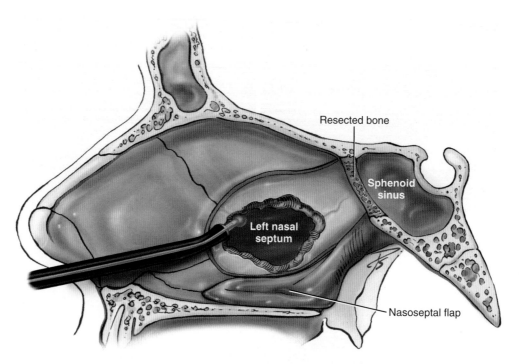

Fig. 28.9. Drawing in sagittal view of the area of the posterior septum removed for exposure.

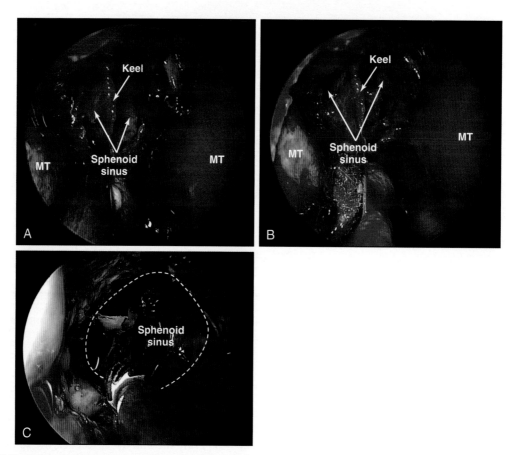

Fig. 28.10. **(A)** Endoscopic view of a posterior septectomy to expose the sphenoid keel. **(B)** Endoscopic view of a bilateral sphenoid antrostomy with exposed keel. **(C)** Endoscopic view of drill-down of the inferior keel and the face of the sphenoid to achieve wide access. *MT,* Middle turbinate.

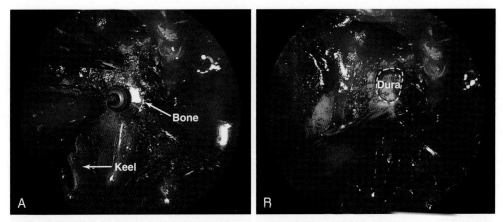

Fig. 28.11. **(A)** Endoscopic view of diamond drilling of bone overlying the dura. **(B)** Endoscopic view of the exposed dura.

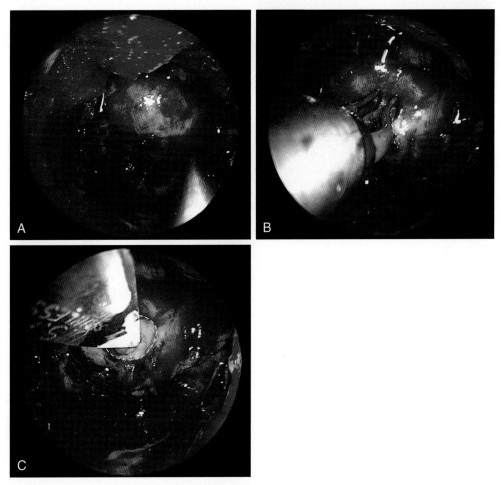

Fig. 28.12. **(A)** Endoscopic view of the exposed sella. **(B)** Endoscopic view of bipolar cauterization of the dura at the point of incision. **(C)** Endoscopic view of incision of the dura with a No. 11 blade.

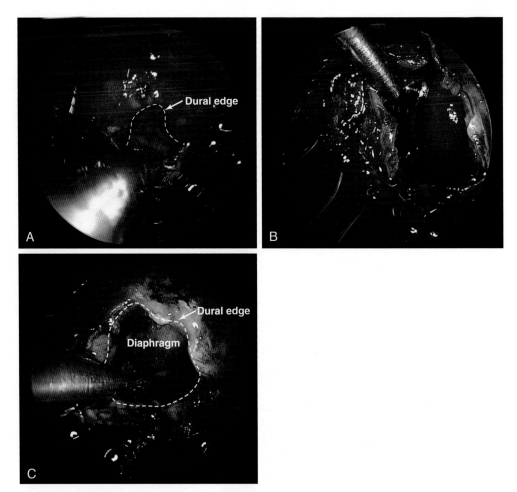

Fig. 28.13. **(A)** Endoscopic view of removal of tumor from the sella. **(B)** Endoscopic view of the curetting of the tumor off the right cavernous sinus with the aid of angled endoscopes. **(C)** Endoscopic view of the descended diaphragm after the tumor is resected.

POSTOPERATIVE CONSIDERATIONS

- The patient is instructed in nasal precautions postoperatively and is asked to avoid nose blowing and strenuous activity. If the need arises, the patient is told to sneeze with the mouth open.
- Once concern for the possibility of a CSF leak has passed, the patient may begin to moisturize the nasal cavities with frequent use of nasal saline and saline irrigations.
- After discharge, the patient is seen as an outpatient and endoscopic débridements are performed similar to those after endoscopic sinus surgery. The surgical sites are surveyed for proper healing and for the development of complications such as infection or CSF leakage.

SPECIAL CONSIDERATIONS

- Any history of nasal, septal, or sinus surgery is elicited from the patient and is part of the surgical planning. Such prior surgery can also affect the approach used or reconstructive options used during surgery.
- A nasoseptal flap is a pedicled flap of septal mucosa based on the posterior septal artery. It is a hardy flap used in CSF leak repair and skull base reconstruction for anterior skull base surgery.[6,7]

REFERENCES

Access the reference list online at ExpertConsult.com.

Endoscopic Transplanum and Sellar Approach

Eric W. Wang, William A. Vandergrift III, Arjun Parasher, Jose Mattos, and Rodney Schlosser

INTRODUCTION

- Endoscopic approaches to intracranial tumors of the planum and sella are increasingly prevalent secondary to improved panoramic visualization, improved tumor resection, increased working angles, and decreased intranasal complications.[1]
- Approaches to the sphenoid planum and sella turcica require an understanding of the anatomic relationships of the sphenoid sinus, optic nerve, carotid artery, sella, planum, and clivus.
- Intracranial dissection requires knowledge and experience of the normal pituitary gland and stalk, cavernous sinus, the carotid artery and its feeding vessels, including the superior and inferior hypophyseal vessels, diaphragma, and optic apparatus.
- A two-surgeon technique allows for an endoscope and two dissecting instruments to be used at all times. Additionally, four-handed surgery is possible, allowing for retraction or suction while continuing dissection.
- The key access to the endoscopic transphenoidal surgery of the sella and planum is wide exposure through the posterior nasal septum, both sphenoid sinuses and the ethmoid sinuses if necessary to provide access through both nares.[1,2]
- Reconstruction of the skull base defect with free grafts and pedicled vascularized flaps is aided by endoscopic visualization and techniques.

ANATOMY

- The natural ostium of the sphenoid sinus can be visualized by identifying and resecting the inferior third of the superior turbinate.
- The sphenopalatine artery (SPA) is a terminal branch of maxillary artery and enters the nasal cavity through the sphenopalatine foramen. The SPA then bifurcates into the posterior lateral nasal artery and the posterior septal artery (PSA). The PSA traverses the rostrum of the sphenoid inferior to the natural ostium and superior to the arch of the choana, and it usually bifurcates into superior and inferior branches. Preservation of this PSA vascular pedicle is essential for a posteriorly based nasoseptal flap that can be used for skull base reconstruction.
- The sella turcica is a saddle-shaped depression in the midline of the sphenoid sinus at the skull base and is the caudal aspect of the hypophyseal fossa, which contains the pituitary gland. The degree of pneumatization of the sphenoid sinus can vary. The sellar pattern results in pneumatization of the clival recess and is the most common variant (Fig. 29.1).
- The planum sphenoidale is the roof of the sphenoid sinus that is immediately anterior to the sella turcica. The slope of the planum varies and may necessitate a posterior ethmoidectomy for improved anterior access (see Fig. 29.1).
- The junction between the sphenoid planum and the sella turcica is the tuberculum sella. This is the approximate level of the limbus of the sphenoid, which corresponds to the axial plane of the optic nerves (see Fig. 29.1).
- Identification of the paraclinoid carotid artery and optic nerve in the lateral aspect of the sphenoid sinus is vital on preoperative imaging and during the endoscopic approach. The lateral opticocarotid recess, a well-established landmark for these structures, is the result of pneumatization of the optic strut (Fig. 29.2).
- The cavernous sinuses form the lateral boundaries of the pituitary gland and are connected anteriorly by superior and inferior intracavernous sinuses (Fig. 29.3). The expansile nature of macroadenomas tends to minimize intracavernous sinus vasculature. However, when

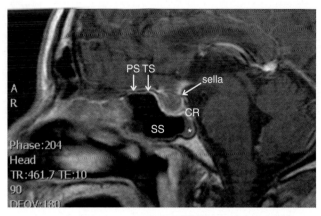

Fig. 29.1. Sagittal T1-weighted magnetic resonance image (MRI) of a pituitary adenoma. The long arrow identifies the sella turcica, containing a pituitary adenoma (sella). Short arrows identify the planum sphenoidale *(PS)* and tuberculum sella *(TS)*. Note that the tuberculum sella is between the planum sphenoidale and the sella turcica. The clival recess *(CR)* is posterior and inferior to the sella and is superior to the clivus *(asterisk)*. SS, Sphenoid sinus. (Courtesy Eric Wang and Rodney Schlosser. © 2010 Medical University of South Carolina, Division of Rhinology, Charleston. With permission.)

operating on secreting microadenomas in normal-sized pituitary glands, these vasculature communications can result in increased bleeding.

■ The sella is bounded posteriorly by the dorsum sella and the posterior clinoids.

■ Superior to the planum sphenoidale lies intracranial vasculature that can be displaced by planum or tuberculum meningiomas and craniopharyngiomas (Fig. 29.4).

PREOPERATIVE CONSIDERATIONS

■ Location and size of the intracranial tumor: Determining the size and anatomic localization of the tumor is essential to providing adequate visual exposure and functional working space to allow for a safe dissection. The size and anterior extension of the tumor may need broader exposure. This would require a posterior or total ethmoidectomy, middle turbinate resection, and extended septectomy. Additionally, the size of the tumor should be considered when planning for the skull base reconstruction. A pedicled flap skull base reconstruction

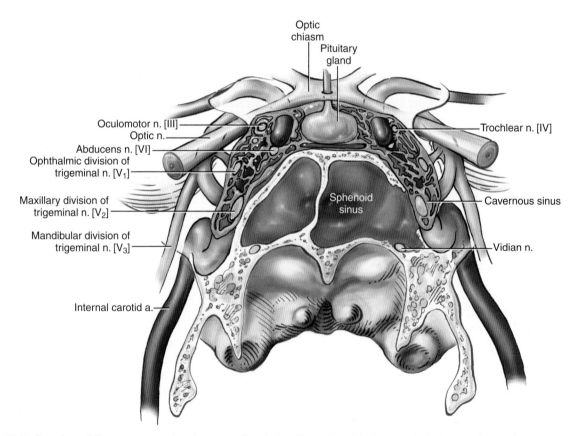

Fig. 29.2. Drawing of the neurovascular structures bordering the sphenoid sinus and pituitary sella. *a.,* Artery; *n.,* nerve.

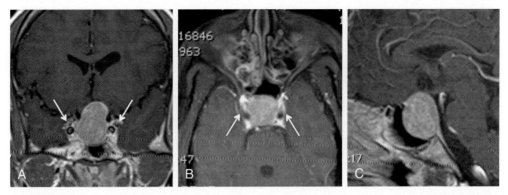

Fig. 29.3. T1-weighted MRIs in coronal **(A)**, axial **(B)**, and sagittal **(C)** planes, which allow a three-dimensional evaluation of the pituitary mass. The arrows identify the cavernous sinuses and the cavernous portion of the carotid arteries. (Courtesy Eric Wang and Rodney Schlosser. © 2010 Medical University of South Carolina, Division of Rhinology, Charleston. With permission.)

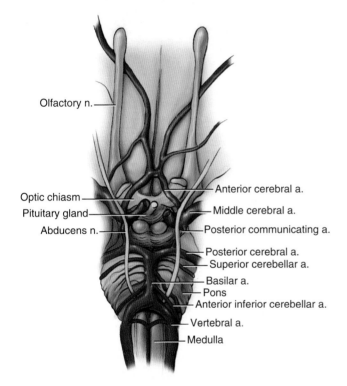

Olfactory n.

Optic chiasm
Pituitary gland
Abducens n.

Anterior cerebral a.
Middle cerebral a.
Posterior communicating a.
Posterior cerebral a.
Superior cerebellar a.
Basilar a.
Pons
Anterior inferior cerebellar a.
Vertebral a.
Medulla

Fig. 29.4. Drawing of the neurovascular structures superior to the pituitary sella. A1, A2 segments of the carotid artery, and the anterior communicating artery lie superior to the optic chiasm and often come into visualization in the removal of anterior skull base meningiomas and craniopharyngiomas. *a.,* Artery; *n.,* nerve.

should be considered for tumors in which the expected defect will be large, particularly anterior skull base and clival lesions, and where the likelihood of a high-flow cerebrospinal fluid (CSF) leak is high.

■ Secreting pituitary tumors may increase the vascularity of the mucosa. Additionally, patients with Cushing disease may have thin nasal mucosa.

■ Evaluation of the nasal septum while taking note of septal deviation and nasal spurs aids in the preoperative planning of the transsphenoidal approach to the sphenoid. Significant septal deviation and nasal spurs can limit visualization of the sphenoid ostium, affect which side of the septum to use for a nasoseptal flap, and necessitate an early septectomy. Care should be taken to not incidentally injure the nasal septal mucosa, as this may be necessary for skull base reconstruction or can result in a postoperative septal perforation.

■ Evaluation of concurrent sinus disease and prior nasal surgeries is important. Active bacterial sinusitis may necessitate staging the procedure. A lack of septal cartilage and bone will require additional care be taken if nasoseptal flaps are raised.

■ Allow for adequate topical decongestion prior to initiating the surgical approach.

Radiographic Considerations

■ Use all three planes on magnetic resonance imaging (MRI) and/or computed tomography (CT) in the preoperative radiographic evaluation.

■ Identify the tumor and the anatomic location. Take note of any anterior and inferior extension into the sphenoid, clivus, and the ethmoid sinuses; the lateral extension and the relationship to the carotid artery; the cavernous sinuses and the temporal lobe; and the suprasellar extension, including extension into the third ventricle (Fig. 29.5). The relationship of the tumor to the optic chiasm and intracerebral vasculature (anterior communicating artery and anterior cerebral arteries) should be examined (Fig. 29.6).

■ Examine the direction of the inner-sinus septum. The size of the sphenoid sinuses and the relationship of each sinus to the sella turcica should be noted. Even an appropriate sphenoidotomy into the smaller

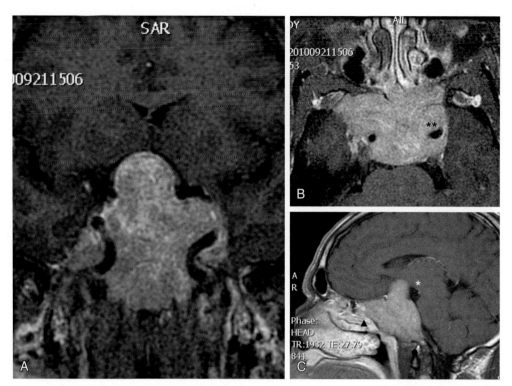

Fig. 29.5. Gadolinium-enhanced T1-weighted MRIs in the coronal **(A)**, axial **(B)**, and sagittal **(C)** planes demonstrating a large pituitary macroadenoma that involves the third ventricle superiorly *(single asterisk)*, the temporal lobe and the bilateral carotid arteries laterally *(double asterisks)*, the sphenoid and posterior ethmoids anteriorly *(triangle)*, and the clivus inferiorly *(circle)*. (Courtesy Eric Wang and Rodney Schlosser. © 2010 Medical University of South Carolina, Division of Rhinology, Charleston. With permission.)

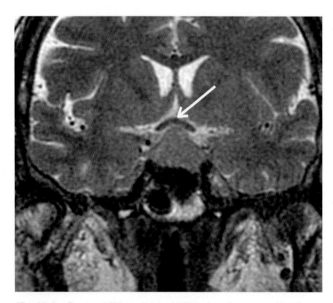

Fig. 29.6. Coronal T2-weighted MRI showing superior displacement of the optic chiasm *(arrow)* caused by a pituitary macroadenoma. (Courtesy Eric Wang and Rodney Schlosser. © 2010 Medical University of South Carolina, Division of Rhinology, Charleston. With permission.)

sphenoid sinus may not allow visualization of the sella if the inner-sinus septum transverses posterolaterally. Special attention to the direction of the inner-sinus septum and the carotid artery is essential. The inner-sinus septum can serve as an important intraoperative landmark. The inner-sinus septum often can be seen attaching to the bony covering of the carotid artery laterally.

- Examine the pneumatization of the sphenoid sinus: Pneumatization of the sphenoid can result in lateral recesses, infrasellar pneumatization into the clival recess, a well-defined opticocarotid recess, and the potential for dehiscence of the carotid artery and optic nerve canal.

- Examine pneumatization of the posterior ethmoid sinuses and vomer. Significant pneumatization of the posterior ethmoid sinuses may result in Onodi cells in direct contact with the optic nerve and displacement of the sphenoid sinus inferiorly. Pneumatization of the vomer may widen the keel appearance of the rostrum and displace the natural sphenoid os laterally.

- The relationship of the planum sphenoidalis and the sella turcica is a good anatomic and radiographic landmark except when the sellar mass has significant anterior extension or the planum is distorted inferiorly.

- The axial plane of the CT scan or MRI can be used to evaluate the nasal septum and inferior turbinate. Deviation of the septum and the size of the inferior turbinates may affect the surgical approach.
- Intraoperative image guidance systems can be utilized as an adjunct to surgical landmarks.

INSTRUMENTATION (FIG. 29.7)

- 0-degree and 45-degree endoscopes with possible use of lens washer
- Straight, angled Beaver blade
- Arachnoid knife
- Curved extended Colorado tip or needle tip monopolar cautery
- High-speed endoscopic drill with a diamond bur
- Intraoperative Doppler
- Image guidance system
- Hemostatic materials (Gelfoam paste, Floseal, Surgifoam, or equivalent)
- Endoscopic sinus surgery instruments and endonasal pituitary instruments should be available.

PEARLS AND POTENTIAL PITFALLS

Pearls

- When endonasal access to the sphenoid is difficult secondary to limited space in the nasal cavity, an early septectomy can prevent injury to the septal mucosa and allow for increased working space. The subperichondrial and subperiosteal plane of the nasal septum can be raised to the rostrum of the sphenoid and allow for identification of the sphenoid os. A resection of the inferior ⅓ to ½ of the middle turbinate may also be indicated to improve access.
- Avoid placing the superior incision of the nasal septal flap too high, as this may compromise olfaction. Attempt to preserve the superior 1 to 2 cm of septal mucosa.
- When raising the nasal septal flap in difficult or revision cases, it may be beneficial to start the elevation of the flap on the floor of the nose, as this is usually an undissected plane that allows for easier identification of the correct plane. Care should be taken during flap elevation near the decussating fibers adjacent to the nasal spine, as this is a frequent site where the flap can be torn. It is helpful to dissect these fibers by elevating from the floor of the nose and sweeping superiorly. This allows the floor tunnel to be connected to a subperiosteal tunnel elevated over the quadrangular cartilage or vomer. Attempting to dissect through the decussating fibers in an anterior to posterior direction often results in tears in the flap, which may compromise a watertight seal for skull

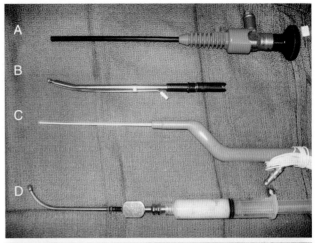
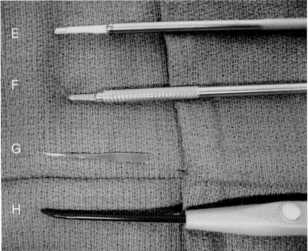

Fig. 29.7. Photographs of instruments used in endoscopic resection of intracranial tumors via a transplanum or sellar approach. **(A)** Endoscope with an Endoscrub lens-cleaning sheath. **(B)** Fifteen-degree endoscopic diamond bur. **(C)** Intraoperative transnasal Doppler imaging probe. **(D)** Gelfoam paste on an olive-tip suction device. **(E)** Straight Beaver blade. **(F)** Angled Beaver blade. **(G)** Arachnoid knife. **(H)** Slightly curved extended Colorado-tip Bovie.

base closure. If a tear occurs, the nasoseptal flap can still be utilized if an underlay material is used.
- Evaluate both nares endoscopically to ensure adequate access to the sella and planum.
- When two surgeons are working in tandem, it is often beneficial to have the endoscopic view offset (the point of dissection off center) to allow for additional working room. This necessitates a broad exposure and a wide cavity to allow adequate access and visualization.
- Identification of the carotid arteries, either endoscopically or by Doppler signal, is vital prior to opening the dura of the sella.
- Removing the bone of the sella or planum without entering the dura improves visualization and safety.

- Meticulous hemostasis should be obtained before opening the dura.
- Gelfoam paste/Floseal/Surgifoam are excellent hemostatic agents. However, care should be taken when using Gelfoam paste during the dissection, as it can obscure the dissection planes, including the pseudocapsule of a pituitary adenoma.
- A multilayer closure can be used when a CSF leak is identified intraoperatively. Abdominal fat-free grafts can be very useful in this reconstruction.
- An angled endoscope can be used in the sella to identify residual anterior and lateral tumor and visually confirm complete tumor removal.

Potential Pitfalls

- Releasing the septum superiorly prior to removal is essential. Rocking the nasal septum can result in an iatrogenic CSF leak.
- When using a nasoseptal flap, approach the decussating fibers of the nasal mucoperichondrium superiorly and laterally. Attempting to elevate this in an anterior to posterior direction will likely result in a tear of the flap.
- At minimum a 1 × 1 cm of the anterior and caudal strut of quadrangular cartilage must be maintained if possible to prevent collapse of the nasal dorsum.
- Take care to sharply resect the inner-sinus septum of the sphenoid with through-cutting instruments or a drill to avoid injury to the carotid artery. The inner-sinus septum can often be attached to the bony canal of the carotid artery. Twisting motions can destabilize the inner-sinus septum and the attached carotid canal, resulting in vascular injury.
- Incomplete removal of the inferior ledge of the sphenoid rostrum can hinder access.
- Inadequate sellotomy can limit visualization and the completeness of tumor resection.

SURGICAL PROCEDURES

- After adequate decongestion with 1:1000 epinephrine or oxymetazoline on neuropatties, 1% lidocaine with 1:100,000 epinephrine is injected into the subperichondrial plane of the nasal septum bilaterally and the superior turbinate.

Step1: Nasal Exposure of the Sphenoid

- When a 0-degree endoscope is inserted into the nose, the important anatomic landmarks—including the nasal septum, choana, middle turbinate, and possibly the superior turbinate—are identified.
- The inferior and middle turbinates are gently outfractured to increase exposure and enlarge the surgical corridor.

- If additional working room is required, the pneumatized portion of the middle turbinate may be resected. This may be particularly important on the side through which the endoscope is placed.

Step 2: Sphenoidotomy

- A standard sphenoidotomy is performed. The inferior 1/3 to 1/2 of the superior turbinate is resected, allowing for visualization of the sphenoid os. The os is entered with a J-curette or probe. After enlarging the os, a Kerrison punch is used to expand the sphenoidotomy laterally and superiorly. The bony sphenoidotomy should not be extended inferiorly until the mucosa between the natural ostium of the sphenoid and the choana is elevated to preserve the sphenopalatine artery. The sphenoidotomy is performed on the contralateral side.

Step 3: Nasoseptal Flap Elevation

- The nasoseptal flap can be raised on either side with a working window on the contralateral side.[3] However, anatomic variability—including tumor sidedness, septal deviation, nasal spurs, and sphenoid anatomy—should be taken into account and dictate the side of a unilateral flap. If a large skull base reconstruction is necessary, bilateral nasoseptal flaps can be raised.
- Using electrocautery, the superior cut of the nasoseptal flap is made from the superior aspect of the sphenoid os posteriorly and carried anteriorly along the axial plane of the midportion of the middle turbinate. Posterior to the middle turbinate, 1 to 2 cm of septal mucosa should be preserved for olfaction. Anterior to the middle turbinate, the flap can be extended superiorly to capture more nasal mucosa and increase the reconstructive surface of the flap. The anterior cut can be made at any point along the coronal plane of the septum, depending on the size of the flap needed. The maximum flap will have an anterior incision at the location of a hemitransfixion incision. Subsequently, the posterior cut is performed by palpating the bony arch of the choana using a curved Beaver blade or needle tip electrocautery. The incision is carried along the arch of the choana (Fig. 29.8A) and proceeds anteriorly and inferiorly along the bone of the vomer until the hard palate is reached (Fig. 29.8B). Depending on the needed size of the flap, the inferior incision can be made at the junction of the nasal septum and nasal floor or it can be extended laterally along the floor of the nose parallel to the junction of the hard and soft palate to the inferior meatus (Fig. 29.8C). The inferior/lateral incision and anterior incision are joined, completing the incision necessary to raise the nasoseptal flap.

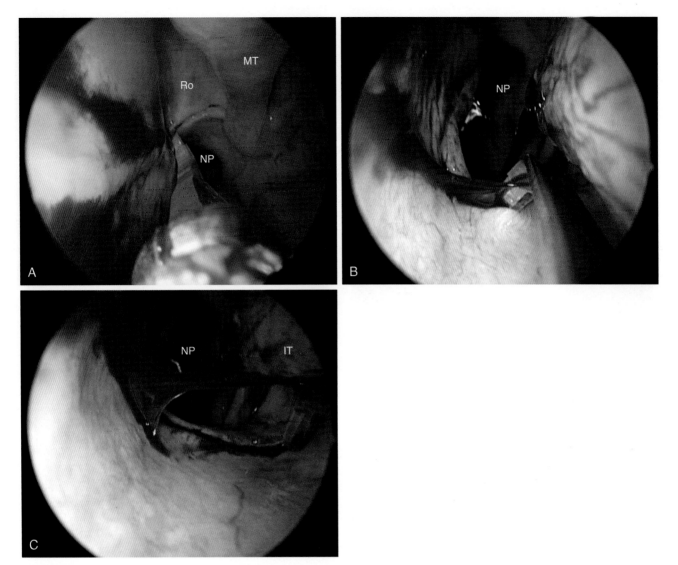

Fig. 29.8. (A) Endoscopic view of the posterior incision of the nasoseptal flap along the arch of the choana. After palpation, a mucosal cut is made with an angled Beaver blade along the arch of the choana to the bone. The rostrum of the sphenoid *(Ro)*, middle turbinate *(MT)*, and nasopharynx *(NP)* are identified. **(B)** Endoscopic view of the posterior incision of the nasoseptal flap proceeding anteriorly and inferiorly along the vomer. The nasopharynx and inferior turbinate *(IT)* are identified. **(C)** Endoscopic view of the posterior incision along the nasal floor parallel to the junction of the hard and soft palate. Note that the incision extends to the inferior meatus. The nasopharynx and inferior turbinate are identified. (Courtesy Eric Wang and Rodney Schlosser. © 2010 Medical University of South Carolina, Division of Rhinology, Charleston. With permission.)

- The nasoseptal flap is then raised from the underlying cartilage and bone of the septum and palate (Fig. 29.9).
- The nasoseptal flap and the vascular pedicle containing the SPA are elevated from the rostrum of the sphenoid (Fig. 29.10). After complete mobilization, the flap is stored in the nasopharynx and protected with a patty.

Step 4: Contralateral Working Window
- A working window is created by resection of a small window of mucosa from the contralateral septal mucosa immediately adjacent to the sphenoid ostium.

By creating the inferior incision parallel to the sphenoid ostium, the vascular pedicle to the nasoseptal flap can be preserved. The mucosa of the posterior septum and anterior sphenoid face between the sphenoid os and the arch of the choana is elevated. This allows for preservation of the contralateral nasoseptal flap if needed (Fig. 29.11).

Step 5: Completion of the Sphenoidotomy and Removal of the Sphenoid Keel
- After preservation of the bilateral SPA pedicles to the nasoseptal flap, a complete removal of the anterior face of the sphenoid is performed using

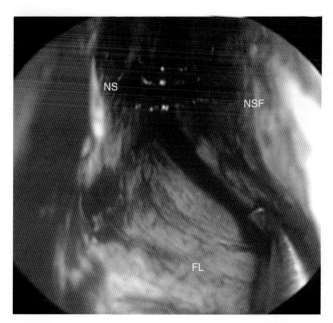

Fig. 29.9. Endoscopic view demonstrating the elevation of the nasoseptal flap *(NSF)* in the submucoperichondrial plane with extension to the floor of the nose *(FL)*. *NS,* Nasal septum.

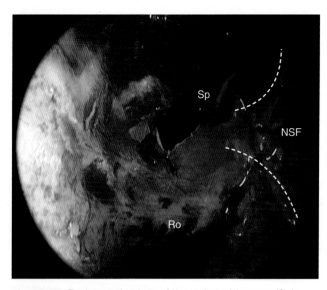

Fig. 29.10. Endoscopic view of the sphenoidotomy *(Sp)* and bony rostrum *(Ro)*. The nasoseptal flap *(NSF)* has been elevated from the rostrum of the sphenoid to protect the vascular pedicle and stored in the nasopharynx. The bony rostrum of the sphenoid is exposed before extension of the sphenoidotomy inferiorly.

Kerrison rongeurs and possibly the endoscopic drill. Care should be taken to remove the entire sphenoid keel and with wide exposure as dictated by the tumor location. It can be helpful to preserve the floor of the sphenoid sinus to support any skull base repairs as long as this does not impair exposure for tumor resection.

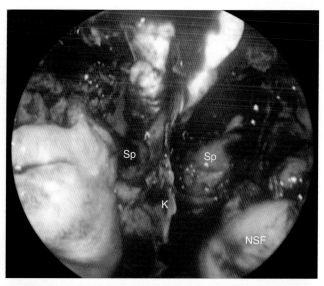

Fig. 29.11. Endoscopic view of the bilateral wide sphenoidotomies *(Sp)*, posterior septectomy, and elevation of a left nasoseptal flap *(NSF)*. The remaining bony keel *(K)* of the vomer is demonstrated. (Courtesy Eric Wang and Rodney Schlosser. © 2010 Medical University of South Carolina, Division of Rhinology, Charleston. With permission.)

Step 6: Removal of the Sphenoid Inner-Sinus Septum

- The inner-sinus septum should be resected with through-cutting instruments or the diamond bur to prevent injury to the carotid canal.
- At the completion of this step, the posterior and lateral walls of the sphenoid, the floor of the sella, the planum superiorly, and clival indentation should be visible. Identification of bony prominences of the paraclinoid internal carotid artery, optic nerve, and opticocarotid recess is possible with adequate aeration of the sphenoid (Fig. 29.12A). Correlate these visual landmarks with preoperative images as well as surgical navigation to ensure correct localization.

Step 7: Removal of the Sella Wall

- With pituitary macroadenomas, the sella wall is often greatly attenuated and careful palpation can reveal bony dehiscences. Once these bony dehiscences are identified, a Kerrison rongeur can be used to remove the sella wall, exposing the dura.
- With a pituitary microadenoma, the sella wall is thicker and may require an initial entry with an endoscopic drill or osteotome.
- Care should be taken to resect only the bony wall of the sella and not enter the dura. The sellotomy is carried laterally to the cavernous segment of the internal carotid artery, superiorly to the tuberculum sella, and inferiorly to the floor of the sella (Fig. 29.12B).

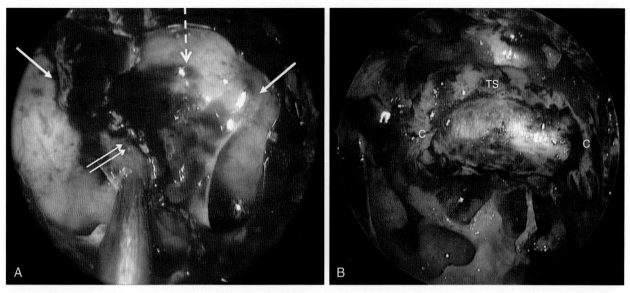

Fig. 29.12. (A) Endoscopic view after bilateral wide sphenoidotomies, posterior septectomy, and removal of the anterior face of the sphenoid. Single arrows identify the carotid artery and its anterior genu. The double arrow identifies the inner sinus septum, now partially resected. The dashed arrow points to the sella wall. **(B)** Endoscopic view after removal of the posterior sphenoid base. The dura is left intact and the sellotomy extends from carotid artery (C) to carotid artery in a lateral dimension and from the tuberculum sella *(TS)* superiorly to the floor of the sella inferiorly. (Courtesy Eric Wang and Rodney Schlosser. © 2010 Medical University of South Carolina, Division of Rhinology, Charleston. With permission.)

Step 8: Resection of the Sella Mass

- Once all bony removal is complete, Doppler can be used to identify any intracranial vessels, to include the internal carotid arteries bilaterally. The arachnoid knife is then used to make a dural incision. The choice of incision can vary. One variation is the creation of superiorly based U-shaped dural flap that is then elevated from the surface of the tumor.
- Blunt dissection is performed around the capsule of the tumor, using a combination of suction, microsurgical dissecting instrument, and angled curettes. This optimizes the chances of a complete tumor removal rather than performing an intratumoral curetting and debulking of the tumor.
- Dissection is typically started inferiorly until the dorsum sella is identified. The dissection then proceeds laterally to clear each medial cavernous sinus wall and the gutter between the cavernous sinus wall and the diaphragm. The final portion of the tumor to be removed is the superior aspect. This allows the majority of tumor removal to occur early in the dissection before the diaphragm descends and impairs visualization.

Transplanum Approach

- Transplanum approaches require broad exposure, which typically mandates bilateral sphenoidotomies, total ethmoidectomies, posterior nasal septectomy, and

middle turbinectomies/maxillary antrostomies, as needed. This larger exposure is usually indicated to limit the restriction of instrument manipulation by bony prominences in both the sinonasal cavity and the skull base (Fig. 29.13).
- After achieving broad exposure, all bony osteotomies are performed before any intracranial dissection begins. This is typically performed using a high-speed diamond bur with irrigation, beginning posteriorly in the midline. Drilling then proceeds laterally over to both optic nerves. Osteotomies are carried slightly anterior to actual tumor extent in order to allow visualization of tissue planes between tumor and normal intracranial structures. By progressing from posterior to anterior, any bleeding that is encountered does not impair visualization. The anterior osteotomy on the planum then connects the two lateral osteotomies. Often, the bone can be separated from the dura in an anterior to posterior fashion (Figs. 29.14 and 29.15).
- Drilling continues until dura is encountered or the skull base is eggshell thin and permits removal with hand instruments.
- The transplanum approach is often used for meningiomas of the tuberculum sella. In these cases, the bony skull base is often thickened and vascularized. Drilling this bone away removes much of the blood supply to these tumors and improves intracranial dissection.

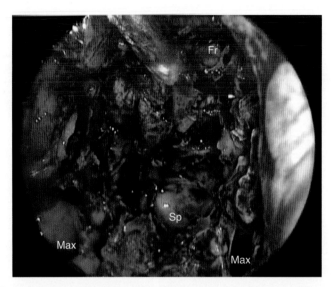

Fig. 29.13. Endoscopic view of a transplanum approach including bilateral sphenoidotomies, total ethmoidectomies, posterior septectomy, middle turbinotomies, and maxillary antrostomies. The maxillary sinuses *(Max)*, sphenoid sinuses *(Sp)*, and frontal recess *(Fr)* are identified. This provides wide exposure for adequate visualization and instrumentation for extended resections. (Courtesy Eric Wang and Rodney Schlosser. © 2010 Medical University of South Carolina, Division of Rhinology, Charleston. With permission.)

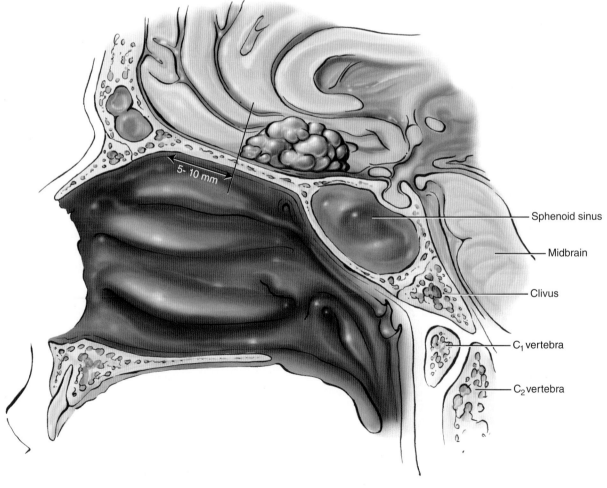

Fig. 29.14. Schematic drawing demonstrating need for anterior access to identify tissue planes. (Courtesy Eric Wang and Rodney Schlosser. © 2010 Medical University of South Carolina, Division of Rhinology, Charleston. With permission.)

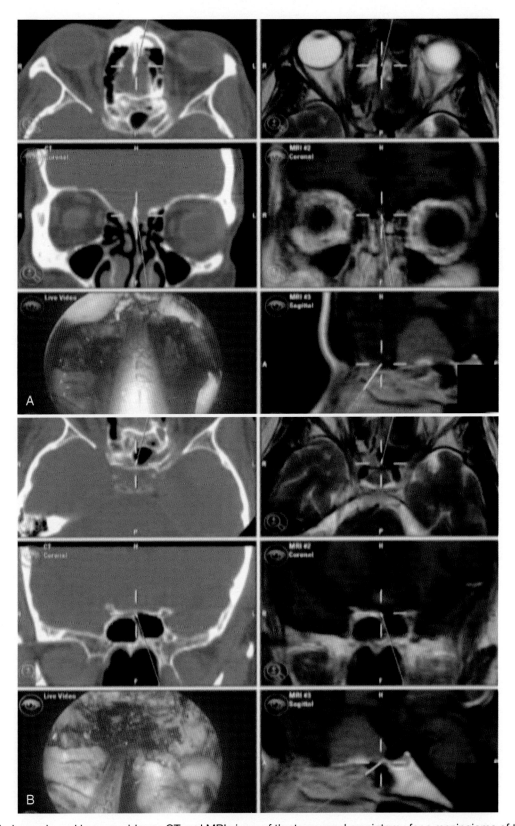

Fig. 29.15. Endoscopic and image guidance CT and MRI views of the transnasal craniotomy for a meningioma of the anterior cranial fossa. The anterior edge of the craniotomy is slightly anterior to the tumor to allow improved visualization of the interface between the tumor and normal tissue. This is clearly delineated on the sagittal MRI [*lower right image* in **(A)**]. The posterior edge of the craniotomy is adjacent to the tuberculum sella, again demonstrated in the sagittal MRI [*lower right image* in **(B)**].

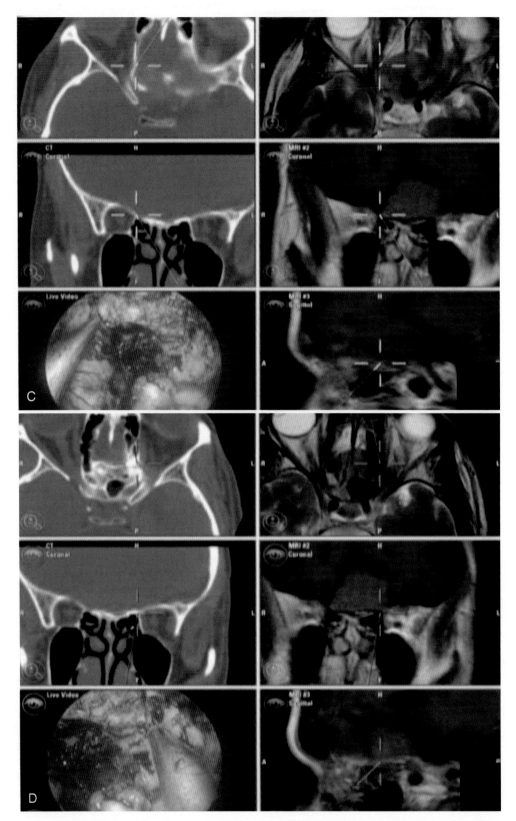

Fig. 29.15, cont'd. The lateral extent of the craniotomy is the orbit bilaterally. This is visualized on the coronal MRI [*middle right images* in **(C)** and **(D)**]. (Courtesy Eric Wang and Rodney Schlosser. © 2010 Medical University of South Carolina, Division of Rhinology, Charleston. With permission.)

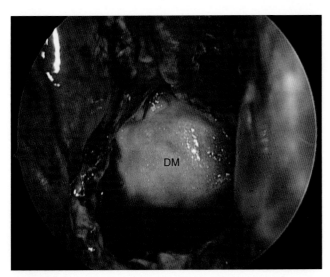

Fig. 29.16. Dural graft matrix *(DM)* reconstruction of a sella defect in a patient without a cerebrospinal fluid leak. (Courtesy Eric Wang and Rodney Schlosser. © 2010 Medical University of South Carolina, Division of Rhinology, Charleston. With permission.)

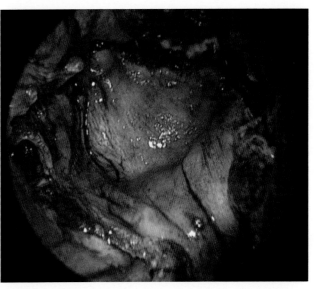

Fig. 29.17. Endoscopic view of a nasoseptal flap covering the sella and skull base defect. (Courtesy Eric Wang and Rodney Schlosser. © 2010 Medical University of South Carolina, Division of Rhinology, Charleston. With permission.)

- After bony osteotomies are complete and hemostasis is achieved with bipolar cautery, intracranial dissection can begin. Doppler can be used if preoperative radiographic studies demonstrate any vessels near the skull base. Dural incisions are made using an arachnoid knife. Tumor removal is then continued using microdissection techniques. Any intracranial vessels or perforators are meticulously preserved and gently elevated from the surface of the tumor. As the tumor is mobilized, it can be dropped into the nasal cavity to minimize retraction of normal frontal lobe. Care should be taken to avoid injury to the pituitary stalk, optic apparatus, and superior hypophyseal arteries arising from the internal carotid artery.

- Hemostasis is obtained during tumor dissection by using bipolar cautery. Once the tumor is removed, hemostasis can be obtained using Gelfoam powder slurry and/or warm water irrigation. We do not typically use this until tumor removal is complete, as it can make identification of tissue planes difficult.

Skull Base Reconstruction

- When no CSF leak occurs, we typically use a dural graft matrix as an underlay graft in the sella. A free mucosal graft may be placed as an overlay (Fig. 29.16) and secured with Gelfoam, nasal packing, or balloon catheter.

- In the presence of CSF leak, a multilayer reconstruction is utilized. A dural graft matrix is used as an underlay graft initially. Abdominal fat grafts can supplement the reconstruction and possible rigid reconstruction.

- For large skull base defects, if a rigid reconstruction is needed, we prefer to use an absorbable PDS plate for an additional layer of reconstruction, which provides a rigid framework and maintains skull base structure.

- A Valsalva procedure is performed to ensure that the skull base reconstruction is water tight and no CSF leak is visualized intraoperatively.

- When indicated, the posteriorly pedicled nasoseptal flap is then used as an overlay graft to support the reconstruction (Fig. 29.17).[3] The flap must lie against the sella and posterior sphenoid walls without redundancy or gap to improve the adherence of the flap. During the postoperative wound healing, the nasoseptal flap will undergo some contracture and the flap should be designed and inset to account for this contracture. The flap is then supported by Gelfoam and possibly nasal packing if indicated for CSF leak or nasal hemostasis.

POSTOPERATIVE CONSIDERATIONS

- Avoid prolonged mask ventilation during emergence from anesthesia, as this can potentially introduce pneumocephalus.

- Avoid any instrumentation of the nose during the immediate postoperative period, including instructions to avoid any nasogastric tubes.

- Instruct the patient to avoid nose blowing or sneezing. Nasal drainage should be carefully blotted.

- Appropriate endocrinology consult is beneficial in the management of postoperative endocrinopathies, including syndrome of inappropriate antidiuretic hormone secretion (SIADH) and hypopituitarism. If no intraoperative steroids are given, cortisol levels can be checked on postoperative day 1.
- During the initial 2 to 3 weeks after surgery, we do not use nasal saline irrigations. CSF leak is the principal concern during the initial postoperative period and saline irrigations can mask symptoms of CSF leak. After this initial period, we recommend the use of saline gels and nasal saline irrigation to help soften nasal crusting.

REFERENCES

Access the reference list online at ExpertConsult.com.

Endoscopic Management of Clival Chordomas and Chondrosarcomas

Jayakar V. Nayak, Andrew Thamboo, Garret Choby, Griffith R. Harsh, and Peter H. Hwang

INTRODUCTION

- Successful management of malignant clival pathology extending into the posterior fossa continues to be a formidable challenge to the skull base surgeon.
- Classically, the clivus and posterior fossa have been approached using lateral and/or transoral-transpalatal routes.
- These approaches often lead to collateral/bystander damage to functional tissue structures uninvolved with the primary disease and are commonly associated with cranial nerve deficits and other significant morbidities.[1,2]

ADVANTAGES TO ENDOSCOPIC RESECTION OF CLIVAL LESIONS

- The endoscopic endonasal approach to the skull base allows access to the entire clivus and early identification of neurovascular structures within the posterior fossa.[3–7]
- This approach avoids cerebral and brainstem retraction to obviate concern of traction/injury to lower cranial nerves via open access to the entire clivus and early identification of neurovascular structure approaches.
- It permits a magnified and highly illuminated view of a typically challenging area, in order to properly visualize the surgical target. Endoscopy allows improved discrimination and verification of tumor borders from normal tissue planes and even edematous/vasogenic brain parenchyma invaded by tumor.

DISADVANTAGES TO ENDOSCOPIC TRANSCLIVAL APPROACHES

- Three-dimensional (depth) appreciation is lost on most two-dimensional monitor systems available today.

This can be particularly challenging for neurosurgeons accustomed to the 3-D neuroanatomy seen through use of operating microscopes for intracranial or spine surgery.
- Lengthy skull base procedures become confined by narrow nostril size and dimensions when performed in an endonasal manner by two surgeons.

CLIVAL CHORDOMAS: BACKGROUND

- The clival chordoma is a malignant tumor arising from remnant cells of the central notochord neuraxis, representing 0.1% of total skull base tumors, although for all chordomas, ⅓ arise at the skull base (compared to the sacrum and general spine).
- Patients present with a wide constellation of symptoms based on route of tumor spread: intracranial extension (headaches, seizures, CN VI palsy) versus inferior spread into the nasopharynx, maxillary sinus, and nose (nasal obstruction, otalgia, and proptosis).[8]
- Represent low-grade malignancies of 3 subtypes: classic, chondroid, and dedifferentiated.
- Classic histologic cell type: physaliferous "soap bubble" cells, which are large cells containing vacuolated cytoplasm.
- Specific stains for cytokeratins, epithelial membrane antigen (EMA), brachyury, and MIB-1 can help to discriminate chordoma versus chondrosarcoma.
- Primary treatment modality is surgical resection followed by adjuvant radiotherapy.
- Although considered a low-grade neoplasm, given its locally aggressive behavior, overall 5-year survival approaches 60% to 70%.[9]

CLIVAL CHONDROSARCOMAS: BACKGROUND

- Malignancy arising from endochondral cartilage; at the skull base, this is found at the petroclival spheno-petrosal, spheno-occipital, and petro-occipital synchondroses.[10]
- Similar to chordomas, ⅓ of chondrosarcomas are noted in association with the clivus.[7,11]
- Patients present with a wide constellation of symptoms related to intracranial and otologic concerns: headaches, seizures, diplopia, otalgia, symptoms associated with eustachian tube dysfunction, and trigeminal cranial neuropathy.
- Histologically divided into 4 major subtypes: conventional (graded 1–3), mesenchymal, clear cell, and dedifferentiated. The most common subtype is seen microscopically as malignant cells admixed within abnormal sheets of cartilage.[10]
- Primary treatment modality is surgical resection followed by adjuvant radiotherapy, although adjuvant chemotherapy appears to be gaining favor in some institutions.

- Five-year survival is reported to be as high as 90%, with a mean survival time of 4.5 years (median 2 years).[12]

ANATOMIC CONSIDERATIONS AND RELATIONSHIPS FOR THE CLIVUS

- The word *clivus*, meaning "slope" in Latin, is the name used for the slanting depression behind the dorsum sellae formed by the junction of the sphenoid bone and the most anterior portion of the basilar occipital bone (Fig. 30.1).
- Functionally, the clivus separates the nasopharynx from the brainstem and posterior cranial fossa and serves to support a portion of the pons.
- The clivus can be considered regionally: the upper clivus faces the nasopharynx anteriorly, and the superior aspect of the clivus includes the posterior clinoid process and dorsum sellae. This extends to the level of the petrous apex.
- Intracranially, the upper ⅔ of the clivus bone is opposite the pons.
- The inferior limit of the clivus is the foramen magnum.

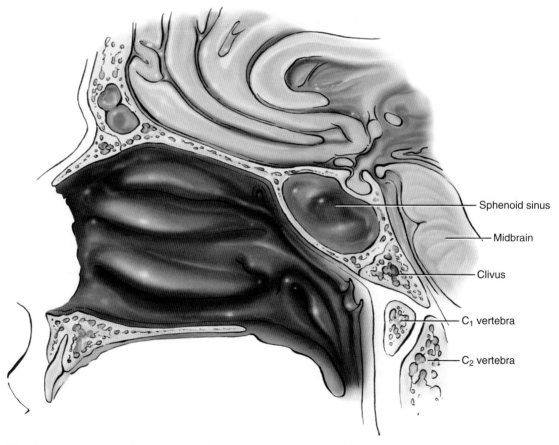

Sphenoid sinus

Midbrain

Clivus

C₁ vertebra

C₂ vertebra

Fig. 30.1. Drawing of bony and soft tissue paraclival anatomy in the sagittal view. The clivus is seen with its surrounding structures: nasopharynx anteriorly, midbrain and brainstem posteriorly, sphenoid sinus and pituitary sella superiorly, and C₁ inferiorly.

- The clival periosteum is closely adherent to the ventral dura overlying the pons (superiorly) and medulla (inferiorly). Between the outer and inner layers of dura are the basilar venous plexus and the abducens nerves (CN VI), both of which are at significant risk during clival procedures.

- The abducens nerve arises medially at the vertebrobasilar junction, then courses laterally before entering the dural plane of the clivus at the Dorello canal, and subsequently passes through the cavernous sinus.

- Several important neurovascular structures lie just deep to the inner (intracranial) layer of clival dura. The basilar artery extends along the midline of the pons and arborizes into multiple paired feeder branches, including the superior cerebellar arteries, anterior inferior cerebellar arteries, and posterior cerebral arteries (Fig. 30.2). Laterally, the intradural portions of cranial nerves III, IV, V, and VI can frequently be visualized.

- The endoscopic surgeon should be familiar with the full course of the internal carotid artery (ICA). The ICA cervical segment extends superiorly from the common carotid takeoff until it enters the carotid canal anterolateral to the jugular foramen and just medial to the styloid process. This petrous portion of the artery then courses along the temporal bone, where it has both a short vertical segment and a longer horizontal segment as the artery courses medially toward the petrous apex. The petrous ICA then passes the superior aspect of the foramen lacerum and gives rise to the vidian artery before the petrolingual ligament, which demarcates the start of the cavernous portion of the carotid. The ICA cavernous segment is quite tortuous as it winds between the dural linings of the cavernous sinus and can be seen endoscopically coursing along the posterolateral wall of the sphenoid sinus. After exiting the cavernous sinus, the ICA courses along the medial aspect of the anterior clinoid process, traverses the dura, and enters the intracranial vault (Fig. 30.3).

PREOPERATIVE CONSIDERATIONS FOR ENDOSCOPIC TRANSCLIVAL WORK

- As with other endoscopic endonasal skull base procedures, operations on clival lesions can typically be addressed by the otolaryngologist/head and neck surgeon with experience and advanced instrumentation in endoscopic skull base procedures. Certain complex lesions and virtually all with intracranial extension will necessitate the involvement of an en doneurosurgeon as well. The two-nostril technique is generally used to allow one or both surgeons to operate through a central corridor.

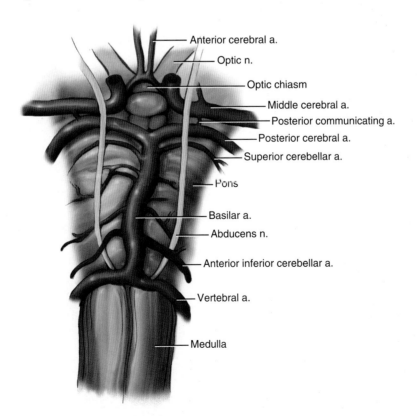

Fig. 30.2. Drawing of the cranial anatomy posterior to the clivus in coronal view. *a.,* Artery; *n.,* nerve.

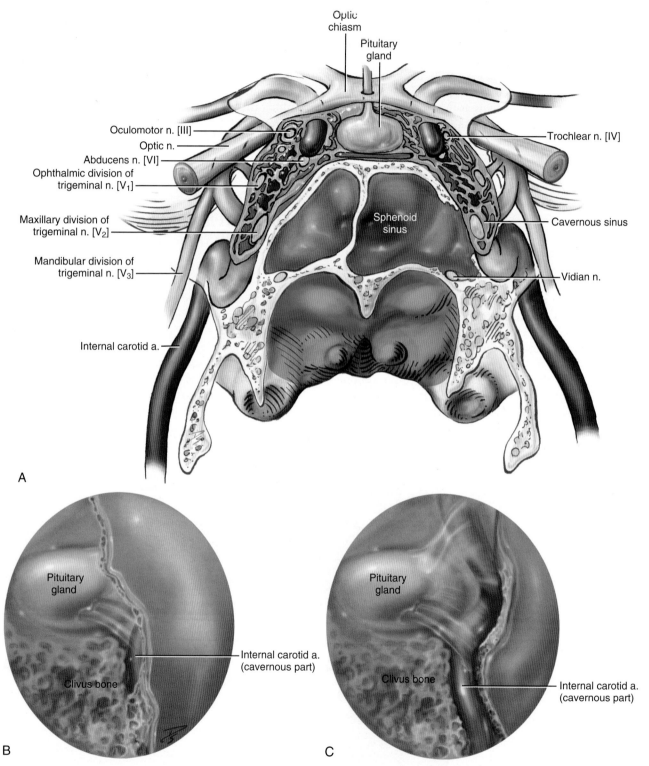

Fig. 30.3. **(A)** Drawing showing the path of the internal carotid artery and its relation to the clivus and other critical neurovascular structures. **(B, C)** Artist's depiction of the unroofing of the bone of the clivus to expose the vertical paraclival and cavernous ICA segments (endoscopic view). *a.*, Artery; *n.*, nerve.

- Appropriate case selection and angle of approach are paramount. A complex relationship between clival tumors and the ICA or vertebrobasilar system may place the patient at significant risk that might be avoided through the use of a lateral or subtemporal approach. Transdural, intracranial extension is rarely a contraindication to the endonasal approach, although it does increase the risks and complexity of the case considerably.
- Monitoring cranial nerves and/or somatosensory evoked potentials (SSEPs) can be helpful; neurophysiologic monitoring use is based on the extent and location of the lesion and surgeon preference.
- Navigation systems have become an essential component of endoscopic skull base procedures. The use of intraoperative navigation guided by fine-cut computed tomographic (CT) or magnetic resonance imaging (MRI) scans allows the surgeon to confirm their localization in the often partially distorted and hemorrhagic operative bed.
- Preoperative placement of a lumbar drain is sometimes indicated, guided primarily by the anticipated size of the dural defect. Intrathecal fluorescein can be administered upon drain placement for intraoperative detection of cerebrospinal fluid (CSF) leaks.
- If a CSF leak is anticipated on tumor extirpation, early in the case, there should be low threshold for elevation and protection of a pedicled intranasal rotational flap (such as the nasoseptal flap) to prevent damage or inadvertent resection of this reconstructive tissue source.

Radiographic Considerations for Transclival Surgery

- CT in combination with MRI are the radiographic studies of choice for evaluating most clival and skull base pathologic processes.
- High-resolution CT scans can be used to evaluate bony erosion and/or confirm involvement of skull base foramina.
- The use of MRIs best assists in differentiating chordoma and chondrosarcoma borders from nasopharyngeal mucosa, dura, or other soft tissue structures.
- The clivus is best assessed via midline sagittal T1-weighted, unenhanced MRIs. The appearance of the clivus changes predictably with patient age, due to increasing proportions of fat-replaced marrow with age (Fig. 30.4). This is important when diagnosing abnormal lesions of the clivus.[13]
- Many skull base neoplasms can be differentiated based on their appearance on CT and T1- and T2-weighted MRIs.

- The course of the ICAs should be closely examined preoperatively. In rare cases, the ICA is situated in a medialized position and is at significant risk during a clival approach.
- Any lateral extension of tumor should be identified early. Significant lateral extension can require additional surgical steps for adequate access, including resection of the medial and lateral pterygoid plates, transpterygoid access, or a cross-court approach. In some cases, far lateral tumor extent may require an alternative surgical approach entirely.
- Some of the more common/classic lesions involving the clivus include:
  - Chordoma (Fig. 30.5)
  - Chondrosarcoma with superior and lateral extension to the temporal lobe (Fig. 30.6)
  - Chondrosarcoma with inferior extension to the foramen magnum (Fig. 30.7)

INSTRUMENTATION FOR ENDONASAL TRANSCLIVAL SURGERY

- 0-, 30-, 45-, and 70-degree rigid, 3-mm, or 4-mm endoscopes
- Mini-Doppler detection for the ICA and vertebrobasilar system (VBS)
- Freer and Cottle elevators
- Sphenoid sinus mushroom punch
- Kerrison punches
- Ring curettes
- Bipolar microforceps with angled tips
- Straight and curved endoscopic scissors
- Cutting and noncutting sinus forceps
- High-speed endoscopic drill with extended-length diamond and fluted burs
- Ultrasonic aspirator with intranasal hand attachments
- Microdébrider tissue shaver
- Endoscope lens clearance system
- Intraoperative computer-assisted navigational system/image guidance platform

PEARLS AND POTENTIAL PITFALLS

- Chordomas and chondrosarcomas of the skull base are challenging lesions to definitively treat at the skull base due to (i) location, especially when ventral to brainstem; and (ii) locally aggressive, invasive behavior.
- During surgery, the patient's head should be positioned in slight flexion. This improves access to the sphenoid sinus and the clivus and marginally decreases bleeding due to dependent blood pooling.

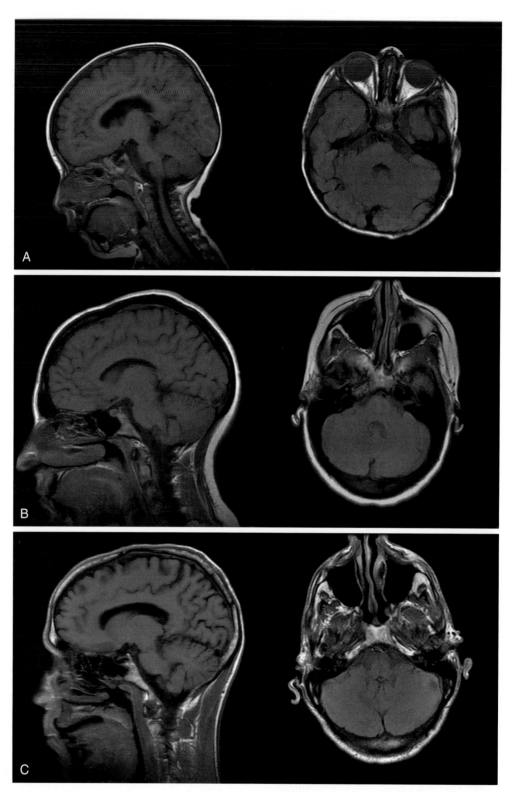

Fig. 30.4. Sagittal and axial T1-weighted noncontrast-enhanced magnetic resonance images illustrating age-dependent changes in the clivus. Images show the appearance of a normal clivus in patients aged 1 year **(A)**, 20 years **(B)**, and 50 years **(C)**. Note the increased signal intensity of the clivus with time, which is caused by an increase in the proportion of yellow (fatty) replacement of the marrow.

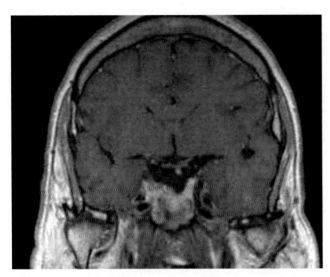

Fig. 30.5. Coronal T1-weighted, contrast-enhanced magnetic resonance image of a clival chordoma demonstrating irregular borders at the clivus-basisphenoid junction and abutting the carotid arteries laterally.

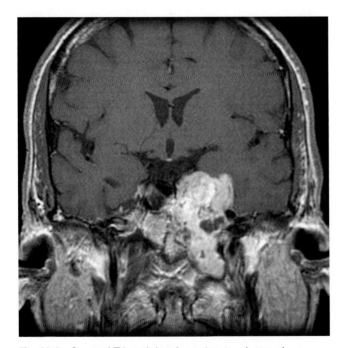

Fig. 30.6. Coronal T1-weighted, contrast-enhanced magnetic resonance image of a skull base chondrosarcoma involving the petroclival synchondrosis with temporal lobe compression. This asymmetric aggressive chondrosarcoma has produced skull base erosion and left internal carotid artery displacement. The petroclival synchondrosis is the typical site of origin of this rare lesion.

- Posterior septectomy is a critical step for this skull base procedure to create a wide surgical corridor to the clivus through both nostrils (binarial) for the introduction of multiple instruments. Complete exposure of the width of the clivus cannot be attained

without partial removal of the bony posterior nasal septum.[14]

- When a nasoseptal flap is desired for reconstruction, this is often harvested upfront and tucked away either in the nasopharynx or the ipsilateral maxillary sinus during the remainder of the procedure.

- When the middle and lower thirds of the clivus are incorporated in the surgical dissection, the approach should be limited laterally by the eustachian tubes. The ICAs run just lateral and posterior to the eustachian tubes and are consequently at risk when dissection is continued beyond this landmark.

- Important landmarks to identify during clival surgery include the floor of the sphenoid sinus, opticocarotid recesses, clivocarotid protuberances, eustachian tubes, vidian canal, and vertical segment of the ICAs.

- Heavy bleeding can be encountered from the clival venous plexus. Adequate hemostasis often requires an extended period of tamponade with hemosealant biomaterials and pledgets combined with patience.

- Surgical planning should be based largely on whether there is any intradural extension of tumor. Great care should be exercised when incising the clival dura, given the proximity of the basilar artery, CN VI, and similar named neurovascular structures directly underneath.

- While knowledge of anatomy verified by image guidance is important, understanding the strategies for tissue management and safe techniques for dissection of chordoma or chondrosarcoma lesions away from dura, brainstem parenchyma, and intracranial tributary feeders is critical to successful surgery and favorable long-term outcomes.

- Chordoma or chondrosarcomas must be meticulously dissected from surrounding brainstem/neural parenchyma while keeping bridging delicate neurovascular structures intact. Collapsing the tumor edges in a centrifugal manner toward the central tumor core is one technique for achieving this.

- CSF leaks at the level of the clivus are among the most difficult to close due to the high-flow basilar cistern present at this region of the skull base and the inability to reliably maintain a water-tight seal. Multilayered reconstruction, predicated on the use of a generous, well-bolstered nasoseptal flap with a hardy pedicle, in concert with ongoing CSF diversion via lumbar drainage, is usually critical to successful skull base reconstruction at this challenging site overlying the posterior fossa.

SURGICAL PROCEDURE

Step 1: Complete the Preoperative Setup

- Ensure availability of appropriate equipment and personnel: image guidance system, radiographic studies, and CT/MRI merge software; SSEP

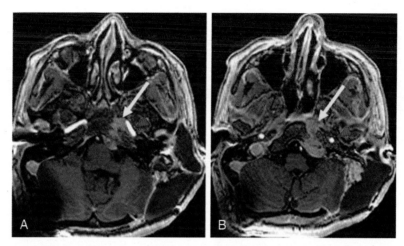

Fig. 30.7. Axial MRI of a left petroclival and petro-occipital chondrosarcoma *(yellow arrows)* in a patient with persistent headaches in the setting of a nonpneumatized (conchal type) sphenoid sinus. In **(A)**, more superiorly, there is a tongue of sarcoma abutting, but not compressing, the left pons, but the lesion is kissing the left internal carotid artery *(red arrowheads)*. In **(B)**, more inferiorly, chondrosarcoma has eroded the clival bone and has crept along the clival dura toward the hypoglossal canal and foramen magnum.

monitoring; extended-length hand and powered instrumentation with diamond and fluted burs in stock; ultrasonic bone aspirator with intranasal handpiece (if available at institution); straight and angled endoscopes with scope cleaner attachments; synthetic dural substitutes and hemostatic biomaterials; high-definition monitors and video recording system.

- After induction of general anesthesia and appropriate IV access is established, position the patient with the head slightly flexed. The head-flexed position improves access to the sphenoid sinus, nasopharynx, and clivus.
- Administer antibiotics and/or corticosteroids at this time, based on personal and institutional preference.
- Using stereotactic equipment, register the patient to the appropriate CT, MRI, or merged CT/MRI image sequences using software applications on navigational systems.
- If involvement of adjacent cranial nerves is a concern, cranial motor nerve and somatosensory monitoring can be implemented.
- Endoscopic endonasal approaches to the clivus can be performed with or without rigid head fixation. The latter is comfortable for the otolaryngologist but can be a point of contention with colleagues from neurosurgery.
- In cases of extradural or small intradural chordomas and chondrosarcomas, a lumbar drain is typically unnecessary. Resection of large intradural tumors will often result in a sizable dural opening; in these cases, multilayered reconstruction and lumbar drain placement is typically indicated.

- Fluorescein (0.1 mL of 10% stock fluorescein diluted into 10 mL CSF or sterile saline) can be injected into the intrathecal space to assist with accurate visualization of CSF leaks during skull base reconstruction.

Step 2: Decongest and Provide Vasoconstriction to the Nasal Cavity

- Under visualization with a 0-degree, 4-mm rigid nasal endoscope, place cottonoids soaked with either 1:1000 epinephrine or oxymetazoline into the nasal cavity; typically 1 or 2 cottonoids are placed both lateral to and medial to the middle turbinate. Adequate decongestion is usually achieved in 3 to 5 minutes.
- Injection of 1% lidocaine with 1:100,000 epinephrine at the attachment of the middle turbinate, sphenoid rostrum, posterior nasal septum, and along the course of the sphenopalatine artery, using a long 25-gauge needle or spinal needle, is often advocated for added hemostasis. A similar 1 to 2 mL transoral injection into the greater palatine foramina is thought to provide added retrograde hemostasis to the posterior nasal cavity.

Step 3: Harvest a Nasoseptal Flap (Optional)

- Harvest a nasal septal flap before performing wide sphenoidotomies and the posterior septectomy to ensure that a large flap pedicle is preserved.[15] The posterior nasal artery (also termed the posterior septal artery) arises between the ostium of each sphenoid sinus (superiorly) and upper arch of each choana (inferiorly). Judicious preservation of the pedicle carrying this axial artery can be important before removal of the clival lesion (Fig. 30.8).

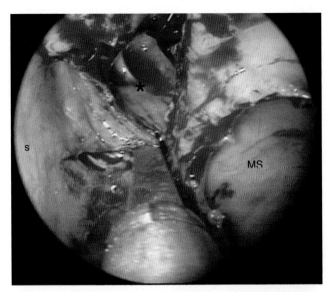

Fig. 30.8. Endoscopic view of harvest of a nasoseptal flap using a straight otologic Beaver blade. Here, an incision is being made along the path of the left septal artery to begin the flap. The asterisk indicates the sphenoid sinus. *MS,* Maxillary sinus; *S,* septum.

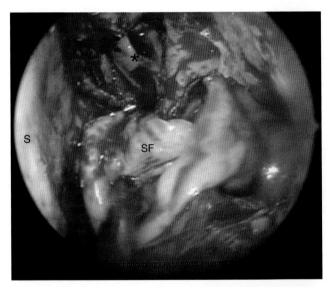

Fig. 30.9. Endoscopic view showing placement of the harvested flap *(SF)* into the maxillary antrostomy for safekeeping until the flap is required during the reconstruction phase of the procedure. The asterisk indicates the sphenoid sinus. *S,* Septum.

- In general, the flap should be harvested on the side contralateral to that with the most lateral extension of tumor.
- The elevated flap can then be placed into the nasopharynx; but to improve subsequent access to the nasopharynx and clivus, it is more appropriately placed into a widely exposed maxillary sinus (Fig. 30.9).

Step 4: Defining the Surgical Corridors to the Sphenoid Sinus and Clivus

- Obtain surgical access to the clivus and surrounding structures. We typically favor a transseptal/medial approach to identify the sphenoid sinuses as a superior landmark and then widen the corridor from this point.
- In most cases, and in our experience, complete removal of the bilateral middle turbinates is unnecessary, as the middle and superior turbinates can be simply lateralized to increase access to the basisphenoid and clivus. If insufficient, partial resection of the inferior portion of the middle turbinates can be performed for atraumatic passage of instruments into the central posterior skull base and clivus during team surgical cases. Also, in selected cases, extended transpterygoid approaches may assist in cases of lateral extension of a clival lesion.

Step 5: Perform Wide Bilateral Sphenoidotomies

- Refer to Chapters 8 and 28 for details on performing a sphenoidotomy.
- The superior turbinate can be partially resected to improve access to the sphenoid ostia, although this step is usually not necessary. Resection of the superior turbinate can result in the concomitant removal of segments of functional olfactory mucosa.
- Once the bilateral sphenoid ostia are identified and widened medial to the superior turbinates, the sphenoid rostrum is widely taken down to expose the lateral wall, opticocarotid recess, and carotid protuberance. Meticulously remove the intersinus septum between the sphenoid sinuses.
- With inferior extension of the sphenoidotomies, the sphenopalatine artery and possibly its posterior septal branches may eventually be encountered. Try to avoid injuring these vessels, as it may compromise health of the nasoseptal flap pedicle. However, coagulation of these vessels with bipolar electrocautery will be needed if they become exposed.

Step 6: Perform a Posterior Septectomy

- Typically, removal of the entire posterior bony septum allows adequate access to the sphenoid sinus and clivus through both nostrils (Fig. 30.10).
- Using the sphenoidotomies as fixed landmarks, perform this step by sharply incising and elevating the mucosa off of the bony septum and/or microdébriding the mucosa directly from the septum.
- Next, safely fracture the posterior septum and intersinus sphenoid septum in a "cross-court" fashion so that the two sphenoidotomies communicate to form a common large sinus. Inferiorly in this keel area of the septum-sphenoid junction, the bone can be quite dense and typically requires use of large bone

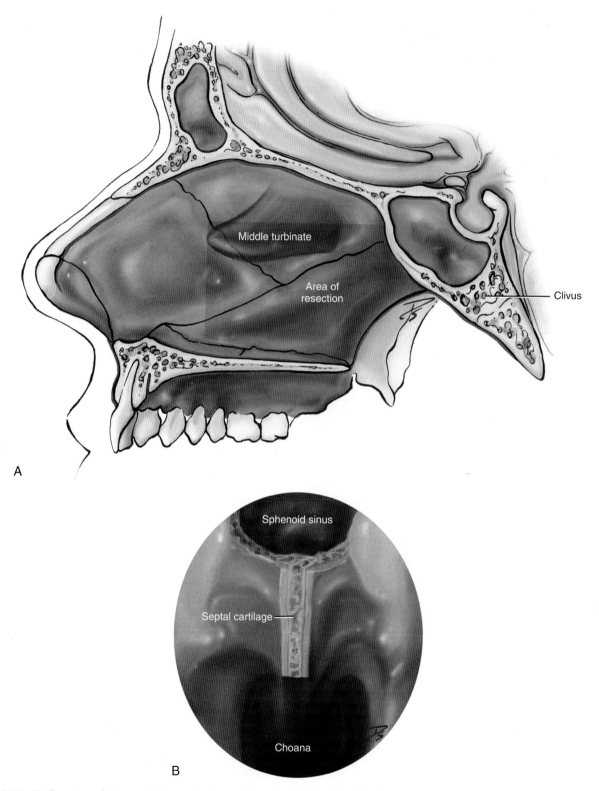

Fig. 30.10. (A) Drawing of the posterior septectomy. The area of resection *(shading)* comes anteriorly to the anterior head of the middle turbinate and posteriorly to the nasopharynx for a complete posterior septectomy. **(B)** Artist's depiction of the endoscopic view after completion of the posterior septectomy.

punches and/or a high-speed drill and cutting bur for removal.

- Avoid removal of bone or mucosa along the superior nasal septum and skull base because this area contains olfactory tissue and a CSF leak can result.

Step 7: Reduce the Floor of the Sphenoid Sinus and Begin Drilling the Superior Clivus

- Reducing the floor of the sphenoid sinus and drilling the superior clivus are important steps for exposure of the superior third of the clivus and early identification of the internal carotid arteries and widening the surgical corridor to improve illumination.
- Once the mucosa is reflected away, the bone in this area, including the sphenoid keel and sphenoid floor, is comprised of dense bone; its removal usually requires high-speed drills with cutting burs and/or heavy rongeurs (Fig. 30.11).
- During bone resection and drilling, the vidian neurovascular bundle can be a useful landmark to note at the lateral roof of the clivus/floor of the sphenoid sinus. While the vidian nerve is comprised of sympathetic and parasympathetic elements, the vidian artery is an anterior extension of, and lies just proximal to, the anterior genu of the ICA (Fig. 30.12).[16]
- If a nasoseptal flap has been previously harvested, great care should be taken not to traverse the vascular pedicle, because the artery courses just below the inferior face of the sphenoid sinus.

Step 8: Identify the Vertical Component of Both Internal Carotid Arteries

- To find the vertical component of an ICA most easily, identify the artery along the posterior wall of the sphenoid sinus/skull base. Then, confirm the course of the ICA into its vertical segment using an intraoperative, mini-Doppler wand. As an alternative, the vertical components of the ICA often stand out on either side of the clivus/clival recess and can be identified in most patients by a vertical bony canal (Fig. 30.13).

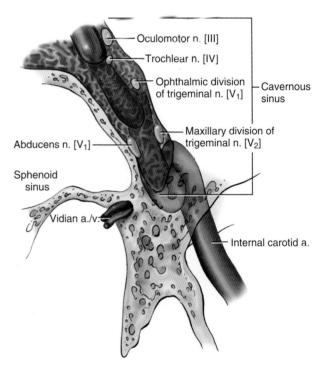

Fig. 30.12. Drawing of the vidian neurovascular bundle and its relation to the internal carotid artery. *a.*, Artery; *n.*, nerve; *v.*, vein.

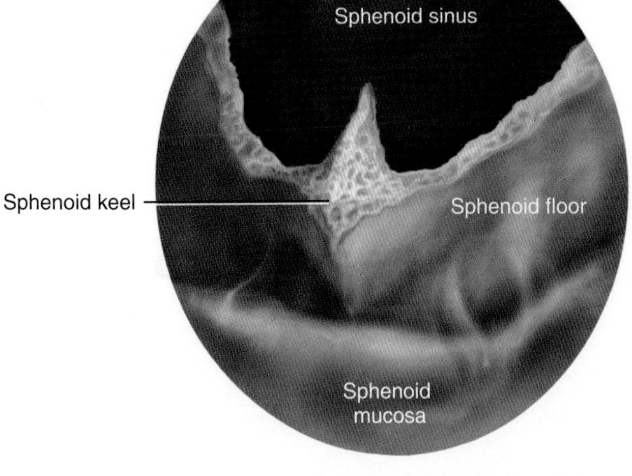

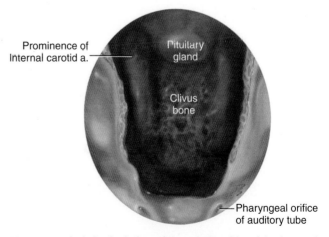

Fig. 30.13. Artist's depiction of the relationship of the internal carotid canals and the arteries' vertical course/impression along the posterior sphenoid skull base (endoscopic view). *a.*, Artery.

Fig. 30.11. Artist's depiction of the sphenoid keel and floor of the sphenoid sinus that must be removed to expose the clivus posteriorly and increase illumination into the surgical corridor (endoscopic view).

- Skeletonize the carotids through takedown of intersphenoid sinus septations if there is extension of the tumor lateral to and behind the arteries.

Step 9: Open the Nasopharyngeal Mucosa and Musculature to Expose the Clivus (Optional)

- The nasopharyngeal mucosa is usually incised sharply, or with extended-tip cautery, and elevated off of the clivus. Alternatively, an inferiorly based flap can be raised and potentially replaced at the end of the procedure, although this flap can be challenging to preserve.
- Resect or detach the buccopharyngeal fascia and longus colli and splenius capitis muscles underlying the mucosal surface to expose the anterior face of the clivus.
- During this portion of the procedure, do not extend the dissection lateral to the eustachian tubes (shown in Fig. 30.13), both to avoid interference with middle ear pressure equalization and prevent injury to the ICAs as they course through the posterolateral nasopharynx.

Step 10: Drill the Clivus Bone Until the Lesion Is Resected or the Clival Dura Is Exposed

- Resect lesions of the clivus, such as chordomas and chondrosarcomas, from the anterior sphenoid-clivus junction using a three-handed, two-nostril technique that combines endoscopy, suction instrumentation, and curettage and computer-assisted, intraoperative navigation (Fig. 30.14).
- The rich vascular channels within the clivus can result in substantial blood loss, requiring repeated need for modern hemostatic agents and cottonoid tamponade.
- In the case of many chordomas, sarcomas, and other related lesions when extradural, removal of the clivus effectively removes the tumor itself. In Fig. 30.15 (same lesion also shown in Figs. 30.7 and 30.14), a hemiclivectomy was required to completely resect broadly invasive, extradural chondrosarcoma from the superior clivus and petrous ICA to the left hypoglossal canal, just superior to the foramen magnum.

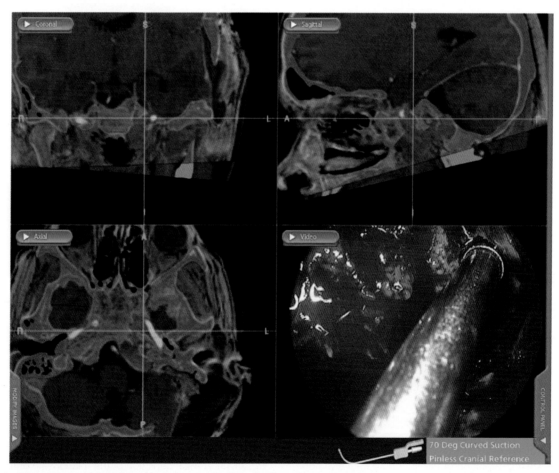

Fig. 30.14. Computer-assisted, intraoperative navigation display with merged/overlayed computed tomography and magnetic resonance studies as well as intraoperative endoscopic view. The crosshairs confirm that the tip of curved suction used here is adjacent to the left petrous internal carotid artery following progressive endoscopic, endonasal resection of extradural chondrosarcoma.

- Once the lesion is resected, the posterior clival recess (inferior to the sella) and pulsations of the brainstem vasculature through the clival dura can be better appreciated.

Step 11: Incise the Dura to Expose the Posterior Fossa for Intracranial Lesions (Optional)

- Lesions such as the chordoma shown in Fig. 30.16 require entry into the posterior fossa.

- Before making any dural incisions, again confirm the course of the ICAs and vertebrobasilar branches using intraoperative image guidance and a mini-Doppler device.
- If durotomy is required, begin it low and medially in the clivus, which may lower the chance of injury to the basilar artery and sixth cranial nerves.
- The dura is often quite vascular; thus, substantial bleeding from the dural venous plexus can be

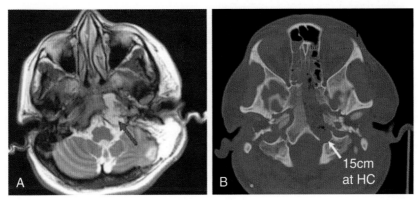

Fig. 30.15. (A) Left petroclival chondrosarcoma *(red arrow),* with differing aspects shown in Figs. 30.7 and 30.14; **(B)** intraoperative computed tomography scan at end of surgery showing the bony tract in the nonpneumatized clival skull base needed to be carved out to achieve complete resection of this lesion from the superior clivus and dura to the hypoglossal canal (HC). The distance from nostril rim to HC within the sloping clivus was 15 to 15.5 cm. This patient remains disease free now 4 years following endonasal skull base surgery and adjuvant radiation therapy.

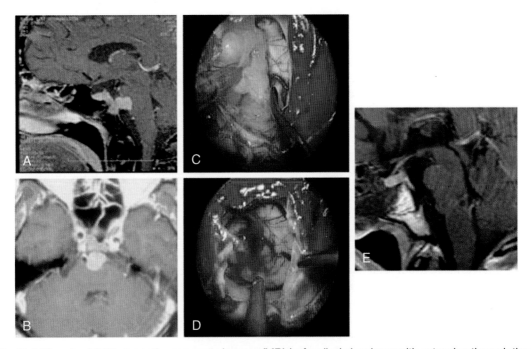

Fig. 30.16. Sagittal **(A)** and axial **(B)** magnetic resonance images (MRIs) of a clival chordoma with extension through the dura, producing central, intraparenchymal brainstem compression. **(C)** Intraoperative images of intracranial clival chordoma resection once the dura is entered; the soft, gelatinous, chordoma is meticulously resected off of the brainstem parenchyma without disturbing the underlying vascular feeders from the vertebrobasilar system. **(D)** Intracranial component of chordoma completely resected with intact brainstem vasculature (basilar artery compressed from tumor) and parenchyma. **(E)** Postoperative sagittal MRI confirming brainstem decompression following tumor resection. (Parts C, D, and E from Lal D, Fischbein NJ, Harsh GR. Surgical treatment of chordomas and chondrosarcomas. In: Laws ER, Sheehan JP, eds. *Sellar and Parasellar Tumors.* New York: Thieme; 2011:155–70.)

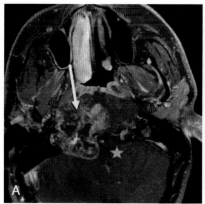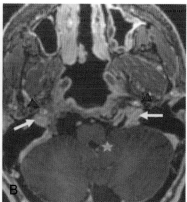

Fig. 30.17. Incomplete resection for some clival malignancies. **(A)** Massive right-predominant, bilaterally invasive, clival tumor *(yellow arrow)* in a 23-year-old male with progressive myelopathy, hoarseness, and dysphagia. Note the lateralized/displaced internal carotid arteries *(red arrowheads)* and the prominent brainstem compression *(green star)* on axial magnetic resonance imaging (MRI). **(B)** Interval postoperative MRI 2.5 status postendoscopic resection, septal flap reconstruction, and adjuvant radiotherapy, showing near-complete surgical excision of the tumor with satisfactory brainstem decompression *(green star)*. However, the retrotubal and retrocarotid *(red arrowheads)* regions bilaterally, nearly impossible to navigate or instrument at the time to endoscopic resection, remain positive for 2 focal sites of chordoma *(yellow arrows × 2)*. These two sites of persistent disease have remained radiographically unchanged for 2.5 years; the patient continues to do well from a neuroclinical standpoint without new sites of fluorodeoxyglucose (FDG)-avid disease by positron emission tomography (PET)-CT.

encountered at this point of the dissection. Hemostasis can usually be achieved via judicious bipolar electrocautery, hemostatic agents, and tamponade.

Step 12: Meticulous Decompression Versus Resection of Intradural Clival Lesions With Neurosurgery

- After confirming depth and lateral landmarks using image guidance, enter the chordoma or chondrosarcoma capsule and decompress the central core of the lesion. The latter can be achieved using suction devices and microcurettes or a two-handed suction technique with Frasier-tip suctions.[7,17]
- Gently and meticulously dissect the decompressed tumor capsule from surrounding brainstem/neural parenchyma while keeping bridging delicate neurovascular structures intact to appropriately decompress the brainstem (see Fig. 30.16).
- In some patients with massive clival tumors, brainstem decompression and clearance of tumor bulk is the main goal, which still allows adjuvant radiation to be dosed more effectively. In many cases, given the slow-growing nature of chordomas, good clinical and radiographic evidence of tumor control can be achieved (Fig. 30.17).
- Ensure local hemostasis using commercial hemostatic compounds underneath damp pledgets, adipose tissue, and bipolar electrocautery.

Step 13: Skull Base Reconstruction of Clival Defects

- Close any dural defect using a multilayer technique. Options include combined use of adipose tissue,

fascia (including fascia lata), porcine mesentery, or synthetic dural substitutes.
- A vascularized nasoseptal flap can be used to successfully reconstruct large skull base defects while achieving a water-tight seal (Fig. 30.18).[18] If unavailable, a gasket seal closure can be used effectively, which employs fascia placed as an underlay graft inside the bony (intracranial) margins of the skull base defect, and then bolstered by a semirigid graft into position using bone, cartilage, or Medpor material.
- Multilayer grafts or vascularized flaps may be kept in position during healing using tissue glues, followed by "break-away layers" of resorbable posterior nasal packing, followed by use of more-rigid packing that may be pulled/removed in the office in 4 to 10 days (surgeon preference). Options for the latter include larger resorbable biomaterial dressings to hardy, finger-length removable sponges (Merocel) to catheter/balloon stents.
- Excellent flap integration and remucosalization can be achieved at the clivus using these reconstructive approaches (see Fig. 30.18).

POSTOPERATIVE CONSIDERATIONS

- Patients should be treated postoperatively with broad-spectrum antibiotics from 7 to 10 days after an extended skull base approach with intranasal packing based on intraoperative findings.
- Possible postoperative complications include synechiae, hematoma, CSF leak (especially challenging

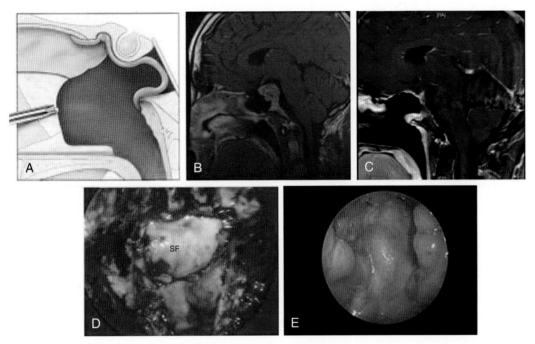

Fig. 30.18. Reconstruction of clival defects. **(A)** Artist's illustration of septal flap posterior inset onlay atop underlay graft for large clival defect with cerebrospinal fluid leak. (Fig 48.2C from Kennedy DW, Hwang PH eds Rhinology, New York, Thieme, p 647 2012.) **(B)** Sagittal MRI of clival chordoma prior to endoscopic resection. **(C)** Sagittal magnetic resonance imaging of the same patient 4 years status postcomplete endoscopic transsphenoidal/transclival resection, showing maintained vascularity to the flap inset illustrated in **(A)**, which closely hugs the lower clivus to planum sphenoidale. **(D)** Intraoperative image of septal flap *(SF)* following placement onto the skull base. **(E)** Same flap in D, now 3 months postoperatively, demonstrating excellent integration of the flap with the surrounding native sphenoid mucosal edges and coverage of the large clival defect.

if originating from high-flow basilar cistern), tension pneumocephalus, meningitis, and cranial neuropathy (most notably affecting orbital muscle movement).

■ When utilized, lumbar drains (and the rare extraventricular drain) are typically kept open 2 to 5 days after transclival approaches in the presence of CSF leak to divert fluid and pressure away from the skull base reconstruction. After resection of clival chordomas, rates of postoperative CSF leak range from 0% to 33%.[15,18]

■ All patients should be seen several times after hospital discharge in routine office follow-up to remove any intranasal bolstering or splint material, verify the absence of sinus infection and/or CSF leak, and carry out the postsurgical débridement of crusts, clot, and fibrinous debris from the nasal cavity to ensure proper mucosal health and sinus ventilation.

SPECIAL CONSIDERATIONS

■ The most catastrophic complication of endoscopic endonasal procedures of the skull base is injury to the ICA. Although this may be managed temporarily via controlled hypotension, packing, crushed muscle plug placement, and blood transfusion, most will ultimately require urgent angiography, intravascular occlusion, and/or intraluminal stenting. Endonasal surgical expertise, instrumentation, and availability of neurointerventional radiology resources should be considered prior to embarking on this type of complex endonasal skull base procedure.

REFERENCES

Access the reference list online at ExpertConsult.com.

Large Skull Base Defect Reconstruction With and Without Pedicled Flaps

E. Ritter Sansoni and Richard J. Harvey

INTRODUCTION

- Advances in endoscopic sinonasal surgical techniques and instrumentation have led to an expansion in the size and diversity of skull base lesions that are amenable to an entirely endoscopic resection. However, one of the requisites for successful removal of skull base lesions is the ability to repair the resultant defect, as failed reconstructions add significant morbidity.[1]

- The ideal endoscopic skull base repair has the following characteristics:
  - Technically feasible as part of an endoscopic procedure
  - Provides a reliable, robust, and long-term separation between the sinonasal and cranial cavities
  - Reconstructs the natural tissue barrier present in the anterior skull base
  - Minimally impacts normal sinonasal and cranial physiology
  - Obliterates dead space following tumor removal
  - Robust during adjuvant treatment
  - Flexible to accommodate skull base defects encountered immediately postresection

- Skull base defects that are small in size, with low-flow intraoperative cerebrospinal fluid (CSF) leaks can be reconstructed with a wide variety of multilayered avascular free grafts or biosynthetic materials with high success rates and limited morbidity.[2,3] However, free grafts have an unacceptably high risk of failure with larger defects for a number of reasons but primarily because the reconstructive bed is nonvascularized (i.e., air on one side and CSF on the other).[4]

- Larger skull base defects (>2–3 cm) and those that are associated with high-flow CSF leaks are best repaired with a multilayered closure technique using a vascularized flap.[4,5] A high-flow leak is created when a CSF cistern is directly opened into the sinonasal cavity.

- There is a wide variety of local and regional vascularized pedicle flaps that the surgeon can use to reconstruct skull base defects with the nasoseptal flap (NSF), first described in 2006, being the workhorse for endoscopic skull base repair.[6–9]

- When choosing the most appropriate reconstructive technique or flap, the surgeon needs to consider the anticipated location, size, and geometry of the bony and dural defects as well as high- versus low-flow CSF leak.[5] Additionally, prior sinonasal surgery, previous or planned radiotherapy, and extent of tumor involvement may limit the available options and should be accounted for.[8]

- Endoscopic skull base reconstruction offers excellent success rates with low perioperative and postoperative morbidity.[10,11] However, predictors of failure have not been entirely defined. There is evidence to suggest that radiotherapy, intraventricular tumor extension, and body habitus (predictive of increased intracranial pressure) may play a role in failed repairs whereas location and tumor histology seem less important.[1,2,12] The most common points of failure of flap repairs are the dependent parts, presumably due to increased pressure, and the most superior parts due to the danger of flap migration or retraction.[7,13]

- Both free and vascularized flap repairs use the theory of multilayered closure to provide a reliable barrier between the skull base and nasal cavity. Early CSF leak closure procedures included attempts at intracranial, but extradural, underlay reconstruction; this was subsequently found to be unnecessary. Underlay materials in multilayer reconstruction are placed subdurally. This forms the water-tight "bath plug" layer, and the pedicled flap is an onlay to provide vascularization.[11,14]

■ The use of allografts has been associated with reasonably high rates of infection, and autologous bone/cartilage grafts have been associated with high rates of resorption.[15]

■ The current philosophy at most major endoscopic skull base centers is to repair large, high-flow defects with one or more local vascularized flaps.[2,4,5,8,13]

■ The focus of this chapter is on the posteriorly based NSF, as this is currently the mainstay of endoscopic skull base repair and adds very little sinonasal morbidity.[5,7,16] Other methods of reconstruction in this chapter are described in the context of adjuncts or alternatives to the NSF when it is not available.

ANATOMY

■ It is essential to assess the location of the lesion, to define which part of the skull base needs to be removed for access, and consequently what the extent of reconstruction is likely to be. These areas have been defined previously in relation to the sagittal or coronal extent of the lesion, as shown in Table 31.1.[17–19] However, much of this is academic, as it is the fixed neurovascular structures that determine the approach and resultant defect. The rule of "avoid crossing neurovascular planes" is equally true via an endoscopic route, as it is for open transcranial approaches. It is therefore important to define the lesion in the sagittal plane as either suprachiasmatic or infrachiasmatic (Fig. 31.1). If the lesion extends lateral to the pterygoids in the coronal plane, the ipsilateral maxillary artery will likely be sacrificed. This will limit available pedicled flaps from the ipsilateral side (see Table 31.1).

TABLE 31.1 Definition of Skull Base Areas

Sagittal Plane	Area	Coronal Plane	Flap Constraints
Transfrontal	1	Transorbital	Contralateral flap needed
Transcribriform	2	Petrous apex (medial transpetrous)	
Transplanum (suprasellar/subchiasmatic) Transsphenoidal (sellar/medial transcavernous)	3	Lateral transcavernous Transpterygoid Transpetrous (superior/inferior)	
Transclival (posterior clinoid/midclivus/foramen magnum) Transodontoid	4	Transcondylar Parapharyngeal space	Contralateral flap not needed

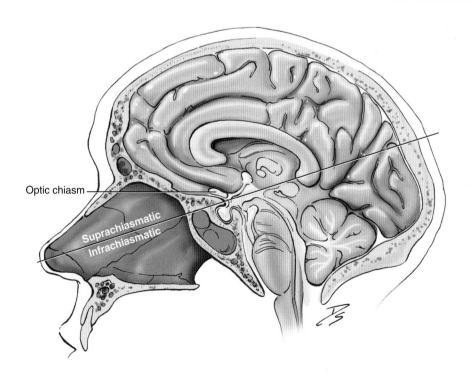

Optic chiasm

Suprachiasmatic

Infrachiasmatic

Fig. 31.1. Suprachiasmatic and infrachiasmatic lesions.

■ Once the extent of skull base removal has been considered, an appropriate repair can be planned. Radiographic analysis shows that a pedicled NSF permits coverage of the entire anterior skull base area from the posterior table of the frontal sinus to the sella with a width from lamina papyracea to lamina papyracea or, alternatively, coverage of a full panclivectomy.[20] An important clinical rule is that coverage of two contiguous skull base areas (e.g., sella and clivus, or cribriform plate and planum sphenoidale) is possible but not three. The units are clival, sella/planum, cribriform, and frontal (see Table 31.1).

■ The rich arterial supply of the sinonasal cavity provides a variety of flaps for skull base reconstruction (Fig. 31.2). Endonasal pedicled flaps with associated vasculature are listed in Table 31.2. The maximum surface area of each flap is approximated and derived from existing literature.[20–29]

PREOPERATIVE CONSIDERATIONS

■ Obtain a detailed history of previous nasal procedures. Prior resection of bone and/or cartilage from the nasal septum or turbinates may make flap harvest more challenging. Prior sphenoid surgery may have compromised the septal branch of the sphenopalatine artery; earlier turbinate surgery may also influence flap options.

■ Carefully note previous systemic or intranasal treatments, especially chemoradiotherapy, which may affect postoperative healing.[30] Consider whether postoperative radiotherapy is likely to be needed, as this will affect the choice of repair.

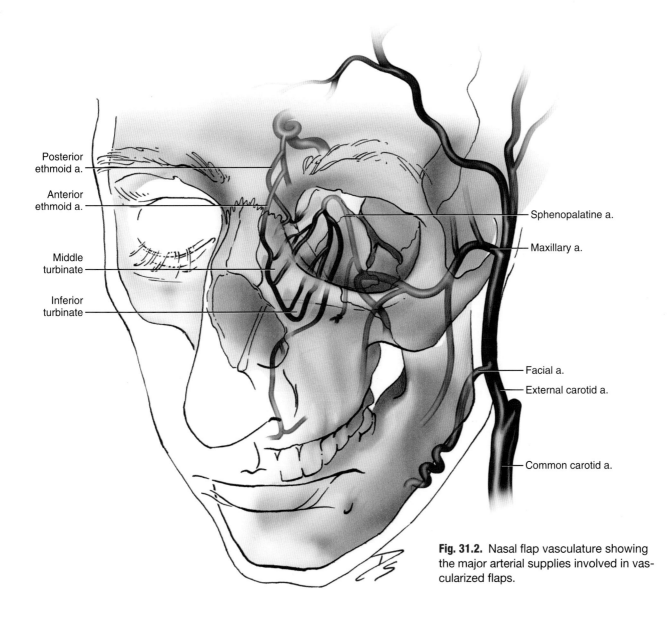

Posterior ethmoid a.
Anterior ethmoid a.
Middle turbinate
Inferior turbinate
Sphenopalatine a.
Maxillary a.
Facial a.
External carotid a.
Common carotid a.

Fig. 31.2. Nasal flap vasculature showing the major arterial supplies involved in vascularized flaps.

TABLE 31.2 Characteristics of Endonasal Pedicled Flaps

Flap	Type	Blood Supply	Midline Range of Coverage	Approximate Maximum Area (cm²)	Comments
Local					
Nasoseptal[7]	Local mucosal	Septal branch of sphenopalatine artery	Transcribriform to transclival	25.1[20]	Mainstay of reconstruction, wide durable flap with long pedicle
Contralateral transposition septal	Local mucosal	Ethmoidal arteries	Transfrontal and transcribriform	NA. Likely similar to nasoseptal flap	Short pedicle, risk of persistent perforation
Inferior turbinate[22,25]	Local mucosal	Inferior turbinate branch of sphenopalatine artery	Transplanum to transodontoid	2.4[47]	Long and narrow flap, anterior reach limited
Nasal floor[23]	Local mucosal	Branches of the sphenopalatine artery and the Woodruff plexus	Transplanum to transodontoid	NA	Technically challenging, short pedicle
Middle turbinate[27]	Local mucosal	Middle turbinate branch of sphenopalatine artery	Transplanum to transsellar	5.6[27]	Technically challenging, very variable dimensions depending on middle turbinate size
Hard palate mucosa[26]	Regional mucosal	Descending palatine artery	Transplanum to transclival	15.25[26]	Long pedicle, risk of oroantral fistula
Regional					
Pericranial (fascial)[29]	Regional fascial	Supraorbital and supratrochlear arteries	Transfrontal to transclival	293[48]	Requires Lothrop procedure to enable flap transposition
Temporoparietal (fascial)[21]	Regional fascial	Anterior branch of superficial temporal artery	Transfrontal to transodontoid	238[21]	Large area, takes time to raise, danger to frontal branch of facial nerve
Facial buccinator[49]	Regional myomucosal	Buccal branch of facial artery	Transcribriform to transplanum	18.75[49]	Risk of epiphora

NA, Not available.

- Undertake a detailed endoscopic examination of the patient's nasal cavity and note any of the following:
  - Evidence of any previous sinonasal surgery, particularly a wide sphenoidotomy
  - Loss of turbinate or septal tissue
  - The presence, location, and extent of any septal deviation
- If there has been previous sinonasal surgery, conduct a pedicle assessment, as provided in Table 31.3.
- Check that endoscopic visualization of the potential defect is going to be possible; this is imperative to permit full closure. It will be necessary to perform a modified endoscopic Lothrop procedure (MELP) if complete resection of the anterior skull base is required.[31]
- The general preoperative health status of the patient is important to consider since comorbid diseases may complicate the patient's recovery. For example, increased body habitus may be associated with increased CSF pressure and obstructive sleep apnea may be more challenging to manage without the use of positive pressure ventilation.

Radiographic Considerations

- Note the potential geometry of the skull base defect that will result after resection. Angles of the skull base surface make placing a graft more difficult and require longer flaps to achieve full coverage and closure.[32] Asian nasal cavities may not have the equivalent septal mucosal flap area available for harvest as compared to the noses of whites.[33]
- Lesions that may involve repair of the posterior table of the frontal sinus will require a MELP, and lateral

TABLE 31.3 Pedicle Assessment

Pedicle	May Be Unavailable Due To	Flaps Excluded If Injured	Flap Alternative
Septal branch of sphenopalatine artery	Extensive tumor involvement Sphenoid surgery Posterior septectomy Tumor/surgery in pteryopalatine fossa Sphenopalatine artery ligation	Posterior septal flap	Contralateral nasoseptal flap Regional flap Turbinate flap for small or posterior cranial fossa defects
Inferior turbinate branch of sphenopalatine artery	Inferior turbinate surgery/tumor Sphenopalatine artery ligation	Inferior turbinate flap	Contralateral nasoseptal flap Regional flap
Descending palatine branch	Surgery/tumor in pterygopalatine fossa Surgery/tumor in infratemporal fossa Cleft palate	Palatal flap	Regional flap
Internal maxillary artery	Surgery/tumor in infratemporal fossa	Posterior septal flap Inferior turbinate flap Nasal floor flap Middle turbinate flap	Contralateral nasoseptal flap Regional flap

frontal sinus floor repair beyond the midpoint of the orbit will require an external approach or orbital transposition.[34,35]

- In younger patients being considered for nasoseptal flap repair, assess the cranium-to-face ratio to ensure that the nasoseptal flap will cover the defect created.[36] The pedicled nasoseptal flap may not be a reliable option for patients under 14 years old.
- If a middle turbinate flap is being considered, note the anatomy and size of the middle turbinate. At least 4 cm middle turbinate length is required for the flap to reach the sella.[27]
- Note whether the arachnoid cisterns, or occasionally ventricles, are likely to be opened. This may influence the need for vascularized repair regardless of the dural defect size, as a high-flow CSF leak will be created.

INSTRUMENTATION

- 0-degree nasal endoscope
- Monopolar needle-tip electrocautery with the tip bent at 45 degrees provides accurate flap incisions with good hemostasis.
- Bipolar electrocautery for accurate control of troublesome hemorrhage
- Blunt dissection instruments, such as a Cottle elevator, for raising the flap over a wide plane
- FESS micro-scissors for fine adjustment of the flap dimensions
- Ball-tip probe for fine nontraumatic manipulation of the flap
- Small curette for fine nontraumatic manipulation of the flap

- Curved olive-tip suction without suction attached for placing the underlay graft material and manipulating the flap
- Straight and angled cutting forceps (large and small) for fine adjustment of the flap dimensions
- Straight and angled grabbing forceps for fine flap adjustment
- Materials
  - Underlay graft
    - Artifical dura mater substitutes: DuraGen, TissuDura, DuraMatrix
    - Autologous option: Fascia (usually tensor fascia lata) and fat (abdominal or left inguinal)
  - Silastic sheeting for coverage of mucosal donor sites and exposed bone
  - Gelfoam dissolvable packing, which helps to support and hold the graft or flap in place
  - Surgiflo gelatin hemostatic matrix NasoPore dissolvable packing, which is more easily removed postoperatively
  - Foley balloon catheter (16 g, 30 mL) for support of dissolvable dressings

PEARLS AND POTENTIAL PITFALLS

- Raising any pedicled flap should occur early in the procedure. This helps to ensure that the vascular supply to the flap remains intact and provides for a speedy reconstruction once the lesion has been removed.
- Any pedicled mucosal flap used should be "oversized" for the defect concerned, as flap length is lost in contouring the flap to the skull base defect. More length is needed for a defect involving skull base angles, and many nasal flaps may need to be raised

as far anteriorly as the mucocutaneous junction. Additionally, making sure that the pedicle is raised will allow for more mobility and greater coverage.

- There are only three versions of NSF harvest currently in use (Fig. 31.3). If the defect is sella and planum only, the flap is raised to the level of the middle turbinate head. The posterior septum and contralateral mucosa are sacrificed. If further coverage of ethmoid, clivus, or rostral skull base is required, the full mucoperiosteum is removed and the contralateral mucosa is brought forward to cover the ipsilateral septal donor site.[37] If more surface area is required, the nasal floor is included in the flap.

- The flap pedicle may itself cause functional problems in the nose, and it may be necessary to skeletonize the pedicle fully to ensure minimal mucosal trapping postoperatively. If problems still occur, it may be possible to divide the pedicle, although this is inadvisable less than 6 months after the repair has taken place.

- Constant awareness of the location of the flap must be maintained throughout the procedure to avoid injury to the vascular pedicle. The flap should be stored in the ipsilateral maxillary sinus or nasopharynx for protection during the resection. Gelfoam may be placed on the exposed periosteum of the pedicle as further protection. If suctioning is required during the placement of the grafts, the use of a neurosurgical patty will avoid displacement of the grafts.

- Special intracranial extradural layers are unnecessary and add nothing to the security of the repair. Underlay materials in a multilayer reconstruction are subdural. This forms the water-tight "bath plug" layer, and the mucosal flap is an onlay flap to provide vascularization[14,38] (Fig. 31.4).

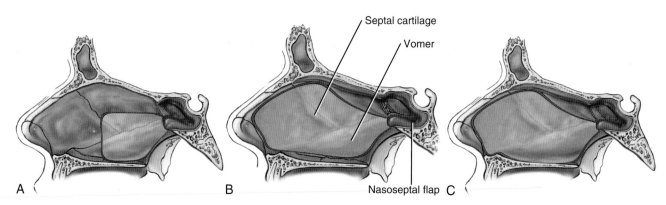

Fig. 31.3. Diagram of septal flap sizes showing basic flap **(A)**, anterior extension **(B)**, and lateral extension **(C)**.

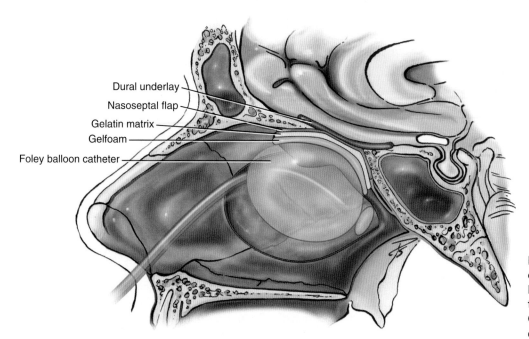

Fig. 31.4. Note the layers of the reconstruction: Dural underlay, nasoseptal flap, gelatin matrix, Gelfoam, Foley balloon catheter.

- Avoid burying functional mucosa under any graft or flap to prevent mucocele formation.
- If the vascularized flap does not cover the entire defect, free mucosal grafts can be used to supplement coverage. It is important to place the vascularized graft at the site that is most likely to leak, such as the most dependent aspect, and the center of the defect where there is no vascular supply.
- Tight packing at the end of the procedure should be avoided to maintain the vascular supply to any pedicled graft.
- When placing the Foley catheter, it is important to recognize that its role is to support and stabilize the absorbable packing rather than to hold up the grafts. Therefore, do not overfill the balloon, as this may inadvertently cause a CSF leak by displacing the grafts intracranially.
- Securing the Foley catheter is an important step in the operation. It must be secure enough that it will not become displaced posteriorly and cause inadvertent airway obstruction. However, it is imperative to not secure it in a manner that puts pressure on the nasal ala, which will lead to necrosis and subsequent notching.
- The routine use of perioperative lumbar drains is not supported and may cause unnecessary morbidity.[39–41] CSF diversion may be considered in selected instances, such as when there is suspected or known intracranial hypertension or in the management of small, early postoperative CSF leaks.[42]

SURGICAL PROCEDURE

- Preoperatively, decide on the preferred flap design to be used for repair of the skull base defect.

- A mixture of 1% ropivacaine with 1:100,000 epinephrine is infiltrated into the area in which the flap will be raised. Topical 1:2000 epinephrine is used for hemostasis throughout the case.

Local Flaps

Posterior Nasoseptal Flap

- After initial approach work, nasal cavity preparation, it is advisable to create a wide ipsilateral maxillary antrum for storage and protection of the flap.
- Define the ipsilateral sphenoid ostium without dissecting too far inferiorly, as this may compromise the vascular pedicle. Also, avoid an initial posterior septectomy if there is a possible need for a septal flap.
- Three possible nasoseptal flap sizes are defined (see Fig. 31.3).

Step 1: Defining the Flap

- The flap is raised unilaterally using a 0-degree nasal endoscope. Use a needle-tip monopolar electrocautery on coagulation mode and setting of 12 to make the mucosal incisions. The boundaries of the flap will vary depending on the design used.
- Starting above the tail of the inferior turbinate, incise the mucosa along the arch of the superior choanae to the posterior free border of the nasal septum (Fig. 31.5A). Turn toward the floor of the nose and move laterally until the desired width is achieved. If the posteroinferior aspect is to remain in place, leave an approximately 1-cm strut of mucosa to help maintain support. Also, make sure to locate the hard palate–soft palate junction so that the

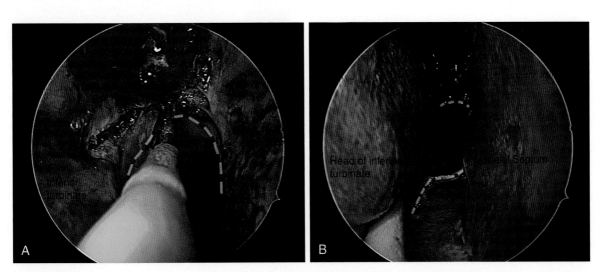

Fig. 31.5. (A) Endoscopic view of the mucosal cut over the superior rim of the choana *(dashed line)*. The cut starts laterally above the tail of the inferior turbinate and below the posterior, horizontal component of the middle turbinate, which has already been resected *(asterisk)*. **(B)** The incision *(dashed line)* is carried anteriorly along the nasal floor until the appropriate length is achieved. The nasopharynx is seen posteriorly *(asterisk)*.

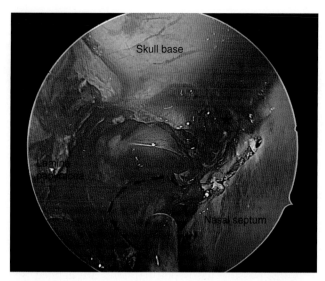

Fig. 31.6. Endoscopic view of the superior mucosal incision, which starts at about the level of the superior aspect of the sphenoid ostium, which has been opened in this case *(dashed line)*. The cut edge of the middle turbinate is seen where it attaches to the skull base *(asterisk)*.

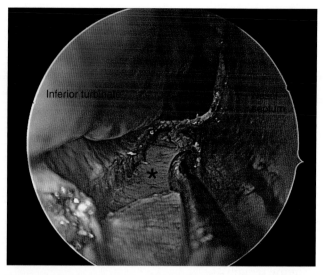

Fig. 31.7. Endoscopic view of initially freeing the septal flap from the nasal floor *(asterisk)* in a subperiosteal plane with a Cottle elevator.

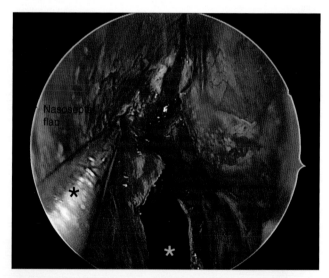

Fig. 31.8. Endoscopic view of raising the nasoseptal flap with a Cottle elevator *(asterisk)*. Leaving it attached superiorly allows for easy dissection to the face of the sphenoid *(dashed line)*. The nasopharynx is seen through the posterior mucosal incision *(white asterisk)*.

soft palate is not injured. Then, cut along the floor from posterior to anterior until the desired length is achieved (Fig. 31.5B). It is critical that the cuts are made down to the bone; otherwise, flap elevation will be significantly more challenging.

- Make the superior mucosal incision starting at the level of the superior aspect of the sphenoid ostium/ superior septal edge and, again, work from posterior to anterior (Fig. 31.6). It is best to leave approximately 1 to 2 cm of superior septum intact to avoid damaging the olfactory fibers if only a sella/planum defect is expected. This is not of concern if a transethmoid resection is required, as olfactory loss will occur as part of the approach. If a more limited flap is needed, take care not to cut through both mucosal layers of the septum. This is easy to do along the superior cut as the bone of the nasal septum is often thin here.
- Mark out the anterior border and connect to the superior and inferior borders. This anterior border is either at the head of the middle turbinate for sella/ planum defects or at the squamomucosal junction if clival, ethmoidal, or frontal reconstruction is required (see Fig. 31.3)

Step 2: Raising the Flap

- Raise the flap using blunt dissecting instruments, such as a Cottle elevator, over a wide area to reduce the risk of tearing the flap. As you work posteriorly, it will be necessary to disconnect the flap inferiorly from the surrounding tissue but leave it attached superiorly (Fig. 31.7). The flap is then raised off the

septum in a subperichondrial/subperiosteal plane, as would be done in an endoscopic septoplasty. Leaving it suspended from the superior septum makes it easier to work with.

- When the flap's pedicle at the superior choana is reached, make sure that elevation continues laterally so that the flap is fully disconnected from the superior rim of the choana (Fig. 31.8). Failure to do this will reduce the extension and maneuverability of the flap and will make it more difficult to protect the flap's pedicle.

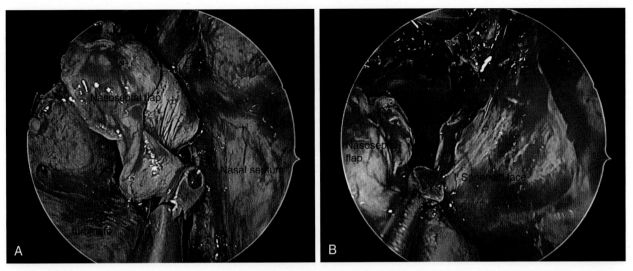

Fig. 31.9. (A) Endoscopic view of the nasoseptal flap being placed into the nasopharynx. **(B)** A Cottle elevator is useful to further elevate the pedicle of the flap laterally over the choana.

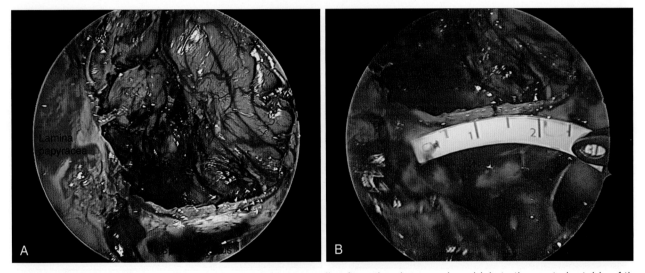

Fig. 31.10. (A) Endoscopic view of the skull base defect extending from the planum sphenoidale to the posterior table of the frontal sinus. **(B)** A cut-down, sterile ruler is useful to accurately measure the defect.

Step 3: Storing the Flap

- Once the flap is fully disconnected inferiorly, anteriorly, and elevated throughout its width and length, disconnect it superiorly and carefully place it in its storage position during the resection (Fig. 31.9A). If necessary, further disconnect the pedicle from the superior rim of the choana and increase the size of the maxillary antrum to enable safe storage (Fig. 31.9B).
- A posterior septectomy can now be performed if required. Throughout the tumor resection, be aware of the location of the flap and protect its pedicle.

Step 4: Reconstruction of Dural Defect

- Once resection is complete, ensure complete visibility of the skull base defect. Remove the nasal mucosa from the bone at the edges of the defect to ensure good apposition of the vascularized flap to that bone and to prevent any functional mucosa from being trapped underneath. This can be done with a Freer elevator or Coblation device.
- Reconstruct the skull base defect in layers. A layer of DuraGen is used as a subdural underlay. If the procedure is combined with an external skull base approach, the graft can be placed from above and adjusted endoscopically. More than one layer of DuraGen can be used if appropriate.
- The underlay layer should be roughly sized to the defect, with an extra 2- to 3-cm border all around to allow for sufficient overlap with the dura and shrinkage (Fig. 31.10).
- If the defect extends anteriorly where the falx cerebri will impede underlay placement, cut "trouser legs" in

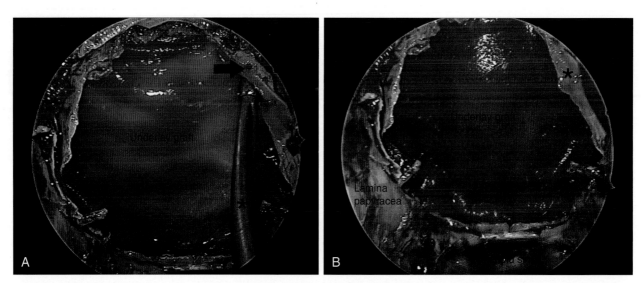

Fig. 31.11. (A) Endoscopic view of a disconnected olive-tip suction *(asterisk)* being used to place the Duragen subdurally *(arrow)*. **(B)** The underlay should completely cover the defect with sufficient overlap with the dura *(asterisk)*.

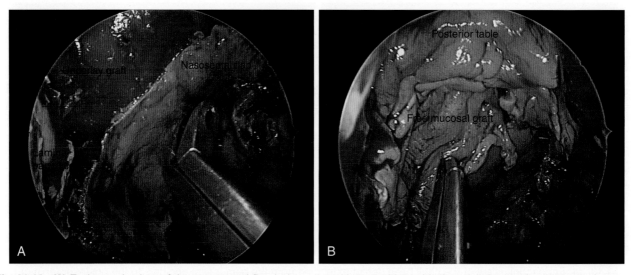

Fig. 31.12. (A) Endoscopic view of the nasoseptal flap being rotated into position with the pedicle attached laterally *(asterisk)*. It is important to place it in the center of the defect to provide vascularization to this area. **(B)** Free mucosal grafts are used to supplement the nasoseptal flap if needed. The medial orbital walls are seen in this view *(asterisks)*.

the DuraGen to straddle the falx. The underlay graft should be carefully manipulated into position using small straight Blakesley forceps and then the edges gently tucked under the exposed skull base edges using an olive-tip suction (disconnected) so that the matrix completely covers the defect (Fig. 31.11).

Step 5: Positioning of Intranasal Flap

- The pedicled mucosal flap should then be retrieved from its storage location and opened out to remove any folds. It should be roughly oriented and turned so that the mucosal side faces into the nasal cavity.
- Once the center of the flap is positioned, work outward and adjust the edges so that the defect is cov-

ered (Fig. 31.12A). Free mucosal grafts can be used at the periphery of the defect if necessary (Fig. 31.12B).
- Ensure that the pedicle is well contoured to the walls of the nasal cavity and skull base. It may be necessary to remove some bone to achieve this.
- Cover the mucosal flap and its edges with small pieces of dissolvable dressing or a gelatin matrix (Fig. 31.13A). Begin at the proximal/lowest aspect of the flap to avoid accidental repositioning.
- NasoPore is used as an additional layer below the gelatin matrix (Fig. 31.13B). This is done largely because NasoPore is easy to remove in the clinic at the first follow-up appointment. Dural sealants are not necessary for the reconstruction.[43]

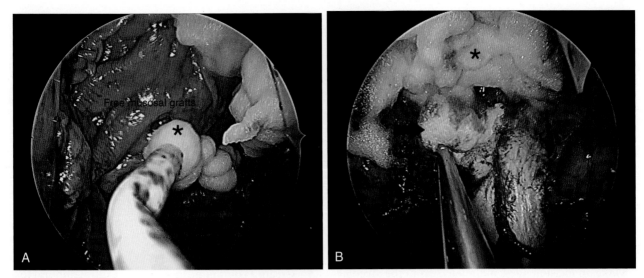

Fig. 31.13. (A) Endoscopic view of a gelatin matrix *(asterisk)* being applied to the reconstructed skull base. **(B)** NasoPore *(arrow)* is placed below the gelatin matrix *(asterisk)* to provide support. (©2017 Stryker. Used with the permission of Stryker.)

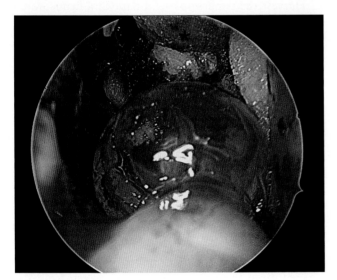

Fig. 31.14. Endoscopic view of a 30-mL Foley balloon catheter being filled below the nasal dressings *(asterisk)*.

- Cover the septal donor site with 0.5-mm Silastic sheeting to aid remucosalization. The Silastic should be left in place for at least 3 weeks.
- Under endoscopic visualization, place a 30-mL Foley catheter into the nasal cavity and fill it with sterile saline until the desired support is achieved (Fig. 31.14). Secure the catheter to the patient's forehead with tape, making sure that there is no retraction or pressure on the alar rim.

Inferior Turbinate Flap
- Create a large maxillary antrostomy for flap storage.
- Incise the superior border of the flap down to bone, from the junction of the vertical palatine bone and posteromedial maxilla horizontally forward to the head of the inferior turbinate at the pyriform aperture.
- Carefully dissect out the mucosa from the inferior turbinate bone underlying it and continue the dissection inferiorly and eventually superiorly to the lateral side of the inferior turbinate bone. Do this in a subperiosteal plane to preserve the underlying pedicled blood supply.
- Continue superiorly to the apex of the inferior meatus and incise and free the mucosa at this point to avoid damage to the lacrimal duct. This will create a narrowing at this point in the flap.
- Further anterior to this, the freeing incision can be more lateral to increase the width of the flap.
- Placement of the flap and multilayered reconstruction should proceed as for the posterior septal flap.

Middle Turbinate Flap
- Before starting, study the imaging to ensure that the flap has adequate dimensions to achieve the desired coverage. The middle turbinate needs to be longer than 4 cm for the flap to reach the sella. Beware of anatomic variations of the middle turbinate, such as a concha bullosa or hypoplasia, which may make dissection more challenging.
- Make a vertical incision at the head of the middle turbinate.
- Make a horizontal incision at the superior medial aspect of the middle turbinate below where it attaches to the lateral lamella of the cribriform plate. There is a danger of CSF leakage if this incision is made too high.
- Elevate the medial and lateral middle turbinate mucosa from the underlying bone in a subperiosteal plane using sharp dissecting instruments.

- Remove the middle turbinate bone piecemeal using through-cutting forceps.
- Incise the mucosa in the axilla of the middle turbinate to detach the lateral mucosa from the wall of the nose. Again, make sure that the incision is placed below the cribriform plate.
- Continue this incision inferiorly and posteriorly to completely free the lateral mucosa.
- The flap should then be unfolded like a book.
- Further careful dissection of the pedicle back to the sphenopalatine foramen will increase the flap length achievable.
- Placement of the flap and multilayered reconstruction should proceed as for the posterior septal flap.

Palatal Floor Flap

- Make an incision a few millimeters from the alveolar ridge anteriorly, extending posteriorly bilaterally to the posterior limit of the hard palate on the oral cavity side.
- Raise the mucoperiosteum over the area, to include the greater palatine neurovascular bundle on one side.
- Enlarge the greater palatine foramen with a drill or Kerrison rongeurs.
- Perform a wide maxillary antrostomy and remove the posterior wall of the maxillary sinus to expose the junction between the sphenopalatine and descending palatine arteries within the pterygopalatine fossa.
- Make a horizontal incision 3 cm posterior to the pyriform aperture and elevate a nasal floor flap to expose the bony pterygopalatine canal. This will enable the descending palatine artery to be released from the canal.
- Pass the freed flap into the nasal cavity to cover the defect.
- Multilayered reconstruction should proceed as for the nasoseptal flap.

Regional Flaps

Pericranial Flap

- Make a bicoronal incision and dissect anteriorly to the supraorbital rim in a subgaleal plane. Then, incise the pericranium down to the underlying calvarium. This incision should be staggered with relation to the coronal incision and it is important to ensure that the flap will be long enough to cover the defect. Elevation of the pericranium to the supraorbital rim can be accomplished with periosteal elevators, Kittners, or with a Ray-Tec sponge. Take care to preserve the supratrochlear and supraorbital arteries. Alternatively, this can be accomplished through a minimally invasive approach.[44]

- Perform a MELP to enlarge the corridor for flap transport and ensure effective functioning of the frontal sinuses.
- Make a bony window through the nasion to enable transport of the flap to the nasal cavity.
- Multilayered reconstruction should proceed as for the posterior septal flap.

Temporoparietal Flap

- Make a large maxillary antrostomy to identify the sphenopalatine artery and the posterior nasal artery.
- Ligate the arteries and dissect them proximally into the pterygopalatine fossa while removing the posterior wall of the maxillary sinus. This maneuverer is often part of the resection or has been previously performed if this option is being considered.
- Create a communication with the infratemporal fossa and remove the anterior aspect of the pterygoid plates to enlarge the tunnel.
- Harvest the temporoparietal flap via a hemicoronal incision by elevating the temporal fascia from the underlying muscle, and separate the temporalis muscle from the lateral orbital wall and the pterygomaxillary fissure.
- Pass a percutaneous tracheostomy cannula over the zygomatic arch and into the infratemporal fossa.
- The resultant tunnel through the infratemporal fossa can be used to transport the temporoparietal flap to the defect.
- Multilayered reconstruction should proceed as for the posterior septal flap.

Free Grafts

- Free grafts should be used for small defects (<1 cm) in low-flow areas where radiotherapy will not be applied and minimal arachnoid disruption has occurred.
- Free mucosal grafts are commonly taken from the inferior turbinate, nasal floor, or remnants from a septectomy.
- Use autologous material where possible for free grafting to the skull base. A variety of materials are commonly used.
- Fascia lata is easily available, and large grafts can be obtained. Also, it has similar characteristics to dura. Comparatively, temporalis fascia is thinner and weaker. These free grafts are best used as adjuncts alongside vascularized flaps rather than as alternatives to them.
- Other materials may be used for free grafting but have certain disadvantages: bone is quickly resorbed, fat is only suitable for small defects, and allografts are associated with higher rates of infection.
- After placement of the free graft material, multilayered reconstruction should proceed as for the posterior septal flap.

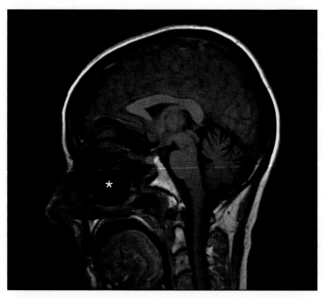

Fig. 31.15. Postoperative T1-weighted MRI scan in the sagittal plane demonstrating the position of the Foley balloon catheter *(white asterisk)*. Note that it is not exerting any direct pressure on the flaps or grafts, but rather it is supporting the dissolvable dressing.

POSTOPERATIVE CONSIDERATIONS

- Use of a Foley balloon catheter in the postnasal space is common practice; these balloons are usually left in place for 2 to 5 days.[7] However, it is unlikely that they provide any actual compressive sealing for the graft. More likely, their role is in protecting the area from any pressure changes that may influence healing and maintaining the dissolvable packing in place for the first 24 to 48 hours (Fig. 31.15).
- Imaging can be performed on the first postoperative day to check for hemorrhage, migration of the flap, and the presence of dead space. An MRI without flap contrast enhancement suggests ischemia and may indicate the need for reexploration.[45] It is also important to note that flap enhancement does not predict or preclude a future CSF leak.[46] Pneumocephalus is normal at this stage.
- The patient should convalesce in a 30-degree head-up position, with 48 hours of bed rest and toilet

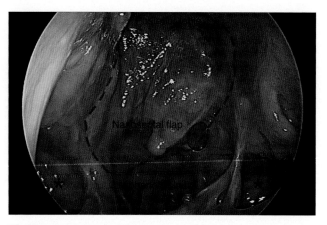

Fig. 31.16. Endoscopic view of a well-healed skull base reconstruction. The approximate outline of the nasoseptal flap *(dashed line)* can be seen extending from the planum sphenoidale posteriorly to cover much of the posterior table of the frontal sinus anteriorly. The maxillary sinuses are also seen in this view *(asterisks)*.

privileges. The patient must be instructed to avoid straining, Valsalva maneuvers, and nose blowing.
- There is no consensus on perioperative antibiotics in skull base surgery. However, it is reasonable to use a third-generation cephalosporin (ceftriaxone), preoperatively and throughout the hospital stay. Patients are then sent home on a 10-day course of amoxicillin/clavulanic acid. Postoperative antibiotics are not prescribed to prevent meningitis but rather to decrease the bacterial burden resulting from the significant sinonasal dysfunction following endoscopic skull base surgery. It is our opinion that this does not violate good antibiotic stewardship.
- Simple nasal saline sprays and 2% mupirocin ointment (water-soluble version) is used in the first 7 days. After this, a large-volume saline squeeze bottle is used in the first few weeks after surgery to optimize healing (Fig. 31.16).

REFERENCES

Access the reference list online at ExpertConsult.com.

Combined Endoscopic and Open Approaches—Frontal Sinus

Frontal Sinus Trephination

Alfred Marc C. Iloreta, Nithin D. Adappa, and Satish Govindaraj

INTRODUCTION

- Modern trephination of the frontal sinus was first described in 1884 by Ogston.[1]
- Since the 1980s, endoscopic sinus surgery has been considered the standard of care for the initial surgical management of frontal sinus disease, except in select cases.[2]
- Despite endoscopic advancements in the field, frontal trephination is an essential part of a sinus surgeon's armamentarium.
- Trephination provides the surgeon with an additional port for dissection, a means of rapid decompression of the frontal sinus via an intersinus septectomy, or resection of tumors that cannot be completely addressed through an endoscopic approach.
- There are a number of indications for frontal trephination alone or in conjunction with an endoscopic procedure.

ANATOMY

- The frontal sinus is a pyramidal structure that resides in the anterior cranial vault and is enveloped by two layers of cortical bone: a thick anterior table and a thinner posterior table.
- The anterior wall of the frontal sinus begins at the nasofrontal suture line and ends below the frontal bone protuberance.
- The anterior wall ranges from 4 to 12 mm in thickness. From superficial to deep, it is covered by layers of skin, subcutaneous fat, the frontalis muscle, and the pericranium.
- The frontal sinus has two extensions:
  - Superior into the squamous portion of the frontal bone
  - Posterior into the orbital part of the frontal bone between the inferior surface of the frontal lobe and the orbital contents

- The intersinus septum is a triangular bony structure that separates the frontal sinus into two independently draining cavities. It can vary in its position so that the frontal sinus cavities may be asymmetric.
- The frontal sinus is lined by a mucosa of pseudostratified ciliated columnar epithelium.
- The frontal recess is part of the frontal sinus outflow tract.
  - The outflow tract has an hourglass shape. The frontal recess is defined as the narrowest part of the tract and is the most inferior aspect of the frontal sinus.
  - The frontal recess is bounded by the following structures:
    - Superior lamina papyracea laterally
    - Vertical lamella of the middle turbinate medially
    - Nasofrontal bone anterosuperiorly
    - Agger nasi cell anteroinferiorly
    - Skull base posteriorly
- The supraorbital and supratrochlear nerves innervate the soft tissue anterior to the frontal sinus and nearby areas.
  - Supraorbital nerve (Fig. 32.1)
    - Branch of the ophthalmic nerve (V1)
    - Passes through the supraorbital foramen (located just above the upper rim of the orbit at the junction of its medial and lateral two-thirds), courses deep to the corrugator muscle, then penetrates superiorly through the frontalis muscle
    - Travels in the dense subcutaneous tissue of the scalp
    - Supplies sensation to the skin of the forehead and upper eyelid
    - Gives a branch to the frontal sinus via the opening for the frontal diploic veins

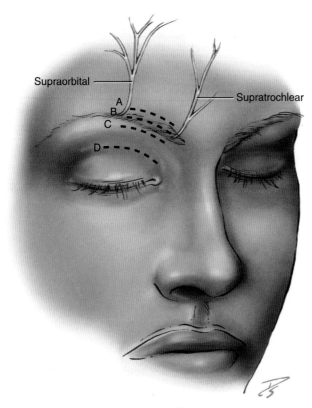

Fig. 32.1. Drawing showing three different incisions that can be made with respect to the brow. **(A)** Suprabrow incision. **(B)** Intrabrow incision. **(C)** Infrabrow incision. **(D)** Upper eyelid crease incision. The supratrochlear and supraorbital neurovascular bundles lie at the medial and lateral limits of the incision. *n.,* Nerve.

  – Supratrochlear nerve (see Fig. 32.1)
    – Passes superior to the trochlea of the superior oblique muscle and exits medially to the supraorbital foramen and passes around the superior orbital rim, deep to the frontalis muscle
    – Penetrates the orbital septum with the supratrochlear artery
    – Penetrates through the body of the corrugator muscle
    – Innervates the skin and conjunctiva of the upper eyelid and the skin of the lower medial forehead

PREOPERATIVE CONSIDERATIONS

■ Frontal sinus trephination is ideal in cases in which a purely endoscopic approach is not feasible and an open osteoplastic flap procedure is too aggressive.

■ If there is any doubt as to whether the frontal sinus can be accessed endoscopically, consent for a trephine procedure should be obtained before surgery.

■ The overall medical condition of the patient should be taken into consideration, since trephination and frontal sinus drainage can often be done faster than

an endoscopic procedure requiring excessive drilling of the frontal recess.

■ Traditionally, the indication for frontal sinus trephination has been acute frontal sinusitis that is refractory to appropriate medical management. This procedure allows immediate drainage and culture of infected material and provides a portal for irrigation of the frontal sinus with catheters or drains.

■ Frontal sinus infection can be addressed acutely through a trephination. Then, once the infection and inflammation have resolved, a staged endoscopic surgery can be performed if frontal recess obstruction persists.[3]

■ Complications of sinusitis—including orbital abscess, intracranial extension, mucopyocele, and Pott puffy tumor—may be avoided with early trephination.[4]

Indications for Trephination

■ Indications for trephination with or without endoscopic frontal sinusotomy include the following:
  – Acute frontal sinusitis with no extrasinus spread not amenable to endoscopic frontal sinusotomy
  – Acute frontal sinusitis with intraorbital or intracranial extension[3]
  – Cerebrospinal fluid leak or encephalocele
  – Frontal osteomyelitis (Pott puffy tumor)
  – Frontal sinus mucopurulence requiring intersinus septectomy for acute decompression
  – Laterally based frontal sinus lesions (e.g., mucocele, inflammatory polyps)
  – Obstruction of the frontal recess secondary to neo-osteogenesis
  – Benign fibro-osseous tumors requiring resection (e.g., osteoma, fibrous dysplasia, soft tissue tumors such as inverted papilloma)
  – Type II, III, or IV frontal cells requiring resection and inaccessible with an endoscopic frontal sinusotomy
  – Rarely: posterior table fracture, meningioma[5]

■ Frontal sinus trephination may also be performed as an adjunct to endoscopic frontal sinusotomy, with the trephination used to irrigate through the frontal sinus to allow identification of the recess from below.

Radiographic Considerations

■ Obtain a computed tomography (CT) scan of the paranasal sinuses before the procedure.

■ During preoperative analysis of the CT, perform a systematic review of the images with attention to the following anatomic features[3,6]:
  – Height and depth (anterior to posterior distance) of the frontal sinus. On average, male patients have deeper frontal sinuses.[7]

TABLE 32.1 Advantages and Disadvantages of Four External Incision Lines

Incision	Scar	Risk of Brow Alopecia	Risk of V1 Numbness	Risk of Infection
Suprabrow	Visible	No	High	Yes
Intrabrow	Not visible	Yes	Low	No
Infrabrow	Not visible	No	Low	No
Upper eyelid crease	Not visible	No	Low	No

- Dehiscence of the superior orbital roof
- Dehiscence of the anterior or posterior table of the frontal sinus
- Presence of frontal sinus cells
- Thickness of the nasofrontal bone
- Thickness of the nasofrontal floor (average is 4 mm)

INSTRUMENTATION

- 0-, 30-, and 70-degree endoscopes
- No. 15 scalpel blade
- Self-retaining retractor or Senn retractors
- Two-pronged skin hook
- Bipolar cautery or Colorado-tip Bovie
- Periosteal elevator or Freer elevator
- 4-mm round cutting bur
- Fine suction device
- Pediatric Kerrison rongeur
- 8F red rubber catheter (if needed)

PEARLS AND POTENTIAL PITFALLS

- The depth of the frontal sinus at several points medial to lateral should be determined before surgery. Some frontal sinuses will not be sufficiently deep to accommodate standard trephine instruments.[7]
- The incision, although described at the medial infrabrow, can be tailored to the location of the lesion.
- An image guidance probe can aid in planning the location of the incision.
- The bone should be saucerized while drilling to avoid sudden entry into the frontal sinus.
- An acutely infected sinus should not be entered through the anterior table to avoid the spread of infection and secondary osteomyelitis.
- The opening should be enlarged only to the size needed.
- A drain or irrigation catheter should be placed in an acutely infected sinus.

SURGICAL PROCEDURE

- Frontal trephination is best performed with the patient under general anesthesia, although in certain situations (e.g., in patients with significant comor-

bidities), it can be done using local anesthesia and intravenous sedation.
- Drape and prepare the patient as is usually done for an endoscopic sinus procedure, with exposure of the entire facial region including the forehead.
- If an image guidance system is being used that requires a guidance headset or headband, place it sufficiently above the eyebrow to allow adequate space for surgical access.
- Image guidance can assist in determining the ideal location for entry into the frontal sinus.

Step 1: Incision

- In general, four different external incision lines have been used: within the eyebrow, below the eyebrow, above the eyebrow, and the upper eyelid crease (see Fig. 32.1). Each approach has certain advantages and disadvantages in terms of the resultant scar, adequacy of drainage, endoscopic assessment, safety of trephination, potential for nerve or vessel injury, and risk of complicating bone infection (Table 32.1).
- The most common approach is the infrabrow incision located at the superomedial aspect of the orbit, immediately below the eyebrow and supraorbital rim, and medial to the supraorbital neurovascular bundle.
- If the entry point is too inferior and medial, the frontal recess may be compromised by scar tissue formation. The ideal point of entry is at the medial floor of the frontal sinus.
- After sterile preparation of the surgical field has been completed, infiltrate lidocaine HCL 1% and epinephrine 1:100,000 injection at the planned incision site. Make the skin incision no longer than 1 to 2 cm, terminating at the medial brow. If the incision is carried medial to the brow margin, a visible scar may result.
- Make the incision with a No. 15 blade. Minimal bleeding will be encountered if an adequate injection is administered before incision. If necessary, use a guarded bipolar cautery in the deeper soft tissue to achieve hemostasis.
- After completion of the skin incision, place a small self-retaining retractor into the incision or, if assistants are available, use small Senn retractors.

- Carry the incision through the periosteum with a No. 15 blade or needle-point Bovie. A blade is preferable so that adequate edges of the periosteum are present for closure.
- Once in the deeper tissues, unipolar or bipolar cautery is permissible to achieve hemostasis. Take care to avoid contact with the retractors and to use guarded cautery devices to prevent thermal injury to the skin.
- The approach through the upper eyelid (blepharoplasty incision) to reach the frontal sinus involves a slightly different dissection[10,11]:
  - Incise the natural upper eyelid skin crease and extend the incision towards the medial and lateral orbital rims.
  - Bluntly dissect parallel to the layers of the orbicularis oculi to identify the preseptal plane above the levator palpebrae. Carry the dissection medial towards the trochlea, lateral to the lacrimal fossa, and superior towards the orbital rim to expose the arcus marginalis.
  - Identify the supraorbital and supratrochlear neurovascular bundles and retract them out of the surgical field to ensure preservation.
  - Once the orbital rim is identified, incise the periosteum parallel to the bony rim.

Step 2: Exposure of Bone

- Once the incision has been made through the periosteum, use a Freer or periosteal elevator to raise the periosteum superiorly and inferiorly until an approximately 1 × 1 cm area of bone is exposed. A wider area can be elevated if the procedure will require the introduction of an endoscope and instruments, such as for tumor removal or encephalocele repair.
- Once bone is exposed, mark the exact point of frontal sinus penetration. The use of image guidance can help confirm the widest and safest point of entry. It is important to penetrate in or near the floor of the frontal sinus, not in the anterior wall.
- The anterior wall contains vertical diploic bone, and entry through the anterior wall is not recommended if the sinus is infected to avoid potential intracranial spread of infection or frontal bone osteomyelitis.

Step 3: Drilling of the Trephination

- Choose a 4-mm round cutting bur to perform the external trephination. The average bone thickness is 4 mm, and the thickness can be measured on the preoperative CT scan as well to estimate the amount of drilling that will be necessary.
- Enter the sinus in a controlled fashion by slowly moving the drill in a circular motion as in saucerizing a mastoid cavity. The goal is to open an anterior window that is approximately 6 to 8 mm with saucerized edges.

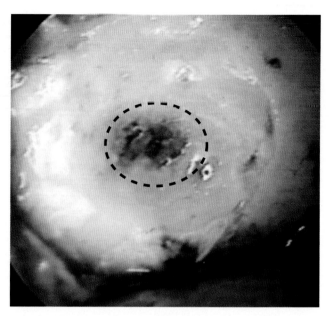

Fig. 32.2. Endoscopic view of the final layer of bone encountered after wide saucerization with a 4-mm round cutting bur. Note the blue hue *(circled)* representing the thin underlying sinus mucosa. At this point, a small curette or image guidance probe can be used to enter the sinus in a safe and controlled manner.

- As the sinus mucosa is approached, a blue hue will be seen through the final layer of bone (Fig. 32.2).
- At this point, use a small curette or image guidance probe to enter the sinus and remove the final layer of bone. This provides a controlled entry into the sinus and tactile feedback to the surgeon. This is critical in the patient with a shallow frontal sinus (small anterior-posterior dimension).
- If the sinus is to be instrumented, enlarge the window with a 2-mm Kerrison rongeur (Fig. 32.3). A bony opening ranging from 5 to 15 mm in diameter is sufficient to accommodate an endoscope and/or instruments (Fig. 32.4).
- Through the trephination, perform dissection and instrumentation based on the indication for the procedure.
- For acute inflammatory disease, the sinus can be irrigated if there is no orbital or skull base dehiscence.
- For chronic inflammatory disease, the sinus can be irrigated with dilute fluorescein or methylene blue to identify the frontal sinus drainage pathway endoscopically.
- Use an endoscope and instruments to remove frontal cells.
- The frontal trephination can be combined with an endoscopic frontal sinusotomy using an above-and-below technique (Fig. 32.5).[12]

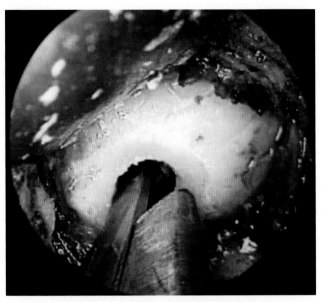

Fig. 32.3. Endoscopic image showing use of a pediatric Kerrison rongeur to widen the opening to an aperture between 5 and 15 mm in diameter.

Step 4: Placement of Drains and Closure

- Red rubber catheters (8F is an ideal size) or silicone tubing can be placed to provide a portal for external irrigation. Sew these catheters in place with a silk or nylon suture to prevent inadvertent removal (Fig. 32.6). Leave external irrigating drains in place for approximately 3 to 5 days.
- When using an upper eyelid approach, a rubber band drain can be used rather than a red rubber catheter. The rubber band drain should be placed laterally.
- Close the skin incision if no drain is to be placed. Use 4-0 polyglactin 910 (Vicryl) suture in an interrupted fashion to reapproximate the periosteum. Close the skin with nonresorbable suture. Use of 5-0 nylon interrupted sutures is recommended. Sutures are removed in 5 to 7 days. Topical antibiotic ointment is applied twice a day until suture removal. No dressing is needed.

POSTOPERATIVE CONSIDERATIONS

- The potential complications of trephination include facial scarring, facial or periorbital cellulitis, paresthesias of the forehead and vertex secondary to trauma to the supraorbital or supratrochlear nerve, eyebrow alopecia, and, rarely, cerebrospinal fluid leak.

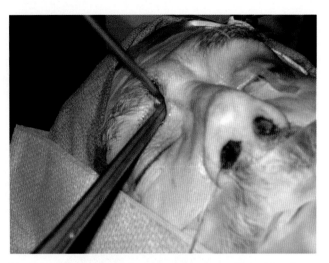

Fig. 32.4. Photograph showing exposure sufficient to allow for placement of endoscopes and/or instruments.

- One potential issue that should be discussed with patients is the potential for trephination failure in the setting of inflammatory disease. In comparison with an osteoplastic flap procedure with or without obliteration, frontal sinus trephination as a definitive procedure has a failure rate as high as 57%.[8]

CONCLUSION

- Frontal sinus trephination is an external approach to the frontal sinus that, despite the advancements in endoscopic techniques, still has a role in the management of frontal sinus disease.
- It is often combined with an endoscopic approach to address inflammatory disease, tumors, and cerebrospinal fluid leaks of the frontal sinus not amenable to a purely endonasal procedure.
- Cosmetic sequelae are minimal, and complications are uncommon.

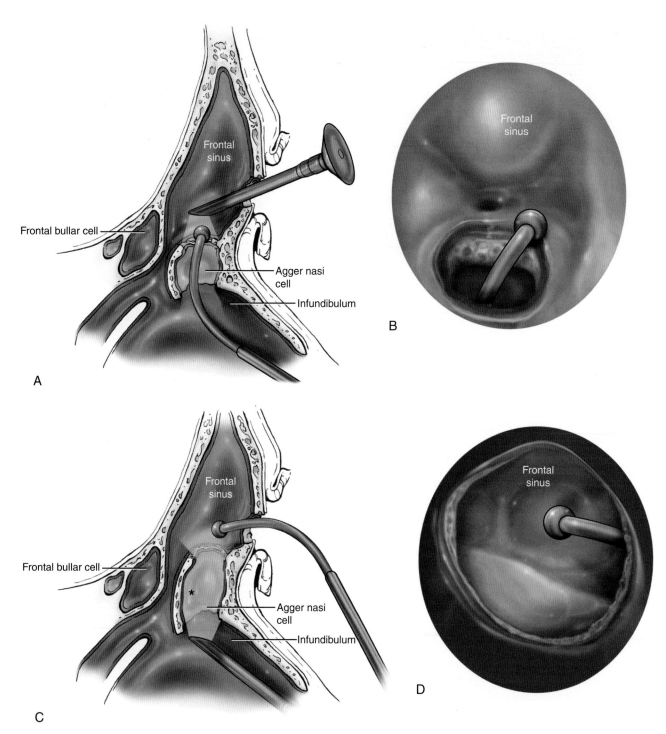

Fig. 32.5. Artist's depiction of the above-and-below technique. **(A, B)** A ball-tip probe is seen at the frontal sinus ostium using a 30-degree endoscope placed through the trephination site. **(C, D)** The trephination port can also be used for instrumentation with the endoscope placed to illuminate the frontal recess from below. This is most often done when a trephination is used to assist in the endoscopic removal of type 3 *(asterisk)* or type 4 frontal recess cells.[13]

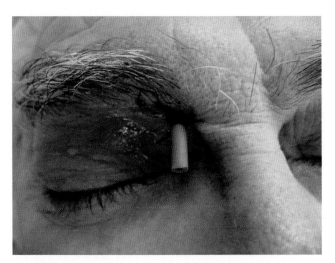

Fig. 32.6. Photograph of an 8F red rubber catheter used for irrigation of the sinus. These drains should be carefully secured in place using silk or nylon sutures. Drains can remain in place for approximately 3 to 5 days.

REFERENCES

Access the reference list online at ExpertConsult.com.

Osteoplastic Flaps With and Without Obliteration

Elisabeth H. Ference and Kevin C. Welch

INTRODUCTION

- The osteoplastic flap with obliteration of the frontal sinus was considered the mainstay of surgical management of the frontal sinus in the 1950s and 1960s.[1]
- The osteoplastic approach to the frontal sinus was first described in 1894 by Schonborn[2] and later modified through the earlier parts of the twentieth century.
- Modern concepts of the osteoplastic approach to the frontal sinus stem from the studies of MacBeth[3] as well as Goodale and Montgomery[4,5] several years later.
- The open approach is now reserved for circumstances in which the endoscopic approach is insufficient or impractical to treat frontal sinus disease.[6]
- Decision making in these cases is still challenging: whether to obliterate, choice of obliteration material, and treatment of the frontal sinus.

ANATOMY

- The mnemonic *SCALP* indicates the layers of the scalp: *S*, skin; *C*, subcutaneous tissue; *A*, aponeurosis and muscle; *L*, loose areolar tissue; *P*, pericranium (periosteum; Fig. 33.1).
- The galea consists of the aponeurosis between the frontalis and occipitalis muscles and is contiguous with the temporoparietal fascia, as well as the superficial aponeurotic system (SMAS) of the face.[7]
- The temporoparietal fascia is the most superficial fascial layer and is an important anatomic landmark. The superficial temporal vessels run along the outer aspect of it, and the frontal branch of the facial nerve runs on its deep surface (Fig. 33.2).[7]
- The temporalis fascia invests the temporalis muscle and is fused with the pericranium at the superior temporal line.

- The temporalis fascia splits at the level of the superior orbital rim, both layers (superficial and deep) continuing inferiorly to straddle the zygomatic arch. A pocket of fat (temporal fat pad) exists between the two layers.[7]
- The frontal sinus develops from small grooves in the cartilage of the lateral nasal wall near the middle meatus during the third and fourth gestational month.
- The phrase *nasofrontal duct* continues to persist in the literature despite the fact that it is anatomically incorrect. A more appropriate description is the frontal sinus outflow tract or frontal recess.
- The frontal recess itself is a space within the anterior ethmoid sinuses. The frontal sinus opens into the anterior part of the middle meatus or directly into the anterior portion of the infundibulum. The natural ostium lies in the posteromedial aspect of the frontal sinus floor.
- The frontal recess is bordered superiorly by the skull base, posteriorly by the second lamella (bulla ethmoidalis), and anteriorly by the first lamella (uncinate and agger nasi).
- The medial border is the vertical attachment of the middle turbinate. The lateral border is the lamina papyracea of the orbit.

PREOPERATIVE CONSIDERATIONS

- The treatment of frontal sinus pathology (neoplastic or inflammatory) that is impractical to treat endoscopically will require an external approach[1]: chronic frontal sinusitis refractory to endoscopic management, recurrent stenosis of the frontal recess, extensive fibro-osseous lesions (fibrodysplasia or ossifying fibroma), defects in the posterior table

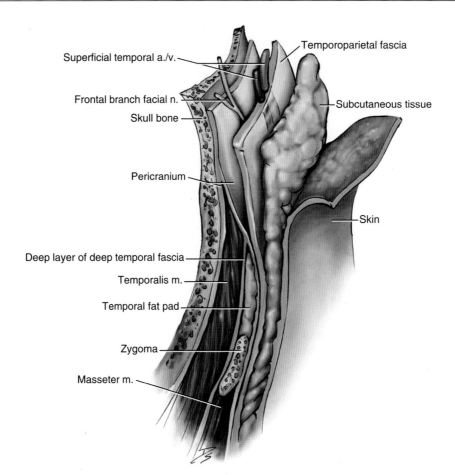

Fig. 33.1. Drawing detailing the layers of the scalp. The mnemonic *SCALP* refers to the various layers. It is important to know where the branches of the facial nerve and vascular structures are located before the coronal flap is elevated. The frontal branch of the facial nerve traverses deep to the temporoparietal fascia but superficial to the pericranium and the superficial layer of the deep temporal fascia. *a.,* Artery; *CN,* cranial nerve; *m.,* muscle; *v.,* vein.

with cerebrospinal fluid (CSF) leak, frontal sinus fractures involving the frontal recess, or obstructing frontal sinus cells.

Radiographic Considerations

- If the surgeon plans on entering the frontal sinus via traditional surgical techniques, a 6-foot Caldwell radiograph is obtained.[8] Two copies are printed, one for reference and one to be used as a sterilized cutout template for surgical planning (Fig. 33.3).
- Alternatively, the frontal sinus can be mapped using stereotactic image guidance.
- A study comparing 6-foot Caldwell radiographs versus transillumination versus image guidance found that image guidance had the least difference between measured and actual values and was statistically superior.[9]
- All patients should receive computed tomography (CT) or magnetic resonance imaging (MRI) evaluation prior to surgical intervention, as these will help to determine whether an endoscopic or an osteoplastic approach is appropriate.

INSTRUMENTATION

- Mayfield headrest
- Soft tissue as well as endoscopic room setup
- Stereotactic guidance instrumentation
- Standard head and neck dissecting instruments
- Scalp hemostatic clips (e.g., Raney clips)
- High-speed drill with cutting and diamond burs
- Oscillating saw
- Trauma implant/instrument plating tray
- Operating microscope
- Osteotomes
- Abdominal fat harvesting setup

PEARLS AND PITFALLS

- Complete removal of all of the sinus mucosa during the obliteration will significantly decrease the risk of postoperative mucocele formation.
- Erosion of the posterior table may be indicative of an underlying dural abnormality and potential rests of sinus mucosa on the dura itself. Obliterating the

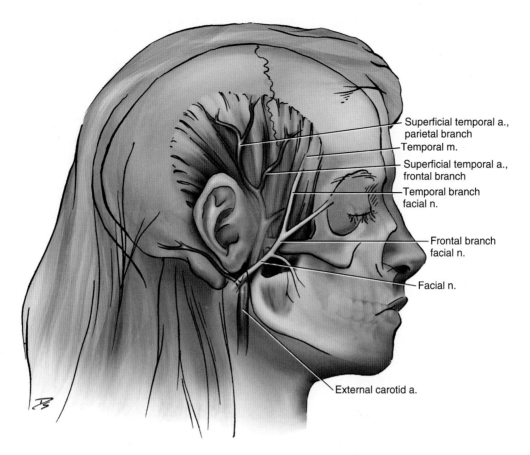

Fig. 33.2. Drawing showing the temporoparietal fascia, the most superficial fascial layer and an important anatomic landmark. The superficial temporal vessel runs along the outer aspect of it and travels vertically in the preauricular space as a terminal branch of the external carotid artery. The frontal branch of the facial nerve runs on its deep surface and travels superior to the supraorbital bony rim. *a.,* Artery; *m.,* muscle; *n.,* nerve.

Superficial temporal a., parietal branch
Temporal m.
Superficial temporal a., frontal branch
Temporal branch facial n.
Frontal branch facial n.
Facial n.
External carotid a.

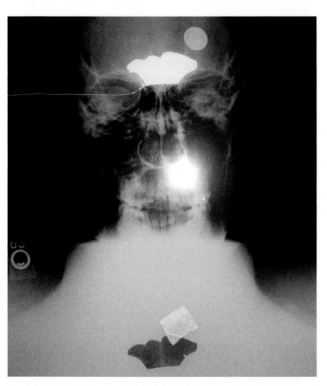

Fig. 33.3. Photograph showing the template of the frontal sinus that has been cut out of the radiograph. The template is soaked in iodine solution and is later placed on the patient before the frontal osteotomies are performed (see Fig. 33.11).

sinus in this case can be problematic during the follow-up period.

- The use of image guidance for mapping the frontal sinus appears to improve intraoperative safety and reduce the rate of complications.[10]
- Fracture of the bone flap can occur due to inadequate osteotomies along the supraorbital ridge or due to excessive thinning or attachment of an osteoma or tumor to the anterior table.[11]

SURGICAL PROCEDURE

- Temporary tarsorrhaphy sutures are placed with monofilament polypropylene sutures or corneal shields are placed to protect the corneas from abrasions.
- The frontal sinus can be approached using multiple incisions: coronal, midforehead, midbrow, or gull-wing incision (Fig. 33.4).
- Reaching the frontal sinus via the coronal incision has advantages over the brow or gull-wing incisions. The planned incision is drawn through the preauricular crease anterior to the tragus to the contralateral side, and the hair is shaved along the incision line.

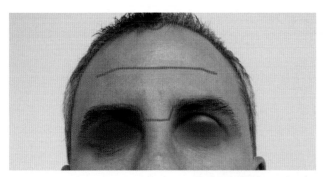

Fig. 33.4. Photograph showing potential incision sites *(red lines)* for accessing the frontal sinus. The midbrow and gull-wing incisions can often leave unsightly scars, whereas the coronal (hairline) incision is frequently more cosmetic.

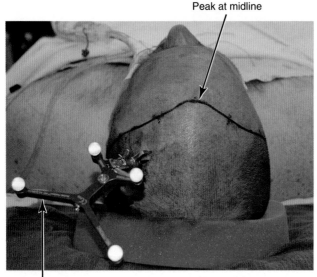

Peak at midline

Skull base array

Fig. 33.5. Photograph showing incision line and skull base array. If stereotactic image guidance is being used to trace the frontal sinus boundaries, the skull reference array is often placed before the sterilization.

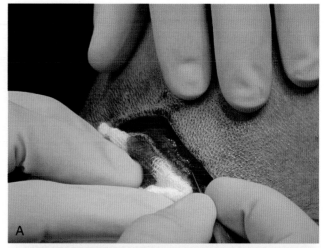

A

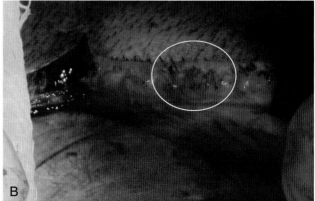

B

Fig. 33.6. (A) Photograph of the beginning of the coronal incision. The incision is started in the midline, with care taken to direct the blade parallel to the follicles so as to minimize alopecia. **(B)** High-power view of the incision line showing hair follicles parallel to the skin incision *(circle).*

- Some surgeons advocate creating a peak in the incision or designing a multiple W-type incision to facilitate realignment at the end of the procedure and to camouflage scarring.
- If a skull reference array is used for stereotactic surgical approaches to the frontal sinus, it can be placed prior to scalp elevation (Fig. 33.5).
- The incision is infiltrated with 1% lidocaine with 1:100,000 epinephrine. Starting in the midline, the skin is incised parallel to the hair follicles to minimize alopecia (Fig. 33.6). Electrocautery should be used sparingly and scalp clips are applied.
- Care must be taken when approaching the tragus as branches of the superficial temporal artery as well as

the frontal branch of the facial nerve may be found in this locale, as described previously.
- The dissection proceeds in either the subgaleal plane or the subperiosteal plane.
- Advocates of preserving the periosteum claim that maintaining the periosteal attachment to the anterior frontal sinus table preserves blood supply.[12] In this instance, the scalp flap is elevated in the subgaleal plane and an incision is made through the periosteum 2 cm posterior to the supraorbital neurovascular bundles to raise them with the scalp flap (Fig. 33.7).
- We typically incise the periosteum and elevate it with the scalp flap for the entire length because this avoids desiccation and inadvertent injury to the periosteum, which might preclude its use in reconstruction if necessary (Fig. 33.8).
- Laterally, the temporoparietal fascia is separated from the superficial layer of the deep temporalis

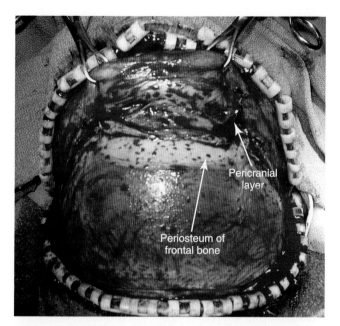

Fig. 33.7. Photograph of the operative field. If the scalp is elevated in the subgaleal plane, an incision is made through the periosteum approximately 2 cm posterior to the supraorbital neurovascular bundles. The osteoplastic flap is raised with the periosteum.

fascia to protect the frontal branches of the facial nerve (Fig. 33.9).

- Anteriorly, the supraorbital and supratrochlear neurovascular bundles are encountered (Fig. 33.10). If notches are present, the neurovascular bundles can be elevated with the entire flap. If foramina are present, a high-speed drill with continuous suction and irrigation can be used to free the neurovascular bundles by removing the inferior portion of the bony foramina.

- Once the frontal sinus is exposed, the previously obtained radiographic template is placed on the bone and the frontal sinus is outlined (Fig. 33.11).

- Alternately, if a skull reference array has been previously attached to the calvarium, the image-guided probe can be used to map out the frontal sinus (Fig. 33.12).

- In both situations, a high-speed drill is used to fashion pilot holes along the course of the outlined frontal sinus, and a beveled osteotomy into the sinus is performed using an oscillating sagittal saw or a piezoelectric bone scalpel.

- Alternatively, a small drill bit can be used to methodically perforate the bone in approximately 0.5- to 1-cm increments; then, these perforations are connected with the drill bit to allow for minimal bone loss so that the flap can lock into place at the conclusion of the procedure without the need for fixation.[13]

- The anterior table is reflected anteriorly if attached to periosteum or removed entirely and stored in sterile saline for replating (Fig. 33.13).

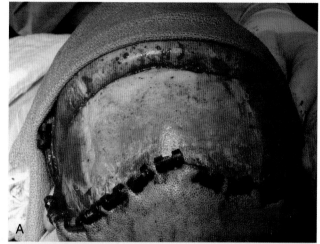

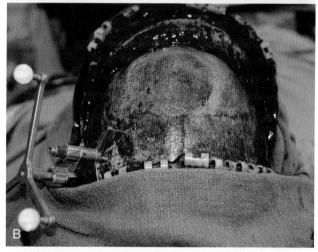

Fig. 33.8. (A) Photograph of a scalp flap raised in the subperiosteal plane. Elevation in this plane may prevent desiccation of and inadvertent injury to the periosteum should it be used to obliterate or cranialize the sinus. (B) Photograph of a scalp flap raised in the subperiosteal plane around the placement of a skull reference array.

- After the frontal sinus lesion is addressed (e.g., excision, ablation), treatment of the frontal sinus itself depends on the underlying pathology and an assessment of the collateral damage to the sinus.

- If the frontal recess is undisturbed or removal of the lesion does not disrupt more than one half of the frontal sinus mucosa, the remainder may be left intact, especially if combined with an endoscopic approach. Otherwise, consideration should be given to obliteration of the frontal sinus.

- If obliterating, all of the mucosa is stripped from the frontal sinus, and the mucosa of the frontal recess is inverted. Under microscopic visualization, a high-speed diamond bur is used to polish the bone.

- It is critical to address all areas of the frontal sinus. The anterior table is also treated in the same manner.

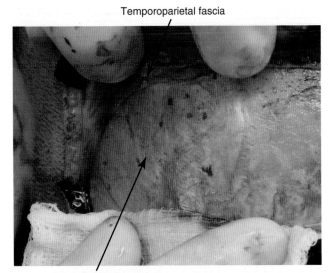

Temporoparietal fascia

Superficial layer of
deep temporal fascia

Fig. 33.9. Photograph after flap elevation in the subperiosteal plane. When the scalp flap is raised in this plane, the temporoparietal fascia is separated from the superficial layer of the deep temporal fascia to protect the frontal branches of the facial nerve.

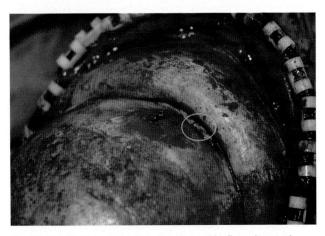

Fig. 33.10. Photograph showing the scalp flap elevated anteriorly and inferiorly so that the supraorbital and supratrochlear neurovascular bundles are identified (circle).

■ Once complete, the frontal recess may be plugged with bone pate, temporalis muscle, or fascia, and the sinus is obliterated with fat (Fig. 33.14). The use of bone cement (hydroxyapatite) for obliteration is not recommended due to the increased risk of infection and need for revision.[14,15]

■ If cranialization is being performed, a pericranial flap can be raised from the coronal flap based on the supratrochlear and supraorbital vessels. This flap can then be laid down into the craniotomy defect and sewn to the dura in order to add a layer of separation of the intracranial and extracranial spaces[16] (Fig. 33.15). Alternatively, if cranialization is planned, the

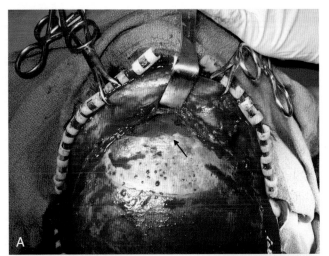

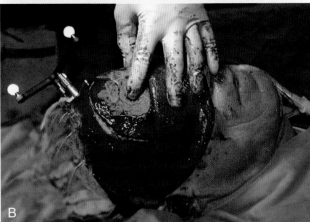

Fig. 33.11. (A) Photograph showing the frontal sinus template (arrow) obtained previously from the Caldwell radiograph, after placement on the frontal sinus. Care must be taken to ensure that the nasofrontal suture and supraorbital rims are aligned with the template before any osteotomies are done. (B) Photograph showing use of the radiographic template to confirm the tracing made by a stereotactic probe.

pericranial flap can be elevated initially when the scalp flap is raised and kept moist during the procedure.

■ The anterior table is replaced and secured to the frontal bone with titanium plates (Fig. 33.16). If a perforation technique was used to create the osteotomy, hardware may not be necessary.[13]

■ The wound is irrigated thoroughly, a drain is placed, and the scalp is closed in at least two layers.

POSTOPERATIVE CONSIDERATIONS

■ It is at the discretion of the surgeon regarding whether perioperative antibiotics are continued.

■ It is the author's opinion that in cases of posterior table fractures, cerebrospinal fluid leak, or dural tears, intravenous antibiotics should be administered prophylactically when performing surgical repair.

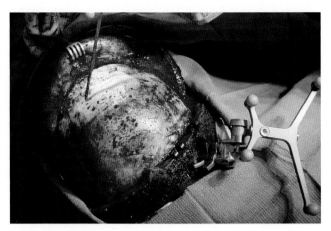

Fig. 33.12. Photograph showing use of an image guidance system, rather than a Caldwell radiograph, to outline the template for the osteoplastic flap.

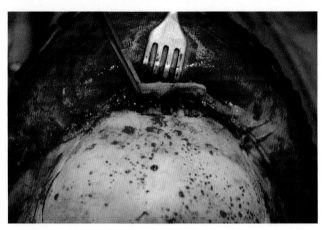

Fig. 33.13. Photograph showing elevation of the anterior table. A series of osteotomies is made with an osteotome or drill. Once the osteotomies are performed, the intersinus septum has to be fractured before the anterior table of the frontal sinus may be elevated.

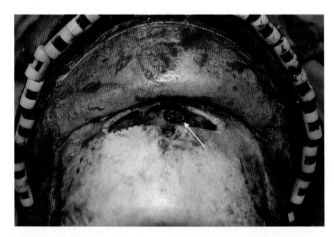

Fig. 33.14. Photograph showing plugging of the frontal recess *(arrow)* once the sinus has been cleared of disease. The recess can be plugged with bone pate, temporalis muscle, and/or fascia.

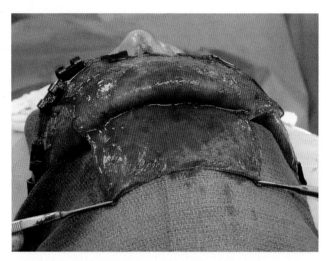

Fig. 33.15. Photograph of a pericranial flap harvested by separating the periosteum from the scalp flap along the subgaleal layer. When flap harvest is done as the final step, often the flap is moist and well vascularized.

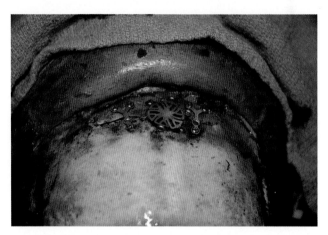

Fig. 33.16. Photograph of the anterior table placed back into position at the end of the procedure. It can be secured with titanium plates or wires.

- In cases of mucopyocele or frontal sinusitis, antibiotics should be directed toward intraoperative cultures obtained during the case.
- Forehead edema and periorbital ecchymosis are common in the immediate preoperative period.
- Infection of the surgical site can occur, especially in cases of obliteration for chronic disease. Infection may lead to cellulitis, abscess, or fistula formation.[11]
- Frontal contour irregularities may be due to areas of bone loss from osteotomy or from resorption due to damage to the overlying periosteum. Embossment of the frontal sinus may occur due to hypertrophy of the bone flap or due to an ill-fitting bone flap that does not contour to its original position.[11]
- Additionally, osteoneogenesis can occur in the bone gap that is created with the sagittal saw cuts and may

cause the anterior plate to be anteriorly displaced. Anterior plate depression can also occur due to excess drilling of the bone and poor plating techniques. It can occur as well as a late complication due to poor healing, bone migration, and bone resorption.[13]

■ MR imaging is the most valuable tool to evaluate the frontal sinus after obliteration with adipose tissue but is limited in its ability to detect small recurrent mucoceles and to differentiate vital adipose tissue from oil cysts due to fat necrosis or granulation tissue.[15]

REFERENCES

Access the reference list online at ExpertConsult.com.

INDEX

Note: Page numbers followed by f indicate figures; t, tables.